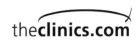

EMERGENCY MEDICINE CLINICS OF NORTH AMERICA

Emergency Department Wound Management

GUEST EDITORS
John G. McManus, MD, MCR
Ian Wedmore, MD
Richard B. Schwartz, MD

CONSULTING EDITOR
Amal Mattu, MD

February 2007 • Volume 25 • Number 1

SAUNDERS

An Imprint of Elsevier, Inc.
PHILADELPHIA   LONDON   TORONTO   MONTREAL   SYDNEY   TOKYO

W.B. SAUNDERS COMPANY
A Division of Elsevier Inc.

1600 John F. Kennedy Boulevard, Suite 1800 • Philadelphia, Pennsylvania 19103-2899

http://www.theclinics.com

EMERGENCY MEDICINE CLINICS	**Volume 25, Number 1**
OF NORTH AMERICA	**ISSN 0733-8627**
February 2007	**ISBN-13: 978-1-4160-4852-7**
Editor: Karen Sorensen	**ISBN-10: 1-4160-4852-9**

The ideas and opinions expressed in *Emergency Medicine Clinics of North America* do not necessarily reflect those of the Publisher. The Publisher does not assume any responsibility for any injury and/or damage to persons or property arising out of or related to any use of the material contained in this periodical. The reader is advised to check the appropriate medical literature and the product information currently provided by the manufacturer of each drug to be administered to verify the dosage, the method and duration of administration, or contraindications. It is the responsibility of the treating physician or other health care professional, relying on independent experience and knowledge of the patient, to determine drug dosages and the best treatment for the patient. Mention of any product in this issue should not be construed as endorsement by the contributors, editors, or the Publisher of the product or manufacturers' claims.

Emergency Medicine Clinics of North America (ISSN 0733-8627) is published quarterly by Elsevier Inc., 360 Park Avenue South, New York, NY, 10010-1710. Months of issue are February, May, August, and November. Business and Editorial Offices: 1600 John F. Kennedy Boulevard, Suite 1800, Philadelphia, PA 19103-2899. Customer Service Office: 6277 Sea Harbor Drive, Orlando, FL 32887-4800. Periodicals postage paid at New York, NY, and additional mailing offices. Subscription prices are $193.00 per year (US individuals), $297.00 per year (US institutions), $259.00 per year (international individuals), $351.00 per year (international institutions), $237.00 per year (Canadian individuals), and $351.00 per year (Canadian institutions). International air speed delivery is included in all *Clinics'* subscription prices. All prices are subject to change without notice. POSTMASTER: Send address changes to *Emergency Medicine Clinics of North America*, Elsevier Periodicals Customer Service, 6277 Sea Harbor Drive, Orlando, FL 32887-4800. **Customer Service: 1-800-654-2452 (US). From outside of the US, call 1-407-345-4000. E-mail: hhspcs@harcourt.com.**

Emergency Medicine Clinics of North America is covered in *Index Medicus, Current Contents/Clinical Medicine, EMBASE/Excerpta Medica, BIOSIS, SciSearch, CINAHL, ISI/BIOMED,* and *Research Alert.*

Printed in the United States of America.

CONSULTING EDITOR

AMAL MATTU, MD, Program Director, Emergency Medicine Residency, and Associate Professor, Department of Emergency Medicine, University of Maryland School of Medicine, Baltimore, Maryland

GUEST EDITORS

LTC JOHN G. McMANUS, MD, MCR, FACEP, US Army Institute of Surgical Research, Fort Sam Houston; Clinical Associate Professor, Emergency Medicine, The University of Texas Health Science Center at San Antonio, San Antonio, Texas

COL IAN WEDMORE, MD, FACEP, Assistant Chief of Emergency Medicine, Madigan Army Medical Center, Tacoma, Washington

RICHARD B. SCHWARTZ, MD, FACEP, Chair and Associate Professor, Department of Emergency Medicine, Medical College of Georgia, Augusta, Georgia

CONTRIBUTORS

DAVID G. BAER, PhD, US Army Institute of Surgical Research, Fort Sam Houston, San Antonio, Texas

TODD BAKER, MD, Associate Director of Emergency Department Ultrasound, Department of Emergency Medicine, Madigan Army Medical Center, Tacoma; Clinical Instructor of Medicine, Division of Emergency Medicine, University of Washington Medical Center, Seattle, Washington

VINCENT BALL, MD, Senior Resident, Department of Emergency Medicine, Madigan Army Medical Center, Tacoma, Washington

ROBERT B. BLANKENSHIP, MD, FACEP, Department of Emergency Medicine, Madigan Army Medical Center, Tacoma; Clinical Instructor of Medicine, Division of Emergency Medicine, University of Washington, Seattle, Washington

DANIEL J. BROWN, MD, SAUSHEC Emergency Medicine, Brooke Army Medical Center, Fort Sam Houston, San Antonio, Texas

MARK F. BUETTNER, DO, ABEM, Medical Director, Great River Wound and Hyperbaric Clinic, Center for Rehabilitation, West Burlington, Iowa

COL LEOPOLDO C. CANCIO, MD, Medical Corps, US Army, US Army Institute of Surgical Research, Fort Sam Houston, San Antonio, Texas

ARJUN CHANMUGAM, MD, MBA, Associate Professor, Department of Emergency Medicine, Johns Hopkins University, Baltimore, Maryland

CHAD S. CRYSTAL, MD, Assistant Program Director, Emergency Medicine Residency Program, Carl R. Darnall Army Medical Center, Fort Hood, Temple, Texas

MOHAMUD DAYA, MD, MS, Associate Professor, Department of Emergency Medicine, Oregon Health & Science University, Portland, Oregon

RYAN H. DeBOARD, MD, Chief Resident Physician, Department of Emergency Medicine, Madigan Army Medical Center, Tacoma, Washington

MAJ MARK DENNY, MD, FACEP, Department of Emergency Medicine, Madigan Army Medical Center, Tacoma, Washington

MARGARET A. FONDER, Medical Student, Johns Hopkins University School of Medicine, Baltimore Maryland

RUBÉN GÓMEZ, MD, PhD, US Army Institute of Surgical Research, Fort Sam Houston, San Antonio, Texas

LTC BENJAMIN HARRISON, MD, Program Director, Emergency Medicine Residency Program, Madigan Army Medical Center, Fort Lewis, Washington

RICHARD S. HARTOCH, MD, Assistant Professor, Department of Emergency Medicine, Oregon Health and Sciences University; Veterans Administration Medical Center, Portland, Oregon

JODY K. HENSON, MD, Texas A&M Health Science Center, Scott and White Hospital, Temple, Texas

JON E. JAFFE, MD, Assistant Professor and Consulting Staff, Department of Emergency Medicine, Texas A&M Health Science Center-College of Medicine, Scott and White Hospital, Temple, Texas

THOMAS RUSSEL JONES, MD, FAAEM, Department of Emergency Medicine, Scott and White Hospital, Texas A&M University College of Medicine, Temple, Texas

ROBERT F. KACPROWICZ, MD, Medical Director, US Air Force Pararescue School, Kirtland Air Force Base, New Mexico

CHRISTOPHER S. KANG, MD, FACEP, Clinical Assistant Professor, University of Washington; Core Faculty Attending Physician, Department of Emergency Medicine, Madigan Army Medical Center, Tacoma, Washington

SHERI KNAPP, FNP, Clinical Instructor, Department of Emergency Medicine, Oregon Health & Science University, Portland, Oregon

GERALD S. LAZARUS, MD, Professor, Department of Dermatology, Johns Hopkins University; Director, Johns Hopkins Wound Center, Johns Hopkins Bayview Medical Center, Baltimore, Maryland

JEREMY D. LLOYD, MD, Faculty, Department of Emergency Medicine, Wilford Hall Medical Center, Lackland Air Force Base, Texas

ADAM J. MAMELAK, MD, Dermatology Resident, Department of Dermatology, Johns Hopkins University, Baltimore, Maryland

MELVIN J. MARQUE III, MD, Faculty, Department of Emergency Medicine, Wilford Hall Medical Center, Lackland Air Force Base, Texas

TODD J. McARTHUR, MD, Resident, Emergency Medicine Residency Program, Carl R. Darnall Army Medical Center, Fort Hood, Temple, Texas

LTC JOHN G. McMANUS, MD, MCR, FACEP, US Army Institute of Surgical Research, Fort Sam Houston; Clinical Associate Professor, Emergency Medicine, The University of Texas Health Science Center at San Antonio, San Antonio, Texas

MICHAEL A. MILLER, MD, FAAEM, Department of Emergency Medicine, Darnall Army Medical Center, Fort Hood; Central Texas Poison Center, Temple, Texas

GREGORY P. MOORE, MD, JD, Attending Physician, Emergency Department, Kaiser, Permanente Sacramento/Roseville; Volunteer Clinical Faculty, Emergency Medicine Residency, University of California Davis School of Medicine, Sacramento, California

YOKO NAKAMURA, MD, Clinical Assistant Professor, Department of Emergency Medicine, Oregon Health & Science University, Portland, Oregon

PARESH R. PATEL, MD, FAAEM, Department of Emergency Medicine, Darnall Army Medical Center, Fort Hood, Temple, Texas

JAMES A. PFAFF, MD, FACEP, FAAEM, Staff Physician, San Antonio Uniformed Health Services Health Education Consortium Emergency Medicine Residency, and Assistant Professor of Emergency Medicine, Uniformed Services University of the Health Sciences, San Antonio, Texas

DAWN F. RONDEAU, ANCP, Instructor, Oregon Health and Sciences University, Portland, Oregon

ALFREDO SABBAJ, MD, MA, Assistant Professor, Oregon Health and Sciences University, Portland, Oregon

RICHARD B. SCHWARTZ, MD, FACEP, Chair and Associate Professor, Department of Emergency Medicine, Medical College of Georgia, Augusta, Georgia

MARGARET K. STRECKER-McGRAW, MD, Department of Emergency Medicine, Scott and White Hospital, Texas A&M University College of Medicine, Temple, Texas

COL IAN WEDMORE, MD, FACEP, Assistant Chief of Emergency Medicine, Madigan Army Medical Center, Tacoma, Washington

DEREK WOLKENHAUER, RRT, CHT, Hyperbaric Safety Officer, Great River Wound and Hyperbaric Clinic, West Burlington, Iowa

MAJ BRADLEY N. YOUNGGREN, MD, FACEP, Assistant Program Director, Department of Emergency Medicine, Madigan Army Medical Center, Tacoma, Washington

CONTENTS

> Wound healing is a complex interchange, orchestrated between cellular components that play their respective parts signaled by and mediated by different cellular instruments of healing. When healing is performed well, the final product is a thing of beauty. When healing is delayed, interrupted, or excessive, then unsightly scars of chronic painful wounds that are frustrating to the patient and physician occur.

> The primary objectives of basic wound management center around promoting optimal wound healing and cosmesis. These objectives may be achieved through the systematic assessment, preparation, and repair of the laceration supplemented with appropriate patient care instructions. The meticulous and methodical management of traumatic wounds described in this article will assist the emergency physician in decreasing overall complication rates and help improve patient satisfaction.

treatment of various complicated wounds. The authors highlight available guidelines, provide the best evidence available, and provide recommendations when data are limited.

Difficult wounds constitute a significant amount of the morbidity and mortality emergency physicians face on a daily basis. There are specific traumatic and atraumatic wounds that are difficult to manage and have a high risk of complications. Emergency physicians must be able to identify these high-risk wounds and patients and take steps to mitigate further morbidity and mortality.

This article makes some introductory comments on the histology of the skin and the pathophysiology of burn injury as these topics pertain to the estimation of the depth of the burn injury. The definition of a major burn and the salient points of its treatment are covered. In addition, some general comments are made about several special injuries for which burn center referral usually is sought. Finally, guidance is given in the selection and treatment of patients who have burns that may be treated on an outpatient basis.

Diligent posttreatment wound care management undoubtedly will improve wound outcome and patient satisfaction. There are limited recommendations in the literature to guide management plans. Nevertheless patients must receive specific instructions to complete wound care. These instructions should include whether a dressing is indicated, which dressing should be used, the duration of use, and the method of application. The plan must explain clearly the reasons for returning for further medical attention, for follow-up, for routine removal of sutures/staples, and an earlier return for possible concerns of infection or dehiscence. Preprinted discharge instruction sheets are useful, and illustrations can be helpful.

The primary goal of wound management is to achieve a functional closure with minimal scarring. Preventing infection is important to facilitate the healing process. Most simple, uncomplicated wounds do not need systemic antibiotics but benefit from the use of topical antibiotics. Judicious use of antibiotics reduces unnecessary adverse events and helps reduce the development of resistance. Although antibiotics can help reduce infection risk and promote healing, they are not a substitute for good local wound care, in particular irrigation and surgical débridement. This article reviews the role of antibiotics in emergency department wound management.

Hyperbaric Oxygen Therapy in the Treatment of Open Fractures and Crush Injuries 177
Mark F. Buettner and Derek Wolkenhauer

This article focuses on the use of hyperbaric oxygen therapy (HBOt) in the treatment of open fractures and crush injuries. Based on the clinical evidence and cost analysis, medical institutions that treat open fracture and crush injuries are justified in incorporating HBOt as a standard of care. Both Medicare and Undersea and Hyperbaric Medical Society guidelines list crush injuries as an approved indication for HBOt. Emergency physicians should familiarize themselves with this emerging treatment modality because of their role in the early management of these injuries.

Reducing Risk in Emergency Department Wound Management 189
James A. Pfaff and Gregory P. Moore

Although substantial dollar amounts are not involved, wound-care litigation constitutes a significant number of lawsuits to emergency medicine physicians, resulting in an increased drain on the physician's time and exposing the physician to all the psychosocial effects involved in the medicolegal process. The procedures outlined in this article-paying attention to wound-care principles, involving patients in the medical decision-making process, and ensuring appropriate medical follow-up-can, it is hoped, reduce the incidence of medical claims.

Emergency Management of Chronic Wounds 203
Richard S. Hartoch, LTC John G. McManus, Sheri Knapp, and Mark F. Buettner

As America's emergency departments witness an increase in care provided to an aging population, the emergency physician increasingly evaluates and treats manifestations of chronic disease. Nonhealing wounds are often a presenting manifestation of chronic disease. They are a source of pain and disability for this population. Emergency physicians should possess a fundamental knowledge in the management of chronic wounds. This article familiarizes the emergency physician with the epidemiology of chronic wounds, the physiology of tissue repair, the pathophysiology involved in wound healing failure, the common types of chronic wounds, and specific management strategies.

FORTHCOMING ISSUES

RECENT ISSUES

The Clinics are now available online!

Access your subscription at
www.theclinics.com

GOAL STATEMENT

The goal of *Emergency Medicine Clinics of North America* is to keep practicing physicians up to date with current clinical practice in emergency medicine by providing timely articles reviewing the state of the art in patient care.

ACCREDITATION

The *Emergency Medical Clinics of North America* is planned and implemented in accordance with the Essential Areas and Policies of the Accreditation Council for Continuing Medical Education (ACCME) through the joint sponsorship of the University of Virginia School of Medicine and Elsevier. The University of Virginia School of Medicine is accredited by the ACCME to provide continuing medical education for physicians.

The University of Virginia School of Medicine designates this educational activity for a maximum of *15 AMA PRA Category 1 Credits™*. Physicians should only claim credit commensurate with the extent of their participation in the activity.

The Emergency Medicine Clinics of North America CME program is approved by the American College of Emergency Physicians for 60 hours of ACEP Category I Credit per year.

The American Medical Association has determined that physicians not licensed in the US who participate in this CME activity are eligible for *15 AMA PRA Category 1 Credits™*.

Credit can be earned by reading the text material, taking the CME examination online at http://www.theclinics.com/home/cme, and completing the evaluation. After taking the test, you will be required to review any and all incorrect answers. Following completion of the test and evaluation, your credit will be awarded and you may print your certificate.

FACULTY DISCLOSURE/CONFLICT OF INTEREST

The University of Virginia School of Medicine, as an ACCME accredited provider, endorses and strives to comply with the Accreditation Council for Continuing Medical Education (ACCME) Standards of Commercial Support, Commonwealth of Virginia statutes, University of Virginia policies and procedures, and associated federal and private regulations and guidelines on the need for disclosure and monitoring of proprietary and financial interests that may affect the scientific integrity and balance of content delivered in continuing medical education activities under our auspices.

The University of Virginia School of Medicine requires that all CME activities accredited through this institution be developed independently and be scientifically rigorous, balanced and objective in the presentation/discussion of its content, theories and practices.

All authors/editors participating in an accredited CME activity are expected to disclose to the readers relevant financial relationships with commercial entities occurring within the past 12 months (such as grants or research support, employee, consultant, stock holder, member of speakers bureau, etc.). The University of Virginia School of Medicine will employ appropriate mechanisms to resolve potential conflicts of interest to maintain the standards of fair and balanced education to the reader. Questions about specific strategies can be directed to the Office of Continuing Medical Education, University of Virginia School of Medicine, Charlottesville, Virginia.

The authors/editors listed below have identified no professional or financial affiliations for themselves or their spouse/partner:
Todd Baker, MD; David G. Baer, MD; Vincent Ball, MD; Robert B. Blankenship, MD, FACEP; Daniel J. Brown, MD; Mark F. Buettner, DO, ABEM; Leopoldo C. Cancio, MD; Arjun Chanmugam, MD, MBA; Chad S. Crystal, MD; Mohamud Daya, MD, MS; Ryan H. DeBoard, MD; Mark A. Denny, MD, FACEP; Margaret A. Fonder, BS; Rubén Gómez, MD, PhD; Benjamin Harrison, MD; Richard S. Hartoch, MD; Jody K. Henson, MD; Jon E. Jaffe, MD; Thomas Russell Jones, MD, FAAEM; Robert F. Kacprowicz, MD; Sheri Knapp, FNP; Gerald S. Lazarus, MD; Jeremy D. Llyod, MD; Adam J. Mamelak, MD; Melvin J. Marque III, MD; Amal Mattu, MD (Consulting Editor); Todd J. McArthur, MD; John McManus, MD, MCR, FACEP (Guest Editor); Michael A. Miller, MD, FAAEM; Gregory P. Moore, MD, JD; Yoko Nakamura, MD; Paresh R. Patel, MD, FAAEM; James A. Pfaff, MD, FACEP, FAAEM; Dawn F. Rondeau, ANCP; Alfredo Sabbaj, MD, MA; Karen Sorensen (Acquisitions Editor); Margaret K. Strecker-McGraw, MD; Ian Wedmore, MD, FACEP (Guest Editor); Derek Wolkenhauer, RRT, CHT; and, Brad Younggren, MD.

The authors/editors listed below have identified the following professional or financial affiliations for themselves of their spouse/partner:
Christopher Kang, MD, FACEP is a stockholder in Calypte Biomedical Corporation and Cardiodynamics.
Richard B. Schwartz, MD (Guest Editor) is the President of, and a patent holder for, AI Medical Devices.

Disclosure of Discussion of non-FDA approved uses for pharmaceutical products and/or medical devices:
The University of Virginia School of Medicine, as an ACCME provider, requires that all faculty presenters identify and disclose any "off label" uses for pharmaceutical and medical device products. The University of Virginia School of Medicine recommends that each physician fully review all the available data on new products or procedures prior to instituting them with patients.

TO ENROLL

To enroll in the Emergency Medicine Clinics of North America Continuing Medical Education program, call customer service at 1-800-654-2452 or visit us online at www.theclinics.com/home/cme. The CME program is available to subscribers for an additional fee of $195.00.

ELSEVIER
SAUNDERS

Emerg Med Clin N Am
25 (2007) xv–xvi

EMERGENCY
MEDICINE
CLINICS OF
NORTH AMERICA

Foreword

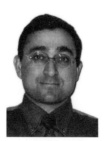

Amal Mattu, MD
Consulting Editor

Wound care is a routine part of the practice of emergency medicine. Millions of traumatic wounds are managed by health care providers every year in the United States, and most of these are treated in emergency departments (EDs) [1]. Despite the routine nature of wound management, the literature indicates that many wounds are initially managed inappropriately [2]. Many of these routine wounds, when initially managed incorrectly, progress to significant complications and morbidity. Up to 20% of all malpractice claims in emergency medicine and up to 11% of malpractice dollars paid by emergency physicians relate to wound care issues [3], oftentimes the result of inappropriate initial management. It would appear, then, that although wound care is a routine part of the practice of emergency medicine, it should also be considered a high-risk part of the specialty.

In this issue of *Emergency Medicine Clinics of North America*, Guest Editors Drs. McManus, Wedmore, and Schwartz have assembled an outstanding group of authors to educate us on this vital aspect of our specialty. Early articles discuss core topics, such as the principles of tissue anatomy and healing, initial evaluation, local anesthesia, basic closure techniques, and post-care of wounds. Later articles address more difficult wounds, including burns, chronic wounds, and complicated lacerations. The authors also address a potpourri of controversial topics, including the use of antimicrobials in wound management, the use of imaging, antimicrobial therapy, and hyperbaric oxygen therapy. A separate article is devoted specifically to risk management in wound care.

0733-8627/07/$ - see front matter © 2007 Elsevier Inc. All rights reserved.
doi:10.1016/j.emc.2007.01.013

This issue of *Emergency Medicine Clinics of North America* represents an important addition to the emergency medicine literature. It should be considered must-reading not only for practicing emergency physicians but also for emergency medicine trainees and for any other health care providers who routinely manage wounds in their daily practice. The principles outlined in this series of articles will undoubtedly reduce medicolegal risk and also improve the routine care of our patients.

Amal Mattu, MD
Emergency Medicine Residency
Department of Emergency Medicine
University of Maryland School of Medicine
110 S. Paca Street, 6th Floor, Suite 200
Baltimore, MD 21201, USA

E-mail address: amattu@smail.umaryland.edu

References

[1] Wedmore IS. Wound care: modern evidence in the treatment of man's age-old injuries. Emergency Medicine Practice 2005;7(3):1–24.
[2] Howell JM, Chisholm CD. Outpatient wound preparation and care: a national survey. Ann Emerg Med 1992;21(8):976–81.
[3] Pfaff JA, Moore GP. ED wound management: identifying and reducing risk. ED Legal Letter 2005;16(9):97–108.

ELSEVIER
SAUNDERS

Emerg Med Clin N Am
25 (2007) xvii–xviii

EMERGENCY
MEDICINE
CLINICS OF
NORTH AMERICA

Preface

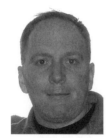 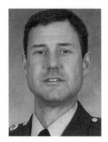 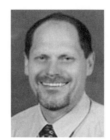

LTC John G. McManus,   COL Ian Wedmore,   Richard B. Schwartz,
MD, MCR, FACEP   MD, FACEP   MD, FACEP
                         Guest Editors

The management of wounds is an essential skill for emergency medicine and acute care physicians. More than 12 million acute care visits a year can be attributed to wounds in the United States alone. Emergency health care providers are faced with an expanding variety of simple and complicated wound types, and it is essential that these clinicians be well versed in the current management of such wounds. Other challenges include the increased incidence of emerging infections and antimicrobial resistance, which adds to the evaluation and treatment challenges. Additionally, multiple new technologies are available for wound management with occasionally conflicting or limited supporting data making their use difficult for the practicing physician.

In addition to the diagnostic and treatment challenges, litigation in wound care is one of the most common areas of emergency medicine malpractice suits. Wound care accounts for 5% to 20% of all emergency department malpractice claims and 3% to 11% of all dollars paid out. The most common reason for litigation in emergency department management of wounds involves failure to diagnose foreign bodies, wound infections, and failure to detect underlying injury to nerves, tendons, or violation of a joint capsule. Proper understanding of wound care is essential for emergency health care providers not only to reduce litigation but also to reduce morbidity and mortality.

This edition of the *Emergency Medical Clinics of North America* will provide information on pathophysiology, epidemiology, management, and

0733-8627/07/$ - see front matter © 2007 Elsevier Inc. All rights reserved.
doi:10.1016/j.emc.2007.01.014   *emed.theclinics.com*

treatment of wounds seen in the acute care setting. A broad spectrum of wound care management is included with management recommendations for acute (routine) wounds along with those for chronic (difficult) wounds. We highlight available guidelines, provide the best evidence available, and provide expert recommendations where data are limited.

The editors are pleased to present a broad range of talented authors to provide an excellent, in-depth review for wound management in the acute health care setting. Our hope is that this text provides readers with an excellent best practice review and valued future reference that will be integrated into clinical practice.

LTC John G. McManus, MD, MCR, FACEP
US Army Institute of Surgical Research
Fort Sam Houston
3400 Rawley Chambers Avenue, Suite B
San Antonio, TX 78234-6315, USA

Emergency Medicine
University of Texas Health and Science Center at San Antonio
7703 Floyd Curl Drive
San Antonio, TX 78229-3900, USA

E-mail address: john.mcmanus@amedd.army.mil

COL Ian Wedmore, MD, FACEP
Madigan Army Medical Center,
Fitzsimmons Drive
Tacoma, WA 98431, USA

E-mail address: ian.wedmore@amedd.army.mil

Richard B. Schwartz, MD, FACEP
Department of Emergency Medicine
Medical College of Georgia
1120 15th Street AF-2026
Augusta, GA 30912-2800, USA

E-mail address: rschwart@mcg.edu

ELSEVIER
SAUNDERS

Emerg Med Clin N Am
25 (2007) 1–22

EMERGENCY
MEDICINE
CLINICS OF
NORTH AMERICA

Soft Tissue Wounds and Principles of Healing

Margaret K. Strecker-McGraw, MD[a],*,
Thomas Russel Jones, MD, FAAEM[a],
David G. Baer, PhD[b]

[a]*Department of Emergency Medicine, Scott and White Hospital, Texas A&M University
College of Medicine, 2401 S. 31st Street, Temple, TX 76504, USA*
[b]*US Army Institute of Surgical Research, 3400 Rawley Chambers Avenue,
Fort Sam Houston, San Antonio, TX 78234, USA*

Basic skin anatomy

Human skin is the largest organ of the body. It provides protection; thermoregulation; and sensory, metabolic, and immune functions and is a dynamic barrier for the underlying organism. Disruption of the skin by wounding can lead to fluid loss, infection, scarring, hypothermia, or compromised immunity [1]. A basic understanding of skin structure will help us understand the extent of injury and will help guide treatment and repair of wounds.

The skin is composed of two major layers: the outermost layer, or epidermis, and the dermis, which are separated by the basement membrane but are mutually dependent upon each other for skin integrity. The subcutaneous tissue that underlies the dermis and consists of adipose cells, fibroblasts, and macrophages and supplies the trunks for blood and nerve supply is termed the hypodermis. Skin appendages arise in the dermis and hypodermis and are derived from embryonic tissue that differentiates into eccrine and apocrine glands, hair follicles, and nails.

Epidermis

The epidermis is derived from ectoderm. It is a stratified epithelial layer that can range in thickness, depending upon the sex and the anatomic location, from approximately 0.05mm to 0.75mm, depending upon the

___

* Corresponding author.
 E-mail address: mkmcgraw@swmail.sw.org (M.K. Strecker-McGraw).

source you read. This layer is avascular, and the classically identified layers are the stratum corneum, stratum lucidum, stratum granulosum, stratum spinosum, and stratum basale.

The outermost layer or stratum corneum is composed of anucleate, keratinized, dead cells surrounded by a cornified envelope called keratinocytes or squames. This layer is several layers thick and is continuously shed, with replacement cells from the underlying layer migrating outward at about the same rate as the dead cells are sloughed form the outermost layer. This layer is resistant to pH changes, temperature, and dehydration. The stratum lucidum underlies the stratum corneum and is an area of remodeling. This is a relatively thin layer and may be absent or patchy upon electron microscopy of thin skin. The stratum granulosum or granular layer underlies the lucidum and is characterized by flat cells with active metabolism. The cells are filled with keratin, and, as they move through this layer, they lose their nuclei and organelles. The stratum spinosum contains cells with spine-like structures that are desmosomes with connections to the surrounding cells. This layer is mitotically active and gives rise to the granulosum as it moves outward. The stratum basale or basal layer is a single cell thick. It is here that keratinocytes divide and begin differentiation. Cells of this layer are pushed outward to give rise to the stratum spinosum. This layer has areas of ingress into the underlying dermis called epidermal ridges, which are intercalated with the dermal ridges. The two layers are separated by a thin basement membrane, which is a semipermeable membrane that regulates the transfer of proteins and other materials across the dermal–epidermal junction. Because the epidermis is avascular, it depends upon diffusion from the capillary beds of the dermis for its blood supply.

Keratinocytes, which are responsible for the production of keratin, are the most populous cell of the epidermis. Langerhans cells, dendritic cells derived from the bone marrow that are part of the reticuloendothelial system, possess an antigen-processing capability and are interspersed among the keratinocytes. Melanocytes arise from neural crest and produce the primary skin pigment melanin. The melanocytes transfer pigment to the surrounding keratinocytes via pinocytosis. Merkel cells for afferent nerve conduction and mechanoreception are found in the basal layer as well.

Dermis

This layer of skin is composed of dense collagenous connective tissue. It is further subdivided into a papillary layer that interdigitates with the epidermal ridges via dermal ridges and secondary dermal papillae and a denser layer termed the reticular layer. Blood supply from the reticular layer enters the papillary layer's dermal ridges to supply blood to the overlying epidermis. The reticular layer supports a vascular plexus that is supplied from the underlying hypodermis. Hair follicles, sebaceous and eccrine glands, and Pacinian corpuscles are present in this layer.

Dermal nerves and vasculature

The cutaneous nerve supply travels along the blood supply to the skin. The source is a single segment of the spinal cord and is the well known "dermatome." The terminal nerve branches along with several specialized sensory structures, including Merkel cells and Meissner corpuscles for light touch, Pacinian corpuscles for pressure detection, Raffini corpuscles for heat detection, thermoreceptors for the detection of heat and cold, and naked nerve endings for the sensation of pain are present in the dermis and basal layers of the epidermis.

Cutaneous vessels arise from underlying vessels derived from septocutaneous or fasciocutaneous perforator vessels or from terminal branches of the musculocutaneous vessels. The terminal branches form the extensive superficial vascular plexus and the deep vascular plexus, which is interconnected to the superficial plexus by vertical dermal vessels and forms a continuous vascular network within the skin. This vascular network is responsible for the thermoregulatory property of the skin. Vasoconstriction and vasodilatation of these vessels are under the control of the hypothalamus. Glomus cells are a specialized vascular structure that is basically an arteriovenous shunt connecting an arteriole and a venule and when open cause and increase in blood flow in the area.

Lymphatics also parallel the blood supply to the skin and are a functioning component of the reticuloendothelial system. Following the pattern of the blood vessels, they become increasingly larger in caliber as they move deeper into the dermis and subcutaneous tissue and ultimately drain into the venous circulation.

Subcutaneous tissue

Mature subcutaneous fat makes up the bulk of the subcutaneous tissue. The lobules that form the subcutaneous layer are separated by thin, fibrous septae through which the vessels and lymphatics course. The septae provide a structural framework that stabilizes the subcutis, compartmentalizing it and connecting the reticular layer of the dermis to the fascial planes that underlie the subcutaneous fat [2]. This layer varies in thickness in various anatomic positions and in individuals.

Epithelial appendages

After injury, reepithelialization is essential to reestablish the barrier function of the skin. This involves cellular migration from wound edge to wound edge and involves epithelial cells derived from the epithelial appendages, such as hair follicles and apocrine and eccrine glands.

Types of wounds

Wounds can be classified as acute or chronic. Acute wounds can be defined as any interruption in the continuity of any tissue of the body [1].

This is in contradistinction to a chronic wound, which can be defined as an interruption in the continuity of any tissue that requires a prolonged time to heal, does not heal, or reoccurs [1].

Acute wounds heal as anticipated and proceed through a normal, orderly, and timely reparative process that results in sustained restoration of anatomic and functional integrity. Chronic wounds do not heal as anticipated and fail to proceed through this process or proceed through the process but fail to establish a sustained anatomic and functional result [3]. Chronic wounds may get stuck in any of the phases of wound healing for greater than 6 weeks [4].

Acute wounds

Lacerations are usually caused by a simple shearing force (eg, from a knife or glass). This is a simple dividing of tissue. There is little kinetic energy imparted to the tissue, so the surrounding tissue injury is minimal, although glass injuries can cause significant damage to soft tissues [5]. Partial avulsion lacerations are complicated lacerations in which the dermis has undergone a significant separation from the superficial fascia, creating a "flap of dermis." This wound can compromise the flap of tissue because its remaining blood supply is derived from the intact dermal portion at the base of the flap. In random flaps, clinical experience has resulted in the observation that the ratio of flap length to width is critical for complete flap survival [6]. This rule varies from anatomic site to anatomic site.

Tension injuries are a result of a blunt or semi-blunt object striking the skin at an angle. Often a triangular flap is created, and the blood supply is interrupted on two sides of the flap [7]. Crushing or compression injuries occur when a relatively blunt object strikes the skin at a right angle [7]. These lacerations often have ragged or irregular edges, and a significant amount of kinetic energy is transferred to the surrounding and underlying tissue. Shearing force is a mechanical force that is parallel rather than perpendicular to an area. This may cause a triangular-shaped flap or tunneling.

Puncture wounds

Puncture wounds account for 3% to 5% of all traumatic injuries presenting to pediatric emergency rooms [8]. Most are on the plantar aspect of the foot. Puncture wounds are commonly caused by nails but can also occur via envenomation; human and animal bites; iatrogenic causes; and foreign bodies such as wood, metal, glass, and plastic. One must be vigilant to suspect a retained foreign body if the mechanism of injury suggests it.

Bite wounds

Bite wounds are one of the most common types of trauma [9]. The majority of such wounds are caused by dogs, cats, and humans and often involve young children. The mechanism of injury can frequently cause crushing, tearing, or avulsion of tissue and cause devitalized tissue with significant bacterial contamination.

Abrasions

Abrasions are skin wounds caused by a tangential force to the epidermis and dermis. The skin surface is forced against a resistant surface and essentially scraped away. Varying thicknesses of epidermis and or dermis can be lost, and deeper abrasions can occur. Abrasions can cover a significant amount of total body surface area and are frequently impregnated with grass, asphalt, and dirt.

Burns

A burn is damage to the skin and underlying structures caused by excessive heat or caustic chemicals. Burns are usually divided into three depths of tissue injury. Superficial or epidermal burns, typified by the common sunburn, are confined to the epidermis. Partial-thickness burns involve the epidermal layer and part of the dermal layer (formerly referred to as second-degree burns). This can further be divided into two depths of partial thickness burns: superficial partial thickness and deep partial thickness. Superficial partial thickness burns involve destruction of the epidermis and the upper one third of the dermis. Blisters form in this type of burn. Deep partial thickness burns destroy epidermis and most of the dermal layer. As a result, the wound is white and dry. Full-thickness burns are burns in which the epidermis, dermis, and epidermal appendages have been destroyed. This burn is waxy and white. Subdermal burns involve destruction of outer epidermis and dermis and extend to the tissue below, including fat, tendon, muscle, and bone.

Burn severity is determined by depth of burn, total body surface area burned in percent, location of burn, and patient age. The rule of nines is a commonly used tool to divide the surface of the body into segments of 9%. Age is a major factor in determining the prognosis of the burn, with infants and elderly individuals at higher risk for a mortal event. The depth of heat or caustic injury depends upon the quantity of heat exposure and depth of heat penetration. Location of the burn with respect to anatomic function and depth of overlying skin also plays a role in the severity of burn. Initial evaluation of a burn patient in the emergency department may underestimate the severity of the burn. The wound may involve deeper structures than can be estimated upon primary evaluation. Burns are dynamic and can evolve into deeper wounds over time depending upon the initial injury and subsequent environmental insults [10].

Chronic wounds

Chronic wounds arise from acute wounding if appropriate interventions are not initiated or if factors known to delay healing predominate. Chronic wounds often occur in individuals who have underlying comorbidities, including advanced age, peripheral vascular disease, malnutrition, diabetes, chronic steroid use, or other chronic diseases that impair tissue healing. Chronic wounds do have differences at the cellular level that distinguish them. Chronic wounds do not have clot formation, which diminishes the growth factors present in platelets and "primes the wound for healing" [1].

Debridement can improve healing by exposing viable tissue [11]. Most chronic wounds are colonized with bacteria and thus require more macrophages and immune response to be mounted to clear away debris, contributing to prolonged healing time [1]. Increased epithelialization, which increases scar friability and the need for increased angiogenesis, can also prolong wound healing. Chronic wounds generally have extensive tissue loss and extensive tissue remodeling.

Pressure ulcers

A pressure ulcer is a disruption of the normal anatomic structure and function of skin that results from an external force associated with a bony prominence that does not heal in an orderly and timely fashion [12]. Pressure ulcers can be categorized according to the National Pressure Ulcer Advisory Panel definitions.

> STAGE 1: An observable pressure-related alteration of intact skin, with indicators such as an adjacent or opposite area on the body, which may include changes in one or more of the following: skin temperature (warmth or coolness), tissue consistency (firm or boggy feel), or sensation (pain, itching). In lightly pigmented skin, the ulcer appears as a defined area of persistent redness, whereas in darker skin tones, the ulcer may appear with persistent red blue or purple hues.
>
> STAGE 2: Partial-thickness skin loss involving the epidermis, dermis, or both.
>
> STAGE 3: Full-thickness skin loss involving damage or necrosis of subcutaneous tissue that may extend down to but not through the underlying fascia.
>
> STAGE 4: Full-thickness skin loss with extensive destruction, tissue necrosis, or damage to muscle, bone, or supporting structures.

Diabetic foot ulcers

Diabetic foot ulcers typically occur on the plantar aspect of the foot in areas prone to excessive pressure. They generally present as symmetric, round, puncture-appearing wound cavities with a clean wound bed and callous around the wound. Atherosclerotic occlusive disease is a factor in the development of malperforate ulcers; however, the combination of autonomic neuropathy, infection, and autonomic dysfunction that produces anhidrosis and hyperkeratosis also contributes to the development of this wound. Diabetic patients typically manifest lesions in the distal popliteal and tibioperoneal arteries, with usual sparing of the dorsal foot.

Venous insufficiency ulcer

Venous insufficiency ulcers are typically partial-thickness wounds resulting from chronic venous insufficiency. They are usually located between the mid calf and malleolus. They have shaggy, irregular borders and often have heavy exudates [13]. There is a brownish pigmentation of the skin secondary to extravasated hemoglobin and loss of subcutaneous fat, leading to lipodermatosclerosis. Although there is unanimous agreement that venous ulcers are due to venous stasis and back pressure, there is less consensus as to the exact pathophysiology that leads to ulceration and impaired healing [14].

Ischemic wounds

Ischemic wounds are generally atrophic and can lead to necrosis of the affected part. The wounds are generally shallow, painful, have a pale base, and are usually caused by a decrement in blood supply to the affected body part. The wounds are commonly present on the most distal portions of the extremities, although more proximal locations are encountered. Other signs of peripheral ischemia, such as dryness of the skin, hair loss, scaling, and pallor, can be present [14]. Occlusive disease is often manifested in the superficial femoral system, often in the adductor hiatus or Hunter's canal.

This brief introduction of the anatomy and types of wounds will help in the evaluation of wounds seen in the emergency department. Knowledge of skin structure can help to define the depth of injury and informs the clinician of the extent of repair that must occur to restore tissue health [1].

Principles of wound healing

Patients presenting to the emergency department commonly have wounds. In a British study of presenting problems, a surprising statistic was reported. Twenty-five percent of the 11 million patients attending Accident and Emergency Departments in England and Wales present with wounds [15]. It behooves the emergency physician to have a thorough working knowledge of principles of wounding, initial wound management, and management of complications from wounds.

In addition, our world seems to be getting smaller, with rapid evacuation from global military conflicts. Due to protective body armor, soldiers may suffer injuries in areas of the body not covered by armor. Frequently these are soft tissue injuries. In combat casualties in Afghanistan during Operation Enduring Freedom, fragments were the most common mechanism of injury (49%), with the extremity as the most common location of injury (58%) [16]. There have been reported unique injury patterns (behind armor blunt trauma) to the victim wearing body armor. These injuries have some of the features of blunt chest trauma and have characteristics of primary blast injury [17].

Physicians should be facile with the management of wounds of any type that present to our care, and it is to the history of this topic we now turn.

History of wound management

Humans have always experienced wounds of some type, whether accidental, from interpersonal trauma, burns from heat sources, or even self-inflicted wounds for attention seeking or for cultic reasons. Wounds readily lend themselves to observation and study. In different ancient societies, there are those who practiced healing arts. The Assyrian cuneiform scripts define laws for practicing wound healers who, like the Egyptians, were definitive in their teaching of the need to drain pus [18]. In some cases, healers felt that different materials were useful to be placed on wounds. Some of these included plant materials or animal feces. Due to this practice, many of their patients contracted tetanus. The first tetanus toxoid (inactivated toxin) was produced in 1924 and was used successfully to prevent tetanus in the armed services during World War II [19]. Before the tetanus vaccine was in use, many patients probably died from inoculation from materials that contained the *Clostridium tetani* endospores.

Hippocrates taught that cleanliness and, to some extent, aseptic technique was important. He realized that wounds could heal primarily but also practiced wound irrigation with antiseptics such as vinegar and wine in preparation for delayed primary or secondary closure [20].

Despite much being known about wounds and wound care, there is much to be learned concerning the intricate interplay and interactions that result in a healed wound. Much is also known about factors that lead to chronic wounds and their clinical manifestations (Box 1), but we still have a great

---

Box 1. Clinical features of nonhealing wounds

Absence of healthy granulation tissue
Presence of necrotic and unhealthy tissue in the wound bed
Excess exudates and slough
Lack of adequate blood supply
Failure of reepithelialization
Cyclical or persistent pain
Recurrent breakthrough of wound
Clinical or subclinical infection

Data from Grey JE, Harding KG. ABC of wound healing; wound assessment. BMJ 2006;332:285–8.

deal to learn about how to convert nonhealing, painful, and resource-taxing wounds into wounds that heal.

Wound healing and phases

Normally, wound healing lasts for up to 2 years, but nutritional and metabolic factors delay healing; hyperalimentation would likely be beneficial under these conditions. Other factors that influence wound healing are the oxygen tension in tissues, the hemodynamic status, and the effects of substances such as cortisone, vitamins A and C, and zinc [21]. Nutrition is a factor that globally affects wound healing. Vitamins and trace minerals can have harmful effects and are discussed in the appropriate section.

To study wounds and to be able to describe phases of healing, various phases have been promoted by different investigators [22,23]. The author prefers to use the phases as described by Jorgensen [24] because the differentiations are most inclusive. Wound healing encompasses coagulation, inflammation, angiogenesis, fibroplasia, contraction, epithelialization, and remodeling. These phases are discussed in detail in the sections that follow.

Hemostasis/coagulation

Excessive bleeding is deleterious to the patient's well-being; however, in the heat of battle in the emergency department and in the transfer process, wounds that seem innocuous, such as digit or scalp wounds, can have significant bleeding. It is beyond the scope of this article to cover techniques that effect hemostasis.

After the injury, the damaged blood and lymphatic vessels undergo vasoconstriction to slow or stop blood loss in the affected area. Norepinephrine secreted by blood vessels and serotonin secreted by platelets and mast cells are responsible for the vasoconstriction of the vessels [25].

As the blood components spill into the site of injury, the platelets come into contact with exposed collagen and other elements of the extracellular matrix. Different tissues that are exposed for contact with platelets activate the extrinsic versus the intrinsic pathway. Exposed tissue plays a dominant role in hemostasis. In the tissues that are exposed from wounds involving the brain, lung, placenta, heart, and uterus, a tissue complex between tissue factor-factor VIIa forms a complex, and hemostasis is achieved using the extrinsic pathway. Skeletal muscle and joint tissue hemostasis involves factor VIIIa and factor IXa complex [26].

Contact between these complexes with platelets causes the release of clotting factors and essential growth factors and cytokines, such as platelet-derived growth factor (PDGF) and transforming growth factor–β (TGF-β) [27]. These growth factors are important triggers not only for hemostasis, but as important messages for the later phases of healing.

It is important for platelets and the coagulation cascade to initiate wound healing. This first phase is much like the moment when the orchestra tunes to begin a performance. The insult has occurred, the platelets and clotting cascade join in and crescendo to form a clot, and then there is silence as the next phase of inflammation begins.

There are clear factors that we can pinpoint that adversely affect clotting and the coagulation cascade. Some patients have hereditary conditions (eg, hemophilia) that affect these clotting factors. The coagulation cascade has numerous components, and there is current scientific interest in controlling these factors in patients who have cerebrovascular, coronary, or atherosclerotic disease. In our current environment, many elderly patients are on aspirin. Platelets that have been exposed to certain medications are ineffective, whether poisoned by aspirin or other agents such as ticlopidine, dipyridamole, and clopidogrel [28].

For most of the wounds we deal with, the vessels have been cut, torn by traction, or abraded. In practice, these vessels heal in what we would understand as a "normal" process. However, electrical injury produces a unique pattern of injury. Vascular injury by electricity is a thermal process extending from the interior to the exterior [29]. This factor should affect the way electrically injured wounds heal.

In the normal patient, the orchestra has come to a crescendo in tune from the interplay with the platelets and the coagulation factors providing hemostasis/coagulation, and chemical signals have been sent to recruit the other factors in healing. Silence prevails for the moment as the conductor turns to the sheet music of wound healing whose first stanza is inflammation.

Inflammation

After hemostasis, the neutrophils enter the wound site and begin the critical task of phagocytosis to remove foreign materials, bacteria, and damaged tissue [27]. This point signals the initiation of the inflammatory phase. There are numerous inflammatory mediators and chemical signals, many of which are probably not delineated yet. Leukemia inhibitory factor, interleukin (IL)-6, IL-11, and possibly other members of this cytokine family are key mediators in various inflammatory processes, such as the acute-phase reaction, tissue damage, and infection [30]. IL-6 and cortisol seem to act synergistically to activate the acute-phase response. A systemic role for IL-1 and tumor necrosis factor is not evident, even if the possibility that these lymphokines may act locally has not been ruled out [31]. Other inflammatory mediators, such as kallikrein kininogen, are present in wounds and kinin receptors, such as kinin-B1 [32].

The inflammatory phase must be temporary. If there is an infection or other inflammatory process active, this retards wound healing. The risk of infection in traumatic wounds is reduced by adequate wound cleansing and debridement with removal of any nonviable tissue and foreign material

[33]. Wound cleansing should be done by solutions that are not tissue toxic or antigenic. The use of povidine-iodine should be discontinued because it is tissue toxic. Better alternatives include nonionic detergents or chlorinated tap water [34]. The goal is to physically remove any foreign material that could lead to increased inflammation and to decrease bacterial counts.

Some suture materials that have been in use for a significant period of time have been found to have excessive inflammatory properties. Catgut should no longer be used because it causes an excessive tissue reaction, which may predispose to infection [33]. Silk can cause an intense tissue reaction, with an increased risk of excessive scarring and of formation of a suture abscess; silk is therefore no longer recommended [33].

Angiogenesis

The next phase of healing involves the creation of vessels and repair of damaged vessels. Any military historian can tell you that the most critical factor in successful military campaigns is the ability to supply troops in the field. The same principle applies to wound healing. The tissues need tissue oxygen and nutrients and removal of carbon dioxide and waste products.

The adhesion of platelets to the denuded subendothelial matrix is the hallmark of the acute phase providing an adhesive substrate for monocytes, whereas chronic monocyte recruitment is regulated by the interaction with neointimal smooth muscle cells and recovering endothelial cells [35]. These monocytes are key players in the process of angiogenesis. In addition, vascular endothelial growth factor (VEGF) is important and is believed to be the most prevalent angiogenic factor throughout the skin repair process [36]. The lack of α_2-antiplasmin markedly causes an over-release of VEGF from the fibroblasts in cutaneous wound lesions, thereby inducing angiogenesis around the area and resulting in an accelerated wound closure [37].

Factors that adversely affect angiogenesis

The dictum "if some is good, more is better" does not apply to the critical process of angiogenesis. The exuberant infiltration with monocytes aggravates neointimal growth and can thereby promote restenosis [35].

Elderly patients heal slower than younger patients. This may be related to delayed angiogenesis. In the aged mice model, a decline in angiogenic growth factor production and a decline in endothelial responsiveness to specific factors may account for the delayed wound angiogenesis. These results indicate that age-related alterations in macrophage function might partially account for the overall delay in the wound repair process [38].

Protamine sulfate given in high doses can inhibit angiogenesis in the granulation tissue generated in an open wound. The abnormal vasoformation that may be initiated by protamine's anticoagulant properties could set the stage for impaired fibroblast synthetic activity [39]. It is to the fibroblasts, which are the agents of collagen construction, that we now turn.

Fibroplasia/fibroproliferation

As part of the inflammatory phase, the macrophages appear and continue to process of phagocytosis and release more PDGF and TGF-β. Once the wound site is cleaned out, fibroblasts migrate in to begin the proliferative phase and deposit new extracellular matrix. The new collagen matrix becomes cross-linked and organized during the final remodeling phase [27].

Nitric oxide in the inducible isoform is synthesized in the early phase of wound healing by inflammatory cells (mainly macrophages) and regulates collagen formation, cell proliferation, and wound contraction [40].

The results are consistent with the hypothesis that control of collagenase (matrix metalloproteinase-1) expression is important for reepithelialization during wound healing and indicate that collagenase regulation is critical to the kinetics of normal wound closure [41].

Factors that adversely affect fibroproliferation

Agents that are toxic to cells that provide the extracellular matrix should not be used in wound care because this can deleteriously affect wound healing. Shur-Clens, SAF-Clens, and saline were found to be the least toxic to fibroblasts (toxicity index 0); Dial Antibacterial Soap and Ivory Liqui-Gel were the most toxic (toxicity index 100,000) [42].

Experimental wounds in aged mice have age-related changes in scar quality and inflammatory cell profile that are similar to those seen in fetal wound healing. Despite an overall decrease in collagen I and III deposition in the wounds of old mice, the dermal organization was surprisingly similar to that of normal dermal basket-weave collagen architecture. By contrast, young animals developed abnormal, dense scars. The rate of healing in young animals seems to be increased at the expense of the scar quality, perhaps resulting from an altered inflammatory response [43].

The nutritional state of the patient has been felt to be important in wound healing. Patients who are malnourished have delayed healing. Proteins and cofactors are required in wound healing. Due to the link with scurvy, physicians have felt that vitamin C in high doses might be useful [44–47]. It is not clear how much vitamin C is helpful, and supplemental ascorbic acid in the seriously ill patient can result in renal failure [48].

Nutrition is linked with promoting wound healing. In a randomized, placebo-controlled, double-arm, crossover study, subjects responding to oral supplements had less redness in the wounds observed that may have been associated with less inflammation, and 70% of normal, healthy subjects studied had accelerated soft-tissue wound healing [49].

Some patients have excessive scar formation, and plastic surgeons or dermatologists want to intervene to decrease the risk of keloid formation. 5-Fluorouracil, a pyrimidine analog widely used in cancer chemotherapy and in glaucoma surgery, has recently shown some efficacy in the treatment of keloids, scars that overgrow the boundaries of original wounds [50].

Other treatments for keloids include silicone gel sheeting, elastic garments, steroids, radiation therapy (1200–2000 gy in five doses), and bleomycin [51].

Beta blockade with propranolol has been shown in male rats to impair wound healing by increased epidermal and connective tissue cell proliferation, polymorphonuclear leucocyte migration, myofibroblast density, and mast cell migration. In propranolol-treated animals, the volume density of blood vessels was increased, and vessels were more dilated [52]. In light of these findings, it is unclear what effect beta blockade has on our elderly patients who frequently are on beta blockers for coronary artery disease.

Vitamin E is a lysosomal stabilizer and is therefore an antiinflammatory compound. Vitamin E fits into the category of aspirin and dexamethasone because these agents have inhibitory effects on collagen synthesis and wound repair, and for this reason vitamin E should probably not be routinely recommended [53].

Contraction/scar formation

The wound next undergoes contraction and scarring as a natural progression. Fibroblasts from the previous phase have laid down collagen, and now the wound contracts. Studies have shown that the orientation of this collagen matrix determines wound attachment and contraction [54]. This phase is hormone dependent, and epidermal growth factor is one of the key chemical signals. In vitro it seems that epidermal growth factor loaded in collagen sponges resulted in significantly increased breaking strength and skin resilience [55]. Other key compounds active in wound contraction are TGF-β, mitogen-activated protein kinase, extracellular signal-regulated kinase, activin-linked kinase 5, and heparin sulfate–containing proteoglycans [56].

Factors that adversely affect contraction

The desired outcome is minimal scarring so that the wound has an excellent cosmetic appearance. There are chemical compounds that can adversely affect wound contraction. In an animal model, the animals on systemic isotretinoin had a significant delay in wound contraction when compared with control animals ($P < .001$). When the isotretinoin was discontinued, all the animals had complete wound healing within a week [57].

In a study with silver sulfadiazine (SSD), the placebo group, which received aqueous cream, healed in a significantly shorter time ($P < .05$) than the control (saline) group. Wound contraction was delayed by saline and SSD. Nystatin and aloe vera, when added to SSD, reversed that effect. These data suggest that a dry wound heals slowly. Infection control without delay of wound healing is appealing, and clinical trials are planned [58].

Isoform nitric oxide is useful in wound healing; however, superoxide levels, as found in excessively high levels of nitric oxide in the wound, impair wound healing [59].

Nutrition is important for this contraction phase because collagen is essentially a protein. In one animal study, open wounds contracted more slowly in the malnourished group. Matching these observations with histopathologic findings based on serial observations in these same animals, the differences between the contraction of open wounds in poorly nourished animals and in the control group seem to be associated with delay in the formation and the poor quality of granulation tissue in the malnourished animals [60].

In some cases, it is desirable that certain wounds do not contract. In an in vitro study using β_2-adrenergic receptor activation, these activators markedly decreased keratinocyte migration and may have some future clinical usefulness in preventing unwanted wound contraction in burn and trauma patients [61].

Wounds that are perpendicular to the lines of Langer are well known to have increased scarring. A novel approach by one author in Cairo, Egypt was to use botulinum toxin type A to prevent widening of perpendicular facial wounds [62].

Epithelialization

This phase is analogous to what occurs in fibroproliferation, with the notable differences being that the main work is done by keratinocytes and not fibroblasts, and the location of the work being done on the surface of the wound. Moist, non-occlusive dressings do not remove the surface that the wound is trying to lay down. Simple gauze moistened by saline or lime solution can serve as dressings but if not remoistened before removal can harm the delicate epithelial layer. It is more advantageous to apply some sort of ointment to prevent drying. Antibiotic ointment is classically used; the antibiotic component is not relevant for wound healing per say but may serve to keep bacterial counts down [63–66].

Factors that adversely affect epithelialization

With respect to keratinocytes, Biolex, Shur-Clens, and Techni-Care, were the least toxic to keratinocytes (toxicity index 0); hydrogen peroxide, modified Dakin's solution, and povidone (10%) were found to be the most toxic (toxicity index 100,000) [42].

Dressings can adversely affect epithelialization by removal of keratinocytes that are attempting to heal the wound. Depending upon the wound and purpose for the dressing, one must remember that wet-to-dry dressings have a place in debriding certain wounds. In vitro experiments reveal that dressings that are silver based have been found to be cytotoxic and should not be used in the absence of infection. Alginate dressings demonstrate high calcium concentrations, markedly reduced keratinocyte proliferation, and affected keratinocyte morphology [67].

We live in a nation in which people are living longer. In healthy humans, aging leads to delayed epithelialization. No effect of age on collagen synthesis was noted, although accumulation of wound noncollagenous protein was decreased. This decrease may impair the mechanical properties of scarring in aged humans [68].

Smokers have been clinically noted to have delayed wound healing. There are deleterious effects of nicotine on wound reepithelialization, and this suggest that smoking may delay wound healing via a nicotinic receptor-mediated pathway [69].

Scar remodeling

Now begins the phase in which the collagen has been synthesized, the wound has contracted, and the wound undergoes remodeling. A role for collagen phagocytosis and intracellular degradation by fibroblasts during remodeling activity has been suggested by studies on several connective tissues characterized by high rates of collagen turnover and remodeling [70]. In addition, myofibroblasts differentiate to remodel the scar. Myofibroblast differentiation is a complex process, regulated by at least a cytokine (TGF-β1), an extracellular matrix component (the ED-A splice variant of cellular fibronectin), and the presence of mechanical tension. The myofibroblast is a key cell for the connective tissue remodeling that takes place during wound healing and fibrosis development [71]. Once remodeling is complete, in a process that occurs over several weeks, the wound achieves its final appearance.

Factors that adversely affect remodeling

Remodeling is dependent on the fibroblast classes, so nutrition and the patient's age should have the most important influence on the finished scar product. The age-associated healing delay in the rat may not be related to the appearance or abundance of distinct myofibroblast or apoptotic cell populations. Proteolysis may have a significant role in delayed wound healing in aged animals [58].

Given its importance in restoring health, it is not surprising that the care of soft tissue wounds is an extremely active area of research and development. Given the above framework of the phases of wound healing, an understanding of these new frontiers will help the clinician to evaluate new products and treatments as they emerge, and thus improve wound care.

Hemostasis

For most wounds, this phase is complete by the time a physician inspects the wound. For the minority of patients with severe wounds, treatments to promote the cessation of bleeding are of upmost importance. Many of these treatments are time honored and, like direct pressure, can be singularly effective [72]. Intensive research into dressings that have improved hemostatic properties as compared with gauze has yielded two excellent candidates, the Hemcon dressing (Portland, OR) and a fibrinogen/thrombin containing dressing. The Hemcon dressing is the only one commercially available

[73]. Although the tourniquet is an ancient medical device, it seems to be poised to make a comeback as a method of emergency hemorrhage control. Extensive use of the Combat Application Tourniquet (North American Rescue Products, Greenville, SC) by the United States military in ongoing conflicts and the positive risk-to-benefit ratio of hemostatic tourniquets suggest that tourniquets will be one of the medical advances that transitions from the military to civilian health care [74]. In addition to improved devices, research into pharmacologic approaches to promoting hemorrhage control has identified recombinant activated factor VII as a potentially useful drug [75]. Ongoing prospective, randomized, blinded, multicenter trials of recombinant-activated factor VII should serve to better inform the use of this drug for patients without inborn errors of the coagulation system.

Tissue oxygenation

The most direct approach to addressing wound ischemia involves the use of hyperbaric therapy to deliver oxygen to wounded tissues. This approach has proven useful, but it is beyond the care typically delivered by emergency physicians. The costs and facilities involved in hyperbaric therapy have driven innovation in direct delivery of oxygen to tissues. Among promising wound treatments in this area is a dressing system that produces molecular oxygen through the enzymatic consumption of hydrogen peroxide solution [76]. Other topical oxygen delivery systems, such as dressings and garments that are designed to be charged with gaseous oxygen and then contain the gas around the wound, have been described. Ambient or low-pressure oxygen is not equivalent to hyperbaric oxygen, and in the absence of evidence of efficacy, these technologies must be considered as unproven.

Edema

The negative effect of edema on wounds is not well understood at a mechanistic level, and hence research in this area is less developed. Until recently, few therapeutic options existed to manage edema directly. More recently, negative pressure therapy has undergone an explosion in interest. The expense and complexity of even the home health care device limits the applicability of this device to only the most challenging of wounds for outpatient care. There exists little experimental evidence for the mechanism of action of topical negative pressure therapy, although there is no shortage of theories. Preclinical and clinical studies of such mechanisms of action offer the potential to greatly inform the development of future approaches to wound care based on a sound understanding of the pathophysiology of edema [77].

Prevention of infection

Perhaps no area of wound care research has remained as active for as long as investigations of treatments to prevent and cure wound infection.

Although high-risk wounds generally indicate systemic antibiotics, research has focused on the application of local treatments to lower risk wounds in the effort to prevent the generally low rate of infection seen in uncomplicated wounds. In general, research has sought to balance the potential for these agents to retard wound healing with the positive effects of reduced bioburden and lower risk of infection [78]. Research has shown povidone-iodine to be of potential use in this respect. In addition, several studies have attempted to quantify the effect of antimicrobial creams and ointments on the incidence of wound infection. Many of these studies do not have sufficient power to make strong statements regarding the slight differences expected in infection rate. A notable exception was a study by Dire and colleagues [79], who found neomycin sulfate/bacitracin/polymyxin B sulfate ointment to be efficacious. Recent work by Anglen [80] highlighted the therapeutic potential of addition of castile soap to irrigation solutions but also highlighted the difficulty in demonstrating efficacy even in injuries where the infection risk is relatively high. Many factors can be considered in the assessment of wounds for risk of infection, leading the decision to deploy topical antimicrobials to be idiosyncratic to the provider. Perhaps the most useful method for prevention of wound infection is a rigorous method for assessing such risk. Lammers and colleagues [81] present an evidence-based decision support tool that may be of use in bringing rigor to this area of clinical judgment.

Inflammatory mediators

In the attempt to improve wound care, significant developmental effort has been focused on the initiation of the inflammatory cascade in response to wounding. For the acute wound, management of inflammation is not necessary. Chronic wounds may benefit from research into the modification of inflammation. Control of inflammation is directly achieved through removal of foreign matter and bacteria that induce such prolonged inflammatory states, but factors that induce transition to reepithelialization and angiogenesis, such as topical growth factors [82], autologous platelet-rich plasma [83], and matrix metalloprotease inhibitors [84], have also shown promise in promoting wound healing. Many of these factors can enhance wound healing in animal models of acute wound healing, although their expense and potential complications usually preclude use when wound healing is expected to progress normally.

Regenerative medicine

Perhaps the last frontier in the treatment of injury and disease is the modification of the process of healing beyond scar formation to tissue regeneration. This regenerative approach (also termed tissue engineering) seeks to recapitulate the generation of tissue that occurs during embryogenesis and development and avoid the process of scar formation. Although research and development of regenerative products has focused on severe wounds and disease states, these approaches will be applicable to wounds of any severity with the decision to deploy regenerative medicine based largely on the associated costs and risks. Research and development addressing regeneration has been focused on three related technologies: extracellular matrix (the acellular components of tissue), growth factors (signaling molecules that direct the actions of cells), and stem cells (cells capable of development into various mature cell types). The most mature of these technologies is extracellular matrix, with commercial products already available. Current research seeks to expand the use of extracellular matrix products, to investigate and optimize the underlying mechanisms of action, and to improve usability of these products [85]. Intermediate in maturity are growth factor products, including the currently available recombinant PDGF. Research is progressing rapidly on an entire alphabet soup of growth factors for application to soft tissue wounds (reviewed in Ref. [82]). Many of these (eg, VEGF and epidermal growth factor) have shown promise in preclinical testing, but FDA approval remains a significant barrier for many of these products.

Much ink has been spilled regarding the application of stem cells to human disease, and the future of this technology is bright. It is important to differentiate between fetal stem cells, with their high potential and controversial status, and adult stem cells, which have less potential but are not controversial from religious, ethical, or moral points of view. Adult mesenchymal stem cells can be derived from various patient tissues and, as autologous cells, avoid the issues surrounding transplant incompatibility. Interest is high in developing stem cells from fat, placenta, and cord blood, and preclinical data exist for the application of bone marrow–derived [86] and muscle-derived [87] cells.

Summary

Wound healing is a complex interchange, orchestrated between cellular components that play their respective parts signaled by and mediated by different cellular instruments of healing. When healing is flawless, the final product is a thing of beauty. When healing is delayed, interrupted, or excessive, then unsightly scars of chronic painful wounds that are frustrating to the patient and physician occur.

References

[1] Wysocki AB. Skin anatomy, physiology, and pathophysiology. Nurs Clin North Am 1999; 34(4):777–97, v.

[2] Elder D, editor. Lever's histopathology of the skin. 9th edition. Philadelphia: Lippincott, Williams, and Wilkins; 2005.

[3] Lazarus GS, Cooper DM, Knighton DR, et al. Definitions and guidelines for assessment of wounds and evaluation of healing. Arch Dermatol 1994;130(4):489–93.

[4] Collier M. Understanding the principles of wound management. J Wound Care 2006; 15(1 Suppl):S7–10.

[5] Provencher MT, Allen LR, Gladden MJ, et al. The underestimation of a glass injury to the hand. Am J Orthop 2006;35(2):91–4.

[6] McCarthy JG, editor. Current therapy in plastic surgery. 1st edition. Philadelphia: Saunders; 2006.

[7] Trott A. Wounds and lacerations: emergency care and closure. 2nd edition. St. Louis (MO): Mosby; 1997.

[8] Baldwin G, Colbourne M. Puncture wounds. Pediatr Rev 1999;20(1):21–3.

[9] Stefanopoulos PK, Tarantzopoulou AD. Facial bite wounds: management update. Int J Oral Maxillofac Surg 2005;34(5):464–72.

[10] DeSanti L. Pathophysiology and current management of burn injury. Adv Skin Wound Care 2005;18(6):323–32.

[11] Steed DL, Donohoe D, Webster MW, et al. Effect of extensive debridement and treatment on the healing of diabetic foot ulcers. Diabetic Ulcer Study Group. J Am Coll Surg 1996;183(1): 61–4.

[12] Margolis DJ. Definition of a pressure ulcer. Adv Wound Care 1995;8(4 Suppl):8–10.

[13] Brown G. Wound documentation: managing risk. Adv Skin Wound Care 2006;19(3): 155–65.

[14] Bruncardi FC, editor. Schwartz's principles of surgery. 8th edition. New York: McGraw-Hill; 2005.

[15] Holborn D, Lester R. Setting standards in traumatic wound care. Proceedings of the Fourth Europeon Conference on Advances in Wound Management. 1994. p. 14–6.

[16] Peoples GE, Gerlinger T, Craig R, et al. Combat casualties in Afghanistan cared for by a single Forward Surgical Team during the initial phases of Operation Enduring Freedom. Mil Med 2005;170(6):462–8.

[17] Cannon L. Behind armour blunt trauma:an emerging problem. J R Army Med Corps 2001; 147(1):87–96.

[18] Leaper DJ. Wounds. Biology and management. History of wound healing. vol. 5. Oxford (UK): Oxford University Press; 1998.

[19] Immunization Action Coalition. Vaccine information for the public and health professionals. Available at: http://www.vaccineinfo.org/tetanus/qandavax.asp. Accessed November 2005.

[20] Littre E. Oeuvres comploetes d'Hippocrate. Wounds. Biology and management. Oxford (UK): Oxford University Press; 1998. p. 5.

[21] Heughan C, Hunt TK. Some aspects of wound healing research: a review. Can J Surg 1975; 18(2):118–26.

[22] Cohen I, Deigelmann R, Lindbald W, editors. Wound healing: biochemical and clinical aspects. Philadelphia: W.B. Saunders Company; 1992.

[23] Dubay A, Franz M. Acute wound healing: the biology of acute wound failure. Surg Clin North Am 2003;83:463–81.

[24] Jorgensen LN. Collagen deposition in the subcutaneous tissue during wound healing in humans: a model evaluation. APMIS Suppl 2003;(115):1–56.

[25] Gogia PP. Physiology of wound healing: clinical wound healing. Thorofare (NY): Slack, Inc.; 1995.

[26] Mackman N. Role of tissue factor in hemostasis, thrombosis, and vascular development. Aterioscler Thromb Vasc Biol 2004;24(6):1015–22.

[27] Diegelmann RF, Evans MC. Wound healing: an overview of acute, fibrotic and delayed healing. Front Biosci 2004;9:283–9.

[28] Tran H, Anand SS. Oral antiplatelet therapy in cerebrovascular disease, coronary artery disease, and peripheral arterial disease. JAMA 2004;292(15):1867–74.

[29] Wang XW, Zoh WH. Vascular injuries in electrical burns: the pathologic basis for mechanism of injury. Burns Incl Therm Inj 1983;9(5):335–8.

[30] Gadient RA, Patterson PH. Leukemia inhibitory factor, interleukin 6, and other cytokines using the GP130 transducing receptor: roles in inflammation and injury. Stem Cells 1999; 17(3):127–37.

[31] Di Padova F, Pozzi C, Tondre MJ, et al. Selective and early increase of IL-1 inhibitors, IL-6 and cortisol after elective surgery. Clin Exp Immunol 1991;85(1):137–42.

[32] Schremmer-Danninger E, Naidoo S, Neuhof C, et al. Visualisation of tissue kallikrein, kininogen and kinin receptors in human skin following trauma and in dermal diseases. Biol Chem 2004;385(11):1069–76.

[33] Leaper DJ. Traumatic and surgical wounds. BMJ 2006;332(7540):532–5.

[34] Angeras MH, Brandberg A, Falk A, et al. Comparison between sterile saline and tap water for the cleaning of acute traumatic soft tissue wounds. Eur J Surg 1992;158(6–7): 347–50.

[35] Schober A, Weber C. Mechanisms of monocyte recruitment in vascular repair after injury. Antioxid Redox Signal 2005;7(9–10):1249–57.

[36] Sayan H, Ozacmak VH, Guven A, et al. Erythropoietin stimulates wound healing and angiogenesis in mice. J Invest Surg 2006;19(3):163–73.

[37] Kanno Y, Hirade K, Ishisaki A, et al. Lack of alpha2-antiplasmin improves cutaneous wound healing via over-released vascular endothelial growth factor-induced angiogenesis in wound lesions. J Thromb Haemost 2006;4(7):1602–10.

[38] Swift ME, Kleinman HK, DiPietro LA. Impaired wound repair and delayed angiogenesis in aged mice. Lab Invest 1999;79(12):1479–87.

[39] McGrath MH, Emery JM 3rd. The effect of inhibition of angiogenesis in granulation tissue on wound healing and the fibroblast. Ann Plast Surg 1985;15(2):105–22.

[40] Witte MB, Barbul A. Role of nitric oxide in wound repair. Am J Surg 2002;183(4):406–12.

[41] Di Colandrea T, Wang L, Wille J, et al. Epidermal expression of collagenase delays wound-healing in transgenic mice. J Invest Dermatol 1998;111(6):1029–33.

[42] Wilson JR, Mills JG, Prather ID, et al. A toxicity index of skin and wound cleansers used on in vitro fibroblasts and keratinocytes. Adv Skin Wound Care 2005;18(7):373–8.

[43] Ashcroft GS, Horan MA, Ferguson MW. Aging is associated with reduced deposition of specific extracellular matrix components, an upregulation of angiogenesis, and an altered inflammatory response in a murine incisional wound healing model. J Invest Dermatol 1997; 108(4):430–7.

[44] Gray M, Whitney JD. Does vitamin C supplementation promote pressure ulcer healing? J Wound Ostomy Continence Nurs 2003;30(5):245–9.

[45] Kaplan B, Gonul B, Dincer S, et al. Relationships between tensile strength, ascorbic acid, hydroxyproline, and zinc levels of rabbit full-thickness incision wound healing. Surg Today 2004;34(9):747–51.

[46] Long CL, Maull KI, Krishnan RS, et al. Ascorbic acid dynamics in the seriously ill and injured. J Surg Res 2003;109(2):144–8.

[47] Ringsdorf WM Jr, Cheraskin E. Vitamin C and human wound healing. Oral Surg Oral Med Oral Pathol 1982;53(3):231–6.

[48] Dylewski DF, Froman DM. Vitamin C supplementation in the patient with burns and renal failure. J Burn Care Rehabil 1992;13(3):378–80.

[49] Brown SA, Coimbra M, Coberly DM, et al. Oral nutritional supplementation accelerates skin wound healing: a randomized, placebo-controlled, double-arm, crossover study. Plast Reconstr Surg 2004;114(1):237–44.

[50] Wendling J, Marchand A, Mauviel A, et al. 5-fluorouracil blocks transforming growth factor-beta-induced alpha 2 type I collagen gene (COL1A2) expression in human fibroblasts via c-Jun NH2-terminal kinase/activator protein-1 activation. Mol Pharmacol 2003;64(3): 707–13.

[51] Mustoe TA. Scars and keloids. BMJ 2004;328(7452):1329–30.

[52] Souza BR, Santos JS, Costa AM. Blockade of beta1- and beta2-adrenoceptors delays wound contraction and re-epithelialization in rats. Clin Exp Pharmacol Physiol 2006;33(5–6): 421–30.

[53] Ehrlich HP, Tarver H, Hunt TK. Inhibitory effects of vitamin E on collagen synthesis and wound repair. Ann Surg 1972;175(2):235–40.

[54] Eichler MJ, Carlson MA. Modeling dermal granulation tissue with the linear fibroblast-populated collagen matrix: a comparison with the round matrix model. J Dermatol Sci 2006; 41(2):97–108.

[55] Lee AR. Enhancing dermal matrix regeneration and biomechanical properties of 2nd degree-burn wounds by EGF-impregnated collagen sponge dressing. Arch Pharm Res 2005;28(11):1311–6.

[56] Chen Y, Shi-Wen X, van Beek J, et al. Matrix contraction by dermal fibroblasts requires transforming growth factor-beta/activin-linked kinase 5, heparan sulfate-containing proteo-glycans, and MEK/ERK: insights into pathological scarring in chronic fibrotic disease. Am J Pathol 2005;167(6):1699–711.

[57] Arboleda B, Cruz NI. The effect of systemic isotretinoin on wound contraction in guinea pigs. Plast Reconstr Surg 1989;83(1):118–21.

[58] Ballas CB, Davidson JM. Delayed wound healing in aged rats is associated with increased collagen gel remodeling and contraction by skin fibroblasts, not with differences in apoptotic or myofibroblast cell populations. Wound Repair Regen 2001;9(3):223–37.

[59] Soneja A, Drews M, Malinski T. Role of nitric oxide, nitroxidative and oxidative stress in wound healing. Pharmacol Rep 2005;57(Suppl):108–19.

[60] Modolin M, Bevilacqua RG, Margarido NF, et al. The effects of protein malnutrition on wound contraction: an experimental study. Ann Plast Surg 1984;12(5):428–30.

[61] Pullar CE, Isseroff RR. Beta 2-adrenergic receptor activation delays dermal fibroblast-mediated contraction of collagen gels via a cAMP-dependent mechanism. Wound Repair Regen 2005;13(4):405–11.

[62] Wilson AM. Use of botulinum toxin type A to prevent widening of facial scars. Plast Reconstr Surg 2006;117(6):1758–66 [discussion: 1767–8].

[63] Campbell RM, Perlis CS, Fisher E, et al. Gentamicin ointment versus petrolatum for man-agement of auricular wounds. Dermatol Surg 2005;31(6):664–9.

[64] Cho CY, Lo JS. Dressing the part. Dermatol Clin 1998;16(1):25–47.

[65] Smack DP, Harrington AC, Dunn C, et al. Infection and allergy incidence in ambulatory sur-gery patients using white petrolatum vs bacitracin ointment: a randomized controlled trial. JAMA 1996;276(12):972–7.

[66] Mahaffey PJ. Something old, something new in wound dressings. BMJ 2006;332(7546):916.

[67] Paddle-Ledinek J, Nasa Z, Cleland H. Effect of different wound dressings on cell viability and proliferation. Plast Reconstr Surg 2006;117(7):110S–8S.

[68] Holt DR, Kirk SJ, Regan MC, et al. Effect of age on wound healing in healthy human beings. Surgery 1992;112(2):293–7 [discussion: 297–8].

[69] Zia S, Ndoye A, Lee TX, et al. Receptor-mediated inhibition of keratinocyte migration by nicotine involves modulations of calcium influx and intracellular concentration. J Pharmacol Exp Ther 2000;293(3):973–81.

[70] McGraw W, Ten Cate A. A role for collagen phagocytosis by fibroblasts in scar remodeling: an ultrastructural sterologica study. J Invest Dermatol 1983;81(4):375–8.

[71] Desmouliere A, Chaponnier C, Gabbiani G. Tissue repair, contraction, and the myofibro-blast. Wound Repair Regen 2005;13(1):7–12.

[72] Naimer SA, Tanami M, Malichi A, et al. Control of traumatic wound bleeding by compres-sion with a compact elastic adhesive dressing. Mil Med 2006;171(7):644–7.

[73] Wedmore I, McManus JG, Pusateri AE, et al. A special report on the chitosan-based hemo-static dressing: experience in current combat operations. J Trauma 2006;60(3):655–8.

[74] Walters TJ, Mabry RL. Issues related to the use of tourniquets on the battlefield. Mil Med 2005;170(9):770–5.

[75] Payne EM, Brett SJ, Laffan MA. Efficacy of recombinant activated factor VII in unselected patients with uncontrolled haemorrhage: a single centre experience. Blood Coagul Fibrinolysis 2006;17(5):397–402.

[76] Wright T, Wyatt G, Francis K, et al. The effects of an oxygen generating dressing on tissue infection and wound healing. The Journal of Applied Research 2003;3(4):363–70.

[77] Venturi ML, Attinger CE, Mesbahi AN, et al. Mechanisms and clinical applications of the vacuum-assisted closure (VAC) device: a review. Am J Clin Dermatol 2005;6(3):185–94.

[78] Ramasastry SS. Acute wounds. Clin Plast Surg 2005;32(2):195–208.

[79] Dire DJ, Coppola M, Dwyer DA, et al. Prospective evaluation of topical antibiotics for preventing infections in uncomplicated soft-tissue wounds repaired in the ED. Acad Emerg Med 1995;2(1):4–10.

[80] Anglen JO. Comparison of soap and antibiotic solutions for irrigation of lower-limb open fracture wounds: a prospective, randomized study. J Bone Joint Surg Am 2005;87(7): 1415–22.

[81] Lammers RL, Hudson DL, Seaman ME. Prediction of traumatic wound infection with a neural network-derived decision model. Am J Emerg Med 2003;21(1):1–7.

[82] Broughton G 2nd, Janis JE, Attinger CE. The basic science of wound healing. Plast Reconstr Surg 2006;117(7 Suppl):12S–34S.

[83] Driver VR, Hanft J, Fylling CP, et al. A prospective, randomized, controlled trial of autologous platelet-rich plasma gel for the treatment of diabetic foot ulcers. Ostomy Wound Manage 2006;52(6):68–70, 72, 74 passim.

[84] Xue M, Le NT, Jackson CJ. Targeting matrix metalloproteases to improve cutaneous wound healing. Expert Opin Ther Targets 2006;10(1):143–55.

[85] Badylak SF. Regenerative medicine and developmental biology: the role of the extracellular matrix. Anat Rec B New Anat 2005;287(1):36–41.

[86] Fu X, Fang L, Li X, et al. Enhanced wound-healing quality with bone marrow mesenchymal stem cells autografting after skin injury. Wound Repair Regen 2006;14(3):325–35.

[87] Bujan J, Pascual G, Corrales C, et al. Muscle-derived stem cells used to treat skin defects prevent wound contraction and expedite reepithelialization. Wound Repair Regen 2006; 14(2):216–23.

ELSEVIER
SAUNDERS

Emerg Med Clin N Am
25 (2007) 23–39

EMERGENCY
MEDICINE
CLINICS OF
NORTH AMERICA

Principles of Basic Wound Evaluation and Management in the Emergency Department

Ryan H. DeBoard, MD[a], Dawn F. Rondeau, ANCP[b],
Christopher S. Kang, MD, FACEP[a,c],
Alfredo Sabbaj, MD, MA[b],
LTC John G. McManus, MD, MCR, FACEP[d,e,]*

[a]Department of Emergency Medicine, Madigan Army Medical Center, Bldg. 9040,
Fitzsimmons Drive, Tacoma, WA 98431, USA
[b]Oregon Health and Sciences University, 3181 SW Sam Jackson Park Road,
Portland, OR 97239-7500, USA
[c]University of Washington, Tacoma, Washington, USA
[d]US Army Institute of Surgical Research, Fort Sam Houston,
San Antonio, TX 78234-6315, USA
[e]Emergency Medicine, The University of Texas Health Science Center at San Antonio,
7703 Floyd Curl Drive, San Antonio, TX 78229-3900, USA

Traumatic lacerations of the skin are one of the most common problems seen and treated in the Emergency Department (ED), accounting for approximately 11 million visits annually [1]. The ED will continue to provide the most available portal to wound care because of 24-hour access and decreasing primary care availability. Provision for effective, safe, and clinically competent wound care will continue to be a priority. Historically, lacerations have been a source of significant litigation against emergency medicine physicians. Because patients and physicians desire the same outcomes of avoidance of infection and an aesthetically appearing repair, a contemporary and disciplined approach to wound management will mitigate such risks and improve patient care and satisfaction [2,3]. This article will review current and fundamental aspects of basic wound management, to include a focused history, methodical physical examination, meticulous wound preparation, effective wound closure techniques, and pertinent postrepair care instructions.

* Corresponding author. US Army Institute of Surgical Research, Fort Sam Houston, San Antonio, TX 78234-6315.

E-mail address: john.mcmanus@medd.army.mil (J.G. McManus).

Wound history

Proper wound management begins with a detailed history of the mechanism of injury as well as the patient's past medical history. Furthermore, the time elapsed from injury is essential in the assessment of possible wound infection, as well as to determine whether or not primary wound repair would be advantageous. Allergies to antibiotics, latex, and local anesthetics should also be documented and considered in wound evaluation and treatment. Obtaining a detailed history will help guide further management, workup, and final patient disposition.

Mechanism of injury

On presentation clinicians should obtain a full understanding of the mechanism of injury to include the time of the injury and the mechanism of the injury (a cut with a knife or a crush suffered when a finger is caught in a door). As with all injuries, it is important to clearly understand the mechanism so as to provide the clues to the magnitude of the injury. If the injury occurred in the setting of an occupational exposure, there may be particular chemicals, acids, or bases that need to be considered. These types of injuries can result in devitalized tissue that may need debridement as well as ongoing assessment as this wound may continue to evolve over time. Furthermore, certain mechanisms may require more extensive evaluation (ie, bites, injections, and so forth) and possible subspecialty consultation. Finally, wounds occurring in contaminated environments may also dictate further treatment and follow-up.

Anatomical location

Anatomically, lacerations are more likely in adults to occur on the head and neck (50%) and upper extremities (35%), followed by trunk and then lower extremities [4]. Children, however, are noted to have a greater percentage of facial lacerations, as compared with adults [5]. Anatomical location of the injury is important because certain sites, such as the lower extremities, are much more prone to infection, especially when compared with lacerations on the face or scalp, which have improved regional blood flow [6,7]. The site of the wound also dictates the repair technique that would provide the best cosmetic result. The wound closure technique ultimately selected is primarily determined by skin tension and dynamics. Skin with less tension and dynamic forces, such as the face, usually result in smaller scars as do wounds that run parallel to the lines of skin tension. This is in contrast to lacerations over joints and those that run perpendicular to skin tension lines. The concern for the final appearance has practical as well as potential medical legal impact.

Underlying medical history

Predisposing medical issues should also be elicited as they may complicate wound healing or have led to the initial wounding (eg, seizure, syncope). Specific factors that may impair wound healing and increase the risk of infection include extremes of age, diabetes mellitus, obesity, malnutrition, chronic renal failure, immunosuppressive medications (ie, steroids or chemotherapy), and inherited or congenital connective tissue disorders [8–10]. A patient's healing response to past traumatic injuries, such as keloid production or a hypertrophic scar, should also be ascertained and discussed with the patient as a possible recurrent outcome and increased morbidity. Patients prone to keloid formation should be made aware that with their heritage, keloid formation from the wound is possible. Asian and African American populations have been most identified with keloid formation [11]. Wounds in these individuals may not achieve a full cosmetically acceptable appearance.

Immunization status

Immunization status should also be obtained and documented. The Advisory Committee on Immunization Practices (ACIP; Centers for Disease Control and Prevention [CDC]) recommendations for tetanus vaccination are displayed in Table 1 [12]. Generally, it is recommended that adults have tetanus toxoid every 10 years. In cases of markedly contaminated wounds and no history of tetanus toxoid in the previous 5 years, then tetanus immune globulin is also indicated. Discussion regarding updating of pertussis for adults is currently ongoing. A newly licensed tetanus-diphtheria-acellular-pertussis vaccine (Tdap) is available for adults. ACIP recommendations for use for tetanus prophylaxis in wound management are

Table 1
Summary guide to tetanus prophylaxis in routine wound management for adults (19 years and older)

History of tetanus immunization	Clean minor wounds		All other wounds[a]	
	Td[b]	TIG	Td	TIG
Fewer than 3 or uncertain doses	Yes	No	Yes	Yes
More than 3 doses				
Last dose within 5 y	No	No	No	No
Last dose within 5–10 y	No	No	Yes	No
Last dose more than 10 y earlier	Yes	No	Yes	No

Note: ACIP recommendations from 3/2/2006 that all adults 19 to 64 receive tetanus-toxoid, diphtheria, and acellular pertussis vaccine (Tdap) for tetanus wound prophylaxis unless previously received. These recommendations are under review by the CDC and not formally approved.

Abbreviations: Td, tetanus-diphtheria toxoid; TIG, tetanus immune globulin.

[a] Such as contaminated wounds (feces, dirt, saliva, soil), puncture wounds, avulsions, burns, crush injuries, and frostbite [13].

[b] Tdap is preferred to Td for adults who have never received Tdap. Td is preferred to TT for adults who received Tdap previously or when Tdap is not available. If TT and TIG are both used, tetanus toxoid absorbed rather then tetanus toxoid for booster use only (fluid vaccine) should be used.

that Tdap should be used if the adult (19–64) has not received this preparation previously [13]. The vaccine is currently not licensed for use in individuals older than 64 years.

Antibiotic coverage

With regard to wound factors obtained in the history that may necessitate antibiotic coverage, high bacterial counts have been seen in animal bites, soil contamination, crush injury, and stellate lacerations, which are all risk factors for infection [4]. In addition, it is also generally accepted that wounds involving normally sterile sites such as tendons, joints, or bones are at increased risk for infection. Finally, puncture wounds, intraoral lacerations, and most mammalian bites are considered to be infection-prone wounds. Prophylactic antibiotics, as recommended in the article by Nakamura and Daya elsewhere in this issue, may then be required because of the increased risk of infection.

Patient's symptoms

Finally, documentation of the patient's symptoms is important. Does the patient experience paresthesia or loss of sensation? These symptoms may represent a neurologic and/or vascular injury. Does the patient complain of severe pain? This complaint may represent an underlying fracture, foreign body, or serious medical condition (eg, compartment syndrome, necrotizing fasciitis). Finally, potential for foreign body exposure to glass, wood, plant, or organic materials should be discussed and documented.

Wound examination

Examination

Careful and meticulous examination of a wound is critical to wound management. Examination begins with an adequate setting to include sufficient lighting to help identify foreign bodies as well as underlying nerve, tendon, vascular, and joint involvement. Typically, if deep structures are involved, the wound may not be a candidate for primary closure in the ED and may necessitate specialty consultation. However, one possible exception is an extensor tendon laceration. Joints with overlying wounds should be completely flexed and extended with examination of the tendons through their full range of motion to assess for possible injury. Joint capsule penetration should also be identified because intraoperative evaluation, irrigation, and repair may be necessary.

Hemostasis

A hemostatic or bloodless field should be established to facilitate adequate visualization of anatomical structures and to assess for the presence of obvious contamination, infection, or devitalized tissue. If, despite persistent direct pressure, the wound continues to bleed, a sphygmomanometer may be inflated proximal to the wound to a level greater than the patient's systolic blood pressure for approximately 20 to 30 minutes at a time. A tightly fitting sterile glove may also be used with digital lacerations to establish hemostasis. For severe hemorrhage, there are now a number of commercial tourniquets [14] and newer hemostatic agents (HemCon Bandage, QuickClot) [15–17] that have recently been used successfully to control life-threatening hemorrhage.

Neurovascular exam

A detailed neurovascular exam should be obtained before the application of anesthesia and repair of the wound. An adequate vascular exam should include presence of pallor or cyanosis, visualization of capillary refill, and the palpation of pulses distal to the wound to assess for adequate perfusion. Motor and sensory function should be evaluated with an accompanying in-depth knowledge of the nerve innervation to the area around and distal to the wound. Muscle groups, including flexor and extensor tendons, near the injury should be evaluated. Two-point discrimination should be used to evaluate and document digital nerve injuries with the normal being 2 to 5 mm over digits and 7 to 12 mm over the palm [18]. An efficient and readily accessible method to perform two-point discrimination is through the use of a calibrated, standard-sized paper clip [19].

Foreign body

Failure to identify foreign bodies may lead to complications such as inflammation, increased risk of infection, delayed wound healing, and loss of function. In a retrospective study of patients with hand wounds, nearly 38% had foreign bodies that were missed by the treating physician on initial wound inspection. As previously mentioned, retained foreign bodies are a source of significant litigation accounting for 14% of lawsuits and 5% of all legal settlements [2].

Once a foreign body has been identified a decision must be made to remove it or not. Extraction is based on the type of object, its location, overall risk of infection, and risk of complications with the removal process. For example, objects that impinge on a neurovascular structure and joints or restrict mechanical function should be considered for removal. This may require surgical consult with possible intraoperative removal. This is in contrast to small, inert foreign objects, such as a minute piece of glass, away from vital structures that may be electively left in place [20,21]. If the foreign body is left in place, the patient should be advised and concur with the clinical decision-making process.

Radiography

Plain radiography has traditionally been the screening method of choice for retained foreign bodies; however, only radiopaque objects, such as metal, rocks, and some types of glass, may be reliably detected. Radiolucent foreign bodies like plastic and wood products are frequently missed, with glass being the most common unidentified foreign body, accounting for 50% of all retained objects [22]. Several studies demonstrated that glass larger than 2 mm can be reliably detected by x-ray [23,24]. Flom and Ellis [25] performed an in vitro study comparing x-ray, CT, and ultrasound and found that ultrasound was better able to detect plastic, wood, and glass when compared with the other two methods. Sensitivities and specificities of foreign body detection with ultrasound have each been reported to be as high as 98% [26]; however, accuracy in this study was found to be dependent on the physical model used, the experience of the sonographer, and the size of the foreign body. CT is able to identify wood splinters and plastic foreign bodies; however, if a wood object is left in the wound for more than 48 hours the wood absorbs water and develops a density similar to soft tissue [27,28]. Finally, MRI, although very accurate in detecting foreign bodies, is not practical for routine use.

Wound preparation

Anesthesia

Once the wound has been examined, adequate anesthesia and pain medication should be administered. Local anesthetic agents are classified into two major groups, amides and esters; dosing is described in Table 2. Patients with an allergy to a member of the ester anesthetic may still be treated with an anesthetic from the amide group, and vice versa. In several studies, patients were primarily allergic to the preservative agent instead of the anesthetic itself as allergies specific to the anesthetic agents are extremely rare [29–33]. Therefore, if available, it may be possible to give an anesthetic without the preservative to these patients. In rare instances, patients may report allergies to both major groups or be unable to specify an allergy to an anesthetic. In such cases, it has been shown that locally injected

Table 2
Local anesthetic properties

Anesthetic, with epinephrine	Class	Maximal dose (mg/kg)	Duration of action
Lidocaine	Amide	5	1–2 h
		7	2–4 h
Bupivacaine	Amide	2	4–8 h
		3	8–16 h
Procaine	Ester	7	15–45 min
		9	30–90 min

diphenhydramine has analgesic properties equivalent to 1% lidocaine; how-ever, disadvantages of diphenhydramine as a local anesthetic include a higher level of discomfort upon initial infiltration as well as a slower onset of action (5 minutes versus 1 to 2 minutes) [34,35]. Benzyl alcohol is another alternative anesthetic for the multi-allergic patient and can be as effective as 1% lidocaine, with less discomfort upon injection when compared with diphenhydramine [36].

Anesthetics may be administered directly into the wound, topically, or via regional nerve blocks. Singer and colleagues [37] describes several ways to reduce pain with local infiltration, including adding sodium bicarbonate, warming the local anesthetic, using smaller gauge needles, injecting the an-esthetic at a slower rate, infiltrating the anesthetic through the edge of the wound, and by pretreating the wound with a topical anesthetic.

Topical anesthetics may also be used for patients with aversions to nee-dles, such as small children, or as an adjunct to pain management. The most common topical anesthetic agents are LET (lidocaine, epinephrine, and tetracaine), TAC (tetracaine, adrenaline, and cocaine), and EMLA (eu-tectic mixture of local anesthetics). LET, a popular agent with a widely ac-cepted safety profile, has been found to be an effective anesthetic in 75% to 90% of cases that occur on the face and scalp [38–40] TAC, on the other hand, is rarely used and has been associated with seizures, cardiac arrhyth-mias, and death [41]. EMLA has been found to be much more effective than TAC, requiring additional injected anesthesia when compared with TAC (15% versus 55%). EMLA, however, has a longer time of onset when com-pared with TAC (55 versus 29 minutes) [42]. Use of a topical anesthetic is dependent on a wound site that is highly vascularized so the agent can be effectively absorbed and distributed. The appearance of blanched skin where the topical analgesic is placed is indicative of effective topical anesthesia.

Epinephrine in combination with a local anesthetic may also be adminis-tered to help obtain hemostasis and to increase the duration of anesthesia; however, sites such as digits and the tip of the nose, ears, and penis should not be anesthetized with epinephrine because of the risk of necrosis secondary to the vasoconstriction of end-arterioles. Supplemental epinephrine has, how-ever, been used safely when anesthetizing the nose and periphery of the ear [43].

A regional nerve block is also another effective method of achieving ad-equate wound anesthesia without distorting wound margins. This method is also useful for large wounds that may require potentially toxic doses of local anesthetic as well as for wounds in which local infiltration may be too pain-ful to tolerate. This technique, as well as procedural sedation, is described by Crystal and Harrison elsewhere in this issue.

Sterile technique

Sterile technique for wound closure has been recommended. In 2004, Perelman and colleagues [44] published their study to look at the use of sterile versus nonsterile gloves. Their study used clean nonsterile gloves in the treatment of uncomplicated wounds and compared the rate of infection. In this cohort of patients, they report there was no significant difference in the incidence of infection. Current recommendations are for sterile nonpowder gloves, which are latex free. Universal precautions would mandate single gloving with all patients and consider double gloving in the situation of a patient with a communicable disease such as the human immunodeficiency virus or hepatitis.

Hair removal

Removal of the hair around wound sites has been associated with increased wound infection rates, thought to be secondary to the damage to intact skin from a razor. Most studies have been done in the preoperative setting for elective surgery. In this setting using a clipper has been thought to cause less skin damage and decrease the tissue injury. Although some references will encourage hair removal to ease wound closure, others suggest that the presence of the hair assists as a guide in approximating wound edges [45]. Eyebrow removal is discouraged because regrowth doesn't consistently occur. In the ED, lubrication with antibacterial ointment to move hair away from the injury will assist in wound visualization and closure.

Irrigation

Proper irrigation can significantly reduce the risk of wound infection. This is achieved through the application of the irrigant in large volumes at a sufficient pressure to reduce or eliminate particulate matter and bacterial loads from the wound. The pressure needed to adequately irrigate a wound should be 5 to 8 psi and may be achieved with a 16- to 19-gauge catheter attached to a 35- to 65-mL syringe [46–48]. Sterile saline remains the most commonly used irrigant. However, tap water may also be used with no significant increase in the incidence of infection [49–51]. Application of povidone-iodine, hydrogen peroxide, or detergents should be avoided because of their tissue toxic properties and because they have not been associated with lower infection rates [52].

Debridement

Debridement is yet another means to improve healing, aesthetic outcome, and to decrease risk of infection. This is performed by removing devitalized tissue that is otherwise unable to resist infection [53]. Methods of mechanical debridement include simple surgical excision as well as previously detailed "high pressure" irrigation. If there is any question as to the extent of tissue devitalization, a "wait-and-see" approach may be considered to limit the amount of tissue excised.

Wound closure

Overview

The art of proper wound closure is a learned skill that is developed and enhanced throughout a career in medicine [54]. Laceration repair in the ED is typically performed using primary closure, which involves immediate approximation of the edges of the wound to improve the rate of healing as well as aesthetic appearance. There are characteristics of the wound that should be accounted for to clinically determine whether or not primary closure can be safely implemented. These factors include location, the degree of contamination, and time from injury to laceration closure, as well as the patient's predisposing medical conditions. A recent study demonstrated that the presence of a foreign body and wounds with increasing widths were at greater risk for infection [8–10,55].

Time since wounding

There is varying literature on when or if to close wounds that are delayed in their presentation to the ED. Lammers and colleagues [56] found that wounds older than 10 hours were at a higher risk for infection (8 hours in the hand). The current American College of Emergency Physicians policy on penetrating extremity wound management recommends that primary closure be completed no more than 8 to 12 hours from the time of injury. Wounds that are at low risk for infection, such as those on the face, scalp, and trunk with minimal contamination, may be safely approximated up to 12 hours after the time of injury. Likewise, wounds that are at moderate risk for infection, such as those on the extremities with poor vascular supply, contaminated wounds, or wounds in an immunocompromised patient, may be closed primarily after thorough cleansing within a 6- to 10-hour period [57].

Clinical judgment, however, may allow the time period for primary repair in certain situations to be extended up to 20 hours from time of injury. One such example would be a clean wound on the face in an otherwise healthy patient without infection risk factors. This is in contrast to a diabetic patient with a 1-hour old, contaminated wound that may not be a candidate for primary closure. The time range ideal for closure therefore depends on each individual situation [58].

Delayed primary closure

On occasion, high-risk wounds may be best treated using a delayed primary closure technique 3 to 5 days after injury, once the risk of infection has decreased. This method is especially suitable for wounds that are large or have a higher potential for poor cosmetic outcome. Delayed primary closure should also be implemented if there is any question as to the extent a patient may develop a wound infection [58]. Further detail will be discussed in the advanced wound management article.

Selection of sutures

Suture placement is the most common method used for primary wound closure and is performed using one of several techniques and different types and sizes of suture material. The appropriate suture material and placement technique used should be based on the location, size, nature, and level of contamination of the wound, as well as the personal preference of the treating health care provider [4,8]. Nonabsorbable suture material, such as nylon and polypropylene, retain most of their tensile strength for more than 60 days and must be removed. This type of suture is relatively nonreactive and used to close the outer layer of the wound.

Absorbable sutures are used to approximate the wound deep to the epidermis. There are two general types of absorbable suture: synthetic (polydixanone and polyglyconate) and natural (cat gut). Synthetic absorbable suture retains its tensile strength for long periods and is useful in areas of high static and dynamic tensions. Because the synthetic absorbable suture lasts longer, it should be designated for approximating deep structures as they may be extruded by the body over time if left too superficial. Absorbable sutures are also useful for subcuticular stitches and to avoid suture removal in children. Equally acceptable cosmetic results were found when absorbable suture was compared with the use of nonabsorbable suture in pediatric facial laceration repair [59]. Synthetic and monofilament sutures are preferred over their braided counterparts as they are less likely to harbor infection.

Deeper sutures reduce skin tension and decrease potential spaces where hematomas may accumulate. Generally, deep sutures improve cosmetic outcome by reducing the overall width of the eventual scar. Caution, however, should be taken to avoid placing deep sutures in highly contaminated wounds because of the associated increase risk of infection [60]. In patients with a history of keloid formation, the wound should be approximated with minimal tension and a pressure dressing placed over the wound for 3 to 6 months to attempt to prevent development of another keloid [11].

Several technical principles should be adhered to achieve the best possible cosmetic outcome. For example, when placing sutures, the wound margins should be slightly everted to promote healing and to reduce the chance of creating a depressed scar. Sutures should be placed snuggly enough to approximate wound edges, but not so tight to cause tissue necrosis. Wound aesthetics are also improved when the knots of deep sutures are adequately buried. The smallest possible size of the chosen suture type capable of approximating the wound should be used to minimize scarring.

Alternative wound-closure techniques

Staples

Staples are a popular method for wound closure in the ED because of their rapid placement, when compared with sutures, and are particularly useful for wounds in the scalp, especially in children [61]. Trunk and extremity wounds may also be closed with staples. However, staples are associated with more noticeable scars, as they are not as meticulously placed as sutures, and more painful removal [37].

Surgical tape

Surgical tape, such as "steri-strips," can be a useful alternative to staples in areas of low skin tension. However, tape alone is usually not effective and should be used in conjunction with adhesives, such as tincture of benzoin. Unfortunately, tincture of benzoin may precipitate a local skin reaction. Surgical tape is typically placed perpendicular to the wound and in strips parallel to each other. It has been noted, however, that in certain wounds on the back and chest, this method can lead to blistering secondary to an increased shearing effect of the surgical tape. Blistering was not present when the surgical tape was placed parallel to the wound edges on wounds in the same anatomical locations [62]. The tape should be left in place until it falls off. Disadvantages with this method of closure include the inability to place the tape on areas with significant hair as well as inability of the patients to get them wet [37]. Recent studies have suggested that steri-strips may be as useful as tissue adhesive for facial lacerations in the pediatric population; however, this topic has not been fully studied leaving this conclusion presently unsubstantiated [63,64].

Cyanoacrylates

Cyanoacrylates are tissue adhesives that were approved by the Food and Drug Administration for use in the United States in August 1998 and allow for the painless and rapid approximation of select simple wounds [65,66]. Removal is not required as the keratinized layer of the epithelium sloughs off with the cyanoacrylate in 5 to 10 days. Tissue adhesives should be placed topically with care taken to avoid placement in the wound or between the wound margins. Applying too much of the tissue adhesive can cause an exothermic reaction. For optimal results, the tissue adhesive should be applied in three to four layers in a dry, bloodless field. Picking, scrubbing, and soaking the area should be avoided. Applying petroleum jelly or antibiotic ointment is not recommended and will actually accelerate removal. If rapid removal of the tissue adhesive is desired, acetone may also be effective [55].

Octyl-cyanoacrylate has one of the greatest tensile strengths of the tissue adhesives and has been found to provide excellent aesthetic outcomes when repairing facial lacerations with similar aesthetic outcomes, infection, and dehiscence rates when compared with sutures 3 months and 1 year after repair [67,68]. Plastic surgeons have observed better long-term aesthetic results with cyanoacrylates after elective facial plastic surgery when compared with sutures [69,70]. Another study found no change in overall cosmetic outcome when tissue adhesive was compared with both nonabsorbable and absorbable sutures [71]. Octyl-cyanoacrylates may be used in other areas of the body with low skin tension, but the wound may require deep absorbable sutures to alleviate surface skin tension. Tissue adhesives should be avoided in wounds overlying sites of repetitive motion such as joints and the hands [72]. Cyanoacrylates are also advantageous because they possess antimicrobial properties toward gram-positive bacteria [73,74]. However, as discussed previously, standard wound preparation and cleansing should still be implemented before repair. Overall, cyanoacrylates are easily applied, thus improving ED efficiency with decreased overall cost when compared with suturing and staples. This technique is also the preferred method of wound closure by most patients [75].

Hair apposition technique

The hair apposition technique (HAT) effectively uses tissue adhesives to rapidly and efficiently approximate the edges of wounds located in the scalp. The wound is closed by twisting together the hair on each side of the scalp laceration. The twist is then secured with tissue adhesive. Despite the nearly painless technique of this procedure, local anesthesia may still be required to adequately examine the wound. Hemostasis is also difficult to achieve with this technique and should not be used in significantly bleeding wounds [76]. The advantages of the HAT include a shorter procedure time, less pain, no need for removal of stitches, and similar or superior wound healing when compared with sutures that is otherwise cost-effective with reported high patient satisfaction [77,78].

Wound care

Postrepair wound care is critical to the overall cosmetic outcome of the wound. Repaired wounds should have a nonadherent dressing placed for 24 to 48 hours to ensure adequate epithelialization and to prevent contamination of the wound. Topical antibiotics may be placed on the wound during this 24- to 48-hour period of re-epithelialization and have been shown to lower infection rates [79]. It should be reiterated that wounds treated with tissue adhesive should not be exposed to antibiotic ointments.

Wounds should be kept clean and dry. Patients should avoid soaking or scrubbing the wound, especially with tissue adhesive, as it may loosen the closure. Gentle blotting of the wound with a towel is recommended over repetitive wiping of the wound. Patients should also be given strict instructions to monitor for signs of infection, to include increased warmth, erythema, pain, swelling, or drainage from the wound.

Prophylactic parenteral antibiotics are not recommended for routine laceration repair as described by Nakamura and Daya elsewhere in this issue.

Table 3
Location and optimal time (days) to suture removal

Location	Days
Scalp	7–10
Face	3–5
Chest/Back/Abdomen	8–12
Extremities	8–12
Hand/Fingers	8–10
Foot	10–12

Clinical concern may govern whether antibiotics should be prescribed based on the degree of wound contamination (such as exposure to soil or fresh water), host risk factors, and the mechanism of injury. It should be reinforced that wound preparation with decontamination will be far more beneficial in preventing infection than antibiotics. Antibiotics should, however, been given to patients with wounds secondary to human bites, cat bites, and some dog bites, as well as wounds with underlying open fractures and exposed joints and tendons [80–82].

Sutures and staples should be removed according to the time frame outlined in Table 3. Scars that may be exposed to sunlight should be protected with sunscreen for at least 6 to 12 months to minimize subsequent hyperpigmentation [4].

Summary

The primary objectives of basic wound management center around promoting optimal wound healing and cosmesis. These objectives may be achieved through systematic assessment, preparation, and repair of the laceration supplemented with appropriate patient care instructions. The meticulous and methodical management of traumatic wounds described in this article will assist the emergency physician in decreasing overall complication rates and help improve patient satisfaction.

References

[1] Markovich V. Suture materials and mechanical after care. Emerg Med Clin North Am 1992; 10:673–88.
[2] Tibbles CD, Pocaro W. Procedural applications of ultrasound. Emerg Med Clin North Am 2004;22:797–815.
[3] Singer AJ, Mach C, Thode HC, et al. Patient priorities with traumatic lacerations. Am J Emerg Med 2000;18(6):683–6.
[4] Hollander JE, Singer AJ. State of the art laceration management. Ann Emerg Med 1999;34: 356–67.
[5] Singer AJ, Thode HC, Hollander JE. National trends in ED lacerations between 1992 and 2002. Am J Emerg Med 2006;24:183–8.
[6] Rogers K. The rational use of antimicrobial agents in simple wounds. Emerg Med Clin North Am 1992;10(4):753–65.

[7] Robson MC. Disturbances of wound healing. Ann Emerg Med 1988;17:1274–8.

[8] Capellan O, Hollander JE. Management of lacerations in the emergency department. Emerg Med Clin North Am 2003;21(1):205–31.

[9] Cruse PJ, Foord R. A five-year prospective study of 23,649 surgical wounds. Arch Surg 1973; 107:206–9.

[10] Howard JM, Barker WF, Culbertson WR, et al. Post-operative study of 23,649 surgical wounds: the influence of ultra-violet irradiation in the operating room and of various other factors. Ann Surg 1964;160:32–81.

[11] Grimes PE, Hunt SG. Considerations for cosmetic surgery in the black population. Clin Plast Surg 1993;20:27–34.

[12] CDC guidelines on tetanus vaccination. Available at: www.cdc.gov/nip/publications/vis. Accessed 13 September, 2006.

[13] Preventing tetanus, diptheria, and pertussis among adults: use of tetanus toxoid, reduced diptheria toxoid and acellular pertussis vaccine. Recommendations of the Advisory Committee on Immunization Practices (ACIP) and Recommendation of ACIP, supported by the Healthcare Infection Control Practices Advisory Committee (HICPAC), for use of Tdap among healthcare personnel. 2006;55(R17):1–33.

[14] Walters TJ, Wenke JC, Kauvar DS, et al. An observational study to determine the effectiveness of self-applied tourniquets in human volunteers. Journal of Prehospital Care 2005;9(4): 416–22.

[15] Wedmore I, McManus J, Pusateri A, et al. The chitosan-based hemostatic dressing: experience in current combat operations, a retrospective review. J Trauma 2006;60(3): 655–8.

[16] Pusateri AE, Modrow HE, Harris RA, et al. Advanced hemostatic dressing development program: animal model selection criteria and results of a study of nine hemostatic dressings in a model of severe large venous hemorrhage and hepatic injury in swine. J Trauma 2003;55: 518–26.

[17] Wedmore I, McManus J, Pusateri A, et-al. The chitosan-based hemostatic dressing: experience in current combat operations. U.S. Army Medical Department Journal. April-June 2005.

[18] Sloan EP. Nerve injuries in the hand. Emerg Med Clin North Am 1993;11(3):651–70.

[19] Finnell JT, Knopp R, Johnson P, et al. A calibrated paper clip is a reliable measure of two-point discrimination. Acad Emerg Med 2004;11(6):710–4.

[20] Lammers RL, Magill T. Detection and management of foreign bodies in soft tissue. Emerg Clin North Am 1992;10(4):767–81.

[21] Weinstock RE. Noninvasive technique for the localization of radiopaque foreign bodies. J Foot Surg 1981;20(2):73–5.

[22] Kaiser WC, Slowick T, Spurling KP, et al. Retained foreign bodies. J Trauma 1997;43(1): 107–11.

[23] Courter BJ. Radiographic screening for glass foreign bodies—what does a "negative" foreign body series really mean? Ann Emerg Med 1990;19(9):997–1000.

[24] Arbona N, Jedrzynski M, Frankfather R, et al. Is glass visible on plain film radiographs? A cadaver study. J Foot Ankle Surg 1999;38(4):264–70.

[25] Ginsburg MJ, Ellis GL. Radiographic evaluation of foreign bodies. Emerg Med Clin North Am 1992;10(1):163–77.

[26] Schlager D, Sanders AB, Wiggins D, et al. Ultrasound for the detection of foreign bodies. Ann Emerg Med 1991;20(2):189–91.

[27] Russell RC, Williamson DA, Sullivan JW, et al. Detection of foreign bodies in the hand. J Hand Surg [Am] 1991;16(1):2–11.

[28] Bauer AR Jr, Yutani D. Computed tomographic localization of wooden foreign bodies in children's extremities. Arch Surg 1983;118(9):1084–6.

[29] Blauga JC. Allergy to local anesthetics in dentistry. Myth or reality? Rev Alerg Mex 2003; 50(5):176–81.

[30] Berkun Y, Ben-Zvi A, Levy Y, et al. Evaluation of adverse reactions to local anesthetics: experience with 236 patients. Ann Allergy Asthma Immunol 2003;91(4):342–5.

[31] Amsler E, Flahault A, Mathelier-Fusade P, et al. Evaluation of re-challenge in patients with suspected lidocaine allergy. Dermatology 2004;208(2):109–11.

[32] Rood JP. Adverse reaction to dental local anesthetic injection—"allergy" is not the cause. Br Dent J 2000;189(7):380–4.

[33] Gall H, Kaufman R, Kalveram CM. Adverse reactions to local anesthetics: analysis of 197 cases. J Allergy Immunol 1996;97(4):933–7.

[34] Ernst AA, Marvez-Valls E, Mall G, et al. 1% Lidocaine versus 0.55 diphenhydramine for local anesthesia in minor laceration repair. Ann Emerg Med 1994;23(6):1328–32.

[35] Xia Y, Chen E, Tibbits DL, et al. Comparison of the effects of lidocaine hydrochloride, buffered lidocaine, diphenhydramine, and normal saline after intradermal injection. J Clin Anesth 2002;14(5):339–43.

[36] Barfield JM, Jandreau SW, Raccio-Robak N. Randomized trial of diphenhydramine versus benzyl alcohol with epinephrine as an alternative to lidocaine local anesthesia. Ann Emerg Med 1998;32:650–4.

[37] Singer AJ, Hollander JE, Quinn JV. Evaluation and management of traumatic lacerations. N Engl J Med 1997;337(16):1142–8.

[38] Ernst AA, Marvez-Valls E, Nick TG, et al. LAT versus TAC for topical anesthesia in face and scalp lacerations. Am J Emerg Med 1995;13:151–4.

[39] Resch K, Schilling C, Borchet BD. Topical anesthesia for pediatric lacerations: a randomized trial of lidocaine-epinephrine-tetracaine solution vs. gel. Ann Emerg Med 1998;32(6):693–7.

[40] Blackburn PA, Butler KH, Hughes MJ, et al. Comparison of tetracaine-adrenaline-cocaine (TAC) with topical lidocaine-epinephrine (TLE): efficacy and cost. Am J Emerg Med 1995; 13:315–7.

[41] Ernst AA, Marvez E, Nick TG, et al. Lidocaine, adrenaline, tetracaine gel versus tetracaine aderenaline cocaine gel for topical anesthesia in linear scalp and facial lacerations in children aged 5 to 17 years. Pediatrics 1995;95:255.

[42] Zempsky WT, Karasic RB. EMLA versus TAC for topical anesthesia of extremity wounds in children. Ann Emerg Med 1997;30:163–6.

[43] Hafner HM, Rocken M, Breuninger H. Epinephrine-supplemented local anesthetics for ear and nose surgery: clinical use without complications in more than 10,000 surgical procedures. J Dtsch Dermatol Ges 2005;3(3):195–9.

[44] Perelman VS, Francis GJ, Rutledge T, et al. Sterile versus nonsterile gloves for repair of uncomplicated laceration in the emergency department: a randomized controlled trial. Ann Emerg Med 2004;43(3):362–70.

[45] Harwood-Nuss A. Harwood-Nuss' clinical practice of emergency medicine. 4th edition. Philadelphia: Lippincott Williams & Wilkins; 2005.

[46] Singer AJ, Hollander JE, Subrananian S, et al. Pressure dynamics of various irrigation techniques commonly used in the emergency department. Ann Emerg Med 1994;24: 36–40.

[47] Owens TB, Bosse M, Hudson M, et al. Does bacteremia occur during high pressure lavage of contaminated wounds? Clin Orthop 1998;1(347):117–21.

[48] Longmire AW, Broom LA, Burch J. Wound infection following high pressure syringe and needle irrigation. Am J Emerg Med 1987;5(2):179–81.

[49] Moscati R, Mayrose MS, Fincher L, et al. Comparison of normal saline with tap water for wound irrigation. Am J Emerg Med 1998;16:379–81.

[50] Riyat MS, Quinton DN. Tap water as a wound cleansing agent in accident and emergency. J Accid Emerg Med 1997;14:165–6.

[51] Bansal BC, Wiebe RA, Perkins SD, et al. Tap water for irrigation of lacerations. Am J Emerg Med 2002;20(5):469–72.

[52] Cooper ML, Laer JA, Hansbrough JF. The cytotoxic effects of commonly used antimicrobial agents on human fibroblasts and keratinocytes. J Trauma 1991;31:775–84.

[53] Calderon W, Chang KN, Mathes SJ. Comparison of the effect of bacterial inoculation in mu-cocutaneous and fasciocutaneous flaps. Plast Reconstr Surg 1986;77:785–92.

[54] Singer AJ, Hollander JE, Valentine SM, et al. Association of training level and short-term cosmetic appearance of repaired lacerations. Acad Emerg Med 1996;3(4):378–83.

[55] Hollander JE, Singer AJ, Valentine SM, et al. Risk factors for infection in patients with trau-matic lacerations. Acad Emerg Med 2001;8:716–20.

[56] Lammers RL, Hudson DL, Seaman ME. Prediction of traumatic wound infection with a neural network-derived decision model. Am J Emerg Med 2003;21(1):1–7.

[57] American College of Emergency Physicians. Clinical policy for the initial approach to patients presenting with penetrating extremity trauma. Ann Emerg Med 1999;33(5): 612–36.

[58] Wedmore IS. Wound care: modern evidence in the treatment of man's age-old injuries. Emerg Med Pract 2005;7(3):1–22.

[59] Karounis H, Gouin S, Eisman H, et al. A randomized control trial comparing long-term cos-metic outcomes of traumatic pediatric lacerations repaired with absorbable plain gut versus non-absorbable nylon sutures. Acad Emerg Med 2004;11(7):730–5.

[60] Mehta PH, Dunn KA, Bradfield JF, et al. Contaminated wounds: infection rates with sub-cutaneous sutures. Ann Emerg Med 1996;27:43–8.

[61] Khan A, Dayan PS, Miller S, et al. Cosmetic outcomes of scalp wound closure with staples in the pediatric emergency department: a prospective, randomized trial. Pediatr Emerg Care 2002;18(3):171–3.

[62] Pushpakumar SB, Hanson RP, Carroll S. Application of steri-strips. Plast Reconstr Surg 2004;113(3):1106–7.

[63] Zempsky WT, Parrotti D, Grem C, et al. Randomized controlled comparison of cosmetic outcomes of simple facial lacerations closed with steri-strip skin closures or dermabond tis-sue adhesive. Pediatr Emerg Care 2004;20(8):519–24.

[64] Mattick A, Clegg G, Beattie T, et al. A randomized controlled trial comparing a tissue ad-hesive with adhesive strips for pediatric laceration repair. Emerg Med J 2002;19:405–7.

[65] Yaron M, Erin MH, Huffer W, et al. Efficacy of tissue glue for laceration in the animal model. Acad Emerg Med 1995;2(4):259–63.

[66] Farion K, Osmond MH, Hartling L, et al. Tissue adhesives for traumatic lacerations in chil-dren and adults. Cochrane Database Syst Rev 2002;3:CD003326.

[67] Quinn JV, Wells GA, Sutcliffe T, et al. A randomized trial comparing octylcyanoacrylate tis-sue adhesive with sutures in the management of lacerations. JAMA 1997;277:1527–30.

[68] Singer AJ, Hollander JE, Valentine SM, et al. Prospective randomized controlled trial of a new adhesive (2-octylcyanoacrylate) versus standard wound closure techniques for lacer-ation repair. Acad Emerg Med 1998;5:94–9.

[69] Torumi DM, Ogrady K, Desai D, et al. Use of 2-octylcyanoacrylate for skin closure in facial plastic surgery. Plast Recontr Surg 1998;102:2209–19.

[70] Simon HK, McLario DJ, Bruns TB, et al. Long-term appearance of lacerations repaired us-ing tissue adhesive. Pediatrics 1997;99(2):193–5.

[71] Holger JS, Wnadersee SC, Hale DB, et al. Cosmetic outcomes of facial lacerations repaired with tissue adhesive, absorbable and non-absorbable sutures. Am J Emerg Med 2004;22(4): 254–7.

[72] Shapiro AJ, Dinsmore RC, North JH. Tensile strength of wound closure with cyanoacrylate glue. Am Surg 2001;67(11):1113–5.

[73] Quinn JV, Osmond MH, Yurack JA, et al. N-2-butylcyanoacrylate: risk of bacterial contam-ination with an appraisal of its antimicrobial effects. J Emerg Med 1995;13:581–5.

[74] Quinn JV, Maw JL, Ramotar K, et al. Octylcyanoacrylate tissue adhesive wound repair ver-sus suture wound repair in a contaminated wound model. Surgery 1997;122:69–72.

[75] Osmond MH, Klassen TP, Quinn JV. Economic comparison of a tissue adhesive and sutur-ing in the repair of pediatric facial lacerations. J Pediatr 1995;126:892–5.

[76] Singer AJ. Hair apposition for scalp lacerations. Ann Emerg Med 2002;40:27–9.

[77] Ong MEH, Ooi BS, Saw SM, et al. A randomized control trial comparing the hair apposition technique with tissue glue to standard suturing in scalp lacerations. Ann Emerg Med 2002; 40:19–26.

[78] Ong MEH, Coyle D, Lim SH, et al. Cost-effectiveness of hair apposition technique compared with standard suturing in scalp lacerations. Ann Emerg Med 2005;46(3):237–42.

[79] Dire DJ, Coppola M, Dwyer DA, et al. A prospective evaluation of topical antibiotics for preventing infections in uncomplicated soft tissue wounds repaired in the ED. Acad Emerg Med 1995;2:4–10.

[80] Cummings P, Del Beccaro MA. Antibiotics to prevent infection of simple wounds: a meta-analysis of randomized studies. Am J Emerg Med 1995;13:396–400.

[81] Thirlby RC, Blair AJ, Thal ER. The value of prophylactic antibiotics for simple lacerations. Surg Gynecol Obstet 1983;156:212–6.

[82] Morgan M. Hospital management of animal and human bites. J Hosp Infect 2005;61(1):1–10.

ELSEVIER
SAUNDERS

Emerg Med Clin N Am
25 (2007) 41–71

EMERGENCY
MEDICINE
CLINICS OF
NORTH AMERICA

Anesthetic and Procedural Sedation Techniques for Wound Management

Chad S. Crystal, MD[a],*, Todd J. McArthur, MD[a], LTC Benjamin Harrison, MD[b]

[a]Emergency Medicine Residency Program, Carl R. Darnall Army Medical Center,
36000 Darnall Loop, Fort Hood, Temple, TX 76544, USA
[b]Emergency Residency Program, Madigan Army Medical Center, Fort Lewis, Bldg 9040,
Fitzsimmons Drive, Tacoma, WA 98431, USA

Local anesthetics

Mechanism of action

Local anesthetics block the conduction of neural messages from the peripheral toward the central nervous system. The primary mechanism of conduction is the sodium channel. These channels are located on the axoplasmic side of the nerve cell and while closed, prevent sodium influx into the cell. This closed channel creates a negative resting potential inside the nerve cell. After a mechanical, chemical, or electrical excitation, these sodium channels open and allow sodium ions into the cell causing depolarization and impulse propagation. Local anesthetic molecules bind to closed sodium channels, preventing activation and cellular depolarization, thus inhibiting propagation of the nerve impulse [1]. This blockade is maintained until the anesthetic wears off, and is displaced from the sodium channel.

Structure of local anesthetics

Local anesthetics consist of an aromatic (hydrophobic) ring structure connected to a tertiary amine (hydrophilic) by an ester or amide linkage. The difference in the linking chain divides the anesthetic into an ester or amide class (Table 1). The hydrophobic ring structure in local anesthetics requires the addition of hydrochloride salt to create a water-soluble injectable medication. In addition to these general features, each local

---

* Corresponding author.
E-mail address: chad.crystal@cen.amedd.army.mil (C.S. Crystal).

0733-8627/07/$ - see front matter. Published by Elsevier Inc.
doi:10.1016/j.emc.2007.01.001

Table 1
Local anesthetics and their properties

Generic (Trade)	Potency	pK$_a$	Duration	Maximum dose (mg/kg)
AMIDES				
Bupivacaine	4	8.1	4	3
Dibucaine	4	8.8	4	1
Etidocaine	4	7.7	4	4
Lidocaine	2	7.8	2	4.5 (7 with epinephrine)
Mepivacaine	2	7.6	2	4.5 (7 with epinephrine)
Prilocaine	2	7.8	2	8
Ropivacaine	4	8.1	4	3
ESTERS				
Chloroprocaine	1	9.0	1	12
Cocaine	2	8.7	2	3
Procaine	1	8.9	1	12
Tetracaine	4	8.2	3	3

Data from Morgan GE, Mikhail MS, Murray MJ, et al. Local anesthetics. In: Morgan GE, Mikhail MS, Murray MJ, et al, editors. Clinical Anesthesiology, 3rd edition. New York: Lange Medical Books; 2002. p. 233–41.

anesthetic has a different chemical composition that determines the potency, duration, and onset of action.

The potency of an individual anesthetic is determined by the lipid solubility of the compound [2]. Highly lipophilic anesthetic agents can more readily cross the cell membrane and create a more effective blockade of nerve conduction. The duration of a local anesthetic is determined by the plasma protein-binding potential [3]. This correlation is thought to exist because the local anesthetic receptor is also a protein [4]. By binding the receptor for a longer period of time, conduction is blocked, and metabolism of the compound is delayed. Two of the more common anesthetics, procaine and bupivacaine, are excellent examples. Procaine binds loosely to the protein and is a shorter acting agent, whereas bupivacaine binds tightly and is used as a longer acting anesthetic [1]. Finally, the onset of action is determined by the pK$_a$ of the particular solution. Only the nonionized form of the anesthetic is able to pass easily through the neural membrane, but only the ionized form (cation) can bind within the sodium channel receptor. The pK$_a$ is the pH at which equal percentages of the drug exists in ionized and nonionized forms. Local anesthetics with pK$_a$ values closer to the physiologic pH produce higher concentrations of nonionized bases. This creates a high level of available drug passing through the membrane, causing a faster onset of action. Because of the pK$_a$, local anesthetics are less effective in acidic situations and more effective in an alkaline environment, which speeds the onset of action by creating a more nonionized anesthetic. For example, the onset of action is decreased in anesthetics containing epinephrine, which require an acidic environment to remain stable. Once inside the neuron, the ionized and nonionized molecules reach equilibrium and allow the ionized form to bind the sodium channel, inactivate it, and prevent propagation.

Toxicity

Toxicity from local anesthetics predominantly results from actions on the central nervous and cardiovascular systems. The severity of toxicity is related to the potency, dose, systemic absorption, protein binding, metabolism, and excretion. Most toxic reactions are related to inadvertent intra-arterial administration. This possibility of intra-arterial administration makes anesthetizing highly vascular sites more prone to systemic toxicity. The absorption rates for different sites from highest to lowest are: intercostals, intratracheal, epidural/caudal, brachial plexus, mucosal, distal peripheral nerve, subcutaneous. Because of its high vascularity, the dosage for intercostal blocks is one tenth of the maximum of peripheral blocks.

Metabolism and excretion also play a key role in an anesthetic's toxicity. These mechanisms differ between the ester and amide classes. Ester anesthetics are rapidly metabolized by plasma pseudocholinesterase. The water-soluble metabolite is then excreted by the urine. Patients who have pseudocholinesterase deficiency (eg, sensitivity to succinylcholine, those taking cholinesterase inhibitors, and patients who have myasthenia gravis) have an increased risk for systemic toxicity. The exception in the ester class is cocaine, which undergoes partial hepatic metabolism while the remainder of the molecule is excreted in the urine unchanged [4]. The amide local anesthetics are metabolized by the liver. Although each agent has a different rate of metabolism, the overall rate of the class is much slower than ester anesthetics. This slowed metabolism mandates smaller doses of the agent over time. Patients who have hepatic dysfunction or poor renal flow are predisposed to a higher risk of systemic toxicity. Care must also be taken with topical application of amide anesthetics such as eutectic mixture of local anesthetics (EMLA) and benzocaine. The metabolites of these agents may induce a methemoglobinemia.

Central nervous system toxicity

The central nervous system (CNS) toxic effects of local anesthetics are directly related to lipid solubility [1]. The gap between the desired clinical effect and systemic toxicity narrows as the lipid solubility of the local anesthetic increases. For example, the high lipid solubility of bupivacaine causes it to have a higher risk for toxicity than lidocaine. In addition to lipid solubility, the protein-binding capacity also contributes to CNS toxicity. Products with higher-protein binding capacity have high concentrations of nonionized molecules, allowing rapid crossing of the blood brain barrier and inducing CNS effects.

CNS toxicity can present as a range of symptoms to include lightheadedness, tongue numbness, metallic taste, and restlessness at low levels, to perioral paresthesias, slurred speech, and excitability or drowsiness at higher levels. Severe toxicity may cause seizures and coma. The etiology of CNS toxicity is unclear, but thought to be due to depression of inhibitory neurons, while leaving the excitatory pathways unopposed [5]. Anesthetic-induced seizures are treated with benzodiazepines, which raise the seizure threshold. A possible complication of using benzodiazepines is the high protein-binding ability of the compound. By administering the drug intravenously, more toxicity could be created by displacing the anesthetic from proteins in the plasma and increasing the free active form [6]. Thiopental 0.5 to 2 mg/kg can be used as an alternate anticonvulsant, but repeat dosing may be needed because of the short duration of action. Careful attention should be given to oxygenation and ventilation because hypoxia, hypercarbia, and acidosis all worsen the toxicity of local anesthetics.

Cardiac toxicity

Cardiac toxicity is caused secondary to blockade of the sodium channels in the cardiac conduction system [1]. The increased activity in reentrant pathways and reduction of the refractory period predisposes the heart to ventricular dysrhythmias. High plasma concentrations also cause depression in myocardial contractility. Dilation of smooth muscle may also cause hypotension. The symptoms of cardiac toxicity can vary from palpitations, cardiac dysrhythmias, hyper- or hypotension, and cardiovascular collapse [7]. Cardiac toxicity usually occurs after the stimulant phase of CNS toxicity. Lipophilic agents such as etidocaine and bupivacaine are most likely to cause cardiac toxicity, but it may result from any of the other local anesthetics. Cardiac toxicity is amplified by the use of epinephrine-combined anesthetics, hypoxia, hypercarbia, and acidosis [3].

As with seizure toxicity, bupivacaine is often associated with increased levels and incidence in cardiac toxicity. A range of effects including hypotension, atrioventricular block, and dysrhythmias has occurred. High degrees of protein-binding and depolarization changes are the proposed reasons for increased toxicity.

Advanced cardiac life support is used to manage cardiovascular collapse for most local anesthetic injections. One exception to advanced cardiac life support guidelines is the use of lidocaine as an antiarrhythmic, because it is also a local anesthetic. Although controversial, high doses of epinephrine have also been effective in bupivacaine-induced cardiac toxicity. Bretylium given at 5 mg/kg and repeated up to 30 mg/kg can occasionally convert ventricular tachyarrhythmias to normal sinus rhythms, or at least facilitate electrical cardioversion. Unfortunately effects from Bretylium may take 30 minutes to occur, so prolonged resuscitation is needed [8].

Allergic reactions

True allergies to local anesthetics are rarely seen. True allergic reactions will usually produce some form of skin or upper airway involvement.

Careful history of the event can allow a physician to discriminate true allergic reactions to anesthetics. Many times the patient will report an uncomfortable drug effect, vagal reaction, or intra-arterial injection of anesthetic as an allergic reaction. True reactions are usually due to the metabolite para-aminobenzoic acid in ester anesthetics and the preservative methylparaben in amide anesthetics. In cases whereby a true allergy is suspected from initial history, a preservative-free agent from the other class should be used. The ester class is responsible for most true allergic reactions. Therefore, if the previous allergic reaction source is in doubt, it is safest to administer a preservative-free amide local anesthetic (eg, cardiac lidocaine). The risk of a hypersensitivity reaction to this agent is extremely low.

Other alternatives for patients who have had prior reactions include benzyl alcohol and diphenhydramine. Benzyl alcohol with saline or epinephrine is the most effective alternative [9]. Diphenhydramine has been shown to cause prolonged analgesia, prolonged rebound hyperesthesia, and severe pain on injection [10]. Furthermore, diphenhydramine carries the additional risk of local irritation and necrosis of the skin when used in the fingertips or areas supplied by the end arteries [11].

Topical anesthetics

Overview

Topical agents have been used since the latter half of the nineteenth century with the advent of cocaine. A century later, there are many safer anesthetic agents that have become available. Repairing lacerations no longer requires a painful injection for anesthetic delivery. In some cases injections may be avoided all together, or performed without pain, through an area treated with a topical anesthetic. In addition to decreasing pain for the patient, topical anesthetics avoid wound edge distortion, which may be produced by subcutaneous infiltrates. There are three main categories of topical anesthetics, based on their location of use: mucosal membranes, nonintact skin, and intact skin.

Topical anesthetics for mucosal membranes

The mucosa of the nose, mouth, and pharynx may be numbed with cocaine or lidocaine. Cocaine is a unique anesthetic in that it also has vasoconstrictive properties, which makes it useful to decrease pain and blood loss. A 4% cocaine solution provides rapid and effective anesthesia for approximately 45 minutes. The maximum dose given should be less than 3 mg/kg. Disadvantages to cocaine are its potential for coronary artery vasoconstriction, hypertension, and tachycardia. Because of these factors, it should not be used in patients who have known or suspected coronary artery disease. Federal regulatory issues and its excessive cost make it a somewhat unattractive agent.

Lidocaine in 1% to 4% concentration is an excellent alternative to cocaine on mucosal surfaces. Although it does not have intrinsic vasoconstrictive properties, additives such as phenylephrine or epinephrine can be added for this effect. Caution must be used to avoid exceeding the maximum weight-based dose because topical application results in a high level of absorption. Calculating the maximum dose before administration can help minimize error. To determine the amount of anesthetic in a given volume, simply multiply the concentration by 10 to determine the milligrams in each 1 mL of solution. For example, 4 mL of 4% viscous lidocaine contains 160 mg of lidocaine. More dilute solutions may be used in situations requiring high volumes.

Application of topical anesthetic to mucous membranes can be accomplished in various methods. Atomizers can be used to create a fine mist for absorption. Lidocaine jelly can be rubbed directly into the mucosa. Cotton swabs or pledgets can be soaked in solution and introduced into the nose to anesthetize an entire surface or selective area. Vaporizers, such as those used for albuterol, can also be used to effectively anesthetize the entire oropharynx, including the vocal cords [12].

Topical anesthetics for intact skin

The three choices available for topical anesthesia to intact skin are: EMLA, LMX-4 (formerly ELA-max), and iontophoretic preparations. EMLA contains a mixture of 2.5% lidocaine and 2.5% prilocaine in a 1:1 ratio by weight. Each gram of cream contains 25 mg of lidocaine and 25 mg of prilocaine, purified water, carboxypolymethylene (thickening agent), and sodium hydroxide (to adjust the pH to 9.4). Initial US Food and Drug Administration (FDA) approval for EMLA cream was for use on intact skin only; however, more recent studies suggest EMLA might be effective and safe for use in open wounds [13,14]. Further studies are needed before EMLA can be recommended for nonintact skin. Because of its high cost (approximately $5.00 per application) and prolonged onset of action, it is not often used in the emergency department (ED).

The suggested dose is 2.5 g on 20 to 25 cm^2 of skin, with a maximum dosage of 2 g on 10 cm^2 of skin. Because of its slow onset of action (45–60 minutes) it should be applied to the intact skin for at least 1 hour, but no longer than 2 hours before the planned procedure. Once applied, it should be covered with an occlusive dressing. The anesthetic penetrates 3 mm in 60 minutes, and 5 mm after a 120-minute application [15]. The effect of the anesthetic will last for 1 to 2 hours. EMLA improves patient comfort during procedures and has a benign profile. Minor complications of EMLA include blanching of the skin, redness at the application site, and contact dermatitis. There is a theoretic risk of methemoglobinemia in infants less than 3 months old because of their low levels of methemoglobin reductase. There is one metanalysis that demonstrated no increased risk of methemoglobinemia when used in neonates, but in general it is not recommended in patients under 3 months old. Although there is a theoretic risk of lidocaine and prilocaine toxicity with EMLA, it should not occur if the product is used as directed. Its application can be advantageous in venipuncture, arterial puncture, lumbar puncture, and arthrocentesis, but its slow onset of action makes it impractical for the large majority of emergency medicine patients.

LMX-4 contains 4% lidocaine cream in a liposomal matrix and is FDA-approved for pain relief from minor cuts and abrasions. Liposomes enhance the action of lidocaine by facilitating the rate and extent of its absorption, allowing it to provide adequate anesthesia in only 30 minutes [16,17]. Unlike EMLA, LMX-4 does not require an occlusive dressing. In limited trials it seems to be a safe topical anesthetic, but some trials have shown little or no improvement over EMLA cream in a 30-minute period [18]. It also does not contain prilocaine, which has been recently implicated in EMLA-induced methemoglobinemia in older children. Thus LMX-4 theoretically should not induce methemoglobinemia—even in young infants.

Lidocaine iontophoresis is another method of dermal anesthesia for intact skin. Iontophoresis allows the introduction of soluble, positively charged lidocaine hydrochloride into the skin by using small external electrical current. Studies have shown this technique to be safe and efficacious [19] with an insignificant systemic absorption of lidocaine [20–22]. Lidocaine iontophoresis achieves anesthesia in 10 to 20 minutes, making it a more rapid alternative to EMLA cream, but some studies suggest EMLA produces better analgesia, which should be borne in mind when selecting for patients [23]. Undesirable effects of this method include the sensation of electrical current flowing through the skin, temporary erythema, blanching, itching, and urticaria at the application site. Iontophoresis devices cost approximately $400, and the one-time use disposable electrodes are $6 to $7.50 each, making this slightly more expensive than EMLA. This cost could theoretically be made up in faster ED turnover.

Topical anesthetics for nonintact skin

TAC (contains tetracaine 0.5%, adrenaline 0.05%, and cocaine 11.8%) and LET (lidocaine 4%, epinephrine 0.1%, and tetracaine 0.5%) are the two primary choices that exist to painlessly provide anesthesia over nonintact skin. Five to 10 mL of TAC is applied to the open wound and securely covered with gauze for 10 to 20 minutes. If securing the gauze with a hand, be sure to use gloves to prevent inadvertent absorption of the medication. TAC can be used anywhere on the body with the exception of the mucous membranes. This will prevent toxicity from the systemic absorption of the agents. It works best on injuries to the face and scalp. There are significant concerns with the use of TAC because of reported cases of respiratory arrest, seizures, and death in children due to its improper application [24]. TAC is expensive, has potential for drug abuse, and also has the regulatory issues involved with dispensing and administering a cocaine-containing medication. These problems have led to most EDs abandoning its use.

An excellent alternative to TAC is LET. Studies have shown LET to be safer, cheaper, and as effective as TAC [25–27]. LET comes in a solution or gel form, which are equally efficacious [28]. However, the gel form may be easier to use because of less run off. To apply LET, place 1 to 3 mL of the agent directly to the wound and leave covered for 15 to 30 minutes. Like TAC, LET should not be applied directly to or near the mucous membranes, the pinna of the ear, the nose, penis, fingers, or toes.

Topical anesthetics have also been effective in relieving pain in burn victims. Some studies have shown a possible healing benefit, with improved blood flow to the affected area. In these studies, application of EMLA has been used within normal limits and has not been associated with systemic toxicity [29,30]. Although treatment of burn relief has been studied, no studies could be found that evaluate the use of topical agents in severe abrasions or "road rash" injuries. Although the mechanism is different, similar tissue damage and pain is expected, and it is not unreasonable to treat these wounds with topical agents, as long as they are applied within dosing recommendations.

Local anesthetics used for subcutaneous infiltration

General

Local anesthetics are classified into either amides or esters (see Table 1). The key differences in these two groups include allergic potential and metabolism. Esters are hydrolyzed in the plasma by pseudocholinesterase, a much more rapid process than the hepatic metabolism of the amides. Due to a slower metabolism, the amides have an increase in possible toxicity, especially in patients who have liver dysfunction. Breakdown of ester compounds by pseudocholinesterase produces para-aminobenzoic acid, a potentially allergenic substance. Because amide metabolism does not create this byproduct, most allergic reactions to local anesthetics are due to esters.

Lidocaine

The most commonly used local anesthetic for intradermal infiltration in the ED is lidocaine. It is effective and has a good safety record. It is available commercially as a 1.0% to 2.0% solution with a pH of 6.5 and a pK_a of 7.9. The onset of action is 4 to 7 minutes after injection. The maximum dose is 3 to 5 mg/kg, up to 300 mg in a single dose. This dose increases with the addition of epinephrine to 7 mg/kg of anesthetic. Solutions without epinephrine provide analgesia for approximately 1.5 hours, whereas those with epinephrine last approximately 3.5 hours. Traditional teaching is that epinephrine should never be used in the hands or feet because of the risk of ischemia from constriction of end arterioles. However, recent literature suggests that with careful screening, epinephrine may be used when performing digital blocks [31–33]. In instances of prolonged ischemia as a result of the injection, arterial vasospasm may be reduced by locally injecting 2 mg of phentolamine near the site or applying topical nitroglycerine.

Bupivacaine

Bupivacaine is a potent local anesthetic whose anesthesia is equivalent to lidocaine. Its high protein binding and pK_a cause its onset of action to occur at 10 to 15 minutes, and its duration of action to be 3 to 6 hours. It is available as either a 0.25% or 0.5% solution. The maximum doses of bupivacaine are 2.0 to 2.5 mg/kg without epinephrine, and 3.0 to 3.5 mg/kg with epinephrine. The dose can be repeated every 3 hours, with the total dose given in 24 hours not to exceed 400 mg. Although bupivacaine provides long patient comfort, the risk of systemic toxicity with bupivacaine is much higher than most other local anesthetics secondary to its high potency and protein-binding properties. This toxic potential has led to the development of newer agents such as ropivacaine and levobupivacaine.

Ropivacaine

Ropivacaine is an amide local anesthetic approved by the FDA in 1996. It is similar to bupivacaine in terms of potency, onset time, and duration of action, but it is 70% less likely to cause the cardio-toxic effects associated with bupivacaine. This agent does have some intrinsic vasoconstrictive properties, so it probably should not be used on end arterial areas. The cost in comparison to bupivacaine is much higher [34].

Levobupivacaine

Levobupivacaine is the S-isomer form of bupivacaine. The pure S-enantiomer has fewer cardiovascular and CNS side effects when compared with regular bupivacaine. Although the potency of the two drugs is similar, the cost of five times more than bupivacaine hinders its use in most EDs [35].

Mepivacaine

Mepivacaine is structurally similar to lidocaine. Its onset of action is similar, but its duration of action is much longer (3 hours). By adding epinephrine, the duration of action is increased by 20% to 30%. Local infiltration solutions come in 0.5% or 1.0%. Mepivacaine does have a reputation for being more toxic than lidocaine, which has limited its clinical use.

Reducing the pain of injection of local anesthetics

There are many techniques that can be used to decrease the pain of injection for local anesthetics. Slow administration in a proximal to distal direction, along with a small needle (27–30 gauge) can decrease the pain of injection [36]. Injecting into tissue that has been exposed by the wound causes less pain than injection through intact skin [37].

Many studies have shown that buffering lidocaine can reduce the pain of infiltration [38–42]. Buffered solutions can be made by adding sodium bicarbonate (44 mEq/50 mL) to lidocaine in a 1:10 ratio (1 mL of bicarbonate is added to 10 mL of lidocaine). However, buffering lidocaine causes an increased rate of biodegradation at room temperature and decreases its shelf life by 7 days. The limiting factor for addition of sodium bicarbonate to local anesthetic is the tendency of more lipid-soluble agents to precipitate. For example, a highly lipid-soluble agent like bupivacaine must be buffered in a 1:50 ratio to avoid precipitation.

Warming of the anesthetic solution has also been shown to reduce pain of administration. However, other studies have shown it to have little or no effect. A reasonable compromise is to ensure that the agent is at least used at room temperature. Lidocaine can be warmed in either dry heat, such as a blanket warmer, or in a temperature-regulated water bath at 37°C. If lidocaine has not been buffered, warming will not shorten shelf life.

Addition of vasoconstrictors to local anesthetics

Adding a vasoconstrictive agent such as epinephrine offers several potential advantages to local agents. Epinephrine can improve a physician's ability for exploration and closure because of increased hemostasis in the surgical field. This effect is especially beneficial because most anesthetics cause smooth muscle relaxation and vasodilation. By constricting the blood vessels, the rate of systemic absorption is decreased. This allows an increase in the maximum dose of anesthetic, reduces systemic toxicity, prevents redistribution of the anesthetic, and prolongs the duration of action.

Commercially prepared solutions of lidocaine and bupivacaine containing epinephrine (1:100,000 to 1:200,000) are available and widely used for subcutaneous infiltration in EDs. These preparations are acidified to a pH of 3 to 4.5 to stabilize the epinephrine component. Because of this acidification, they have a slower onset of action and can be associated with more pain on injection than single agents.

Regional anesthesia

General indications and contraindications

Regional anesthesia is indicated in areas that are amenable to the blockade of a specific peripheral nerve (or nerve group) and provides a possible advantage over other techniques. As always, the method of anesthesia chosen is a decision made between the physician and the patient. The factors influencing the decision may include patient preference, physician comfort with a particular technique, and time constraints in busy EDs. The risks and benefits of each proposed procedures(s) must be explained to the patients, so they may consent after making a fully informed decision. Multiple nerve blocks are discussed in the following section, and indications for each block are explained within.

Generally, nerve blocks are contraindicated in uncooperative patients and in those who are unable to communicate severe pain on injection. Severe pain with injection is a good indicator of an intraneural injection, which may cause ischemic nerve injury. Other general contraindications include infection over the site, distortion of anatomic landmarks, and an allergy to the local anesthetic being used [43]. Contraindications to specific procedures are discussed (see later discussion).

Advantages

Emergency physicians have multiple methods of reducing discomfort and pain during procedures. Peripheral nerve blocks have multiple benefits over local infiltration during anesthesia. First, lower levels of anesthetic may be used to produce a greater effect and avoid risks of systemic toxicity. Second, regional blocks are often less painful to perform than subcutaneous injections and help result in less anxiety for the patient. Lastly, regions of injury that have great cosmetic significance (such as the lip and face) can be distorted by local injection and hinder the physician's ability to approximate wound edges properly. By using a regional block in these injuries, tissue distortion is avoided, and a less edematous field for repair is created.

Disadvantages

Patient selection in regional anesthesia is important, because success is guided by high levels of patient cooperation to detect subtle paresthesias during the procedure. There is a risk of systemic toxicity (approximately $7.5/10,000$), most of which is due to inadvertent intravascular injection, and a small risk of peripheral nerve damage ($1.9/10,000$) [44]. Failure of a nerve block is also a risk, because the procedure is usually performed without a stimulator in the ED. This risk of failure is likely related to the clinical experience of the physician, but requires the patient be informed that further anesthesia may be necessary.

General techniques

Peripheral nerve blocks should be performed in an area with adequate monitoring and resuscitation equipment because of the risk of systemic toxicity. Accidental intravascular injection of the anesthetic is responsible for immediate toxicity. Multiple techniques can be used in attempts to prevent vascular injection. Careful aspiration of the syringe before injection is generally used, and the use of an "immobile needle" technique can also be useful. This technique is performed by connecting a syringe to the needle by a piece of flexible tubing. This flexible tubing allows the operating physician to use both hands for needle localization and stabilization while an assistant aspirates and injects the agent with a syringe. Delays in toxicity may occur when excessive amounts of local anesthetic are absorbed into the systemic circulation. The different properties of each anesthetic agent will alter the timing of delayed toxicity. A high index of suspicion is needed to diagnose the fist signs of both immediate and delayed toxicity.

Patients who have severe pain or anxiety before a procedure may be premedicated with a systemic benzodiazepine or opioid to reduce anxiety and pain of injection. However, sedation must be light to facilitate adequate patient cooperation with the procedure. Skin preparation should involve antiseptic fashion before needle insertion. Providone–iodine is a traditional agent, but there are now multiple agents that are acceptable.

Knowledge of local anatomy and adequate patient cooperation are required for a successful block. Most procedures are performed with "blind" techniques, which rely on production of paresthesia in the nerve's sensory distribution when contacted by the needle. Successful blocks require local anesthetic to be injected in proximity to the nerve (perineural) but not directly within it (intraneural). Intraneural injection can cause elevated pressures in the sheath and may produce ischemia. Pain intensity and duration serve as clues to the injection site of the agent. Perineural injections cause a brief increase in the paresthesia, whereas intraneural injections produce an intense and prolonged pain. Immediate termination of the injection is indicated if intraneural positioning is suspected, and the needle should be repositioned for adequate anesthesia [38].

Wrist blocks

Although effective, wrist blocks have a slow time or onset and can be time consuming if a total block is required. For many injuries to the hand, digital blocks or local infiltration could be more effective. In certain situations wrist blocks are indicated and seem to be the best choice. Examples of the injuries amenable to a wrist block include: road rash, thermal burns requiring debridment, hydrofluoric acid burns, injury to more than one finger, and lacerations to the palm.

Radial nerve

Landmarks for the radial nerve include the radial artery and the radial styloid. Once these landmarks are located, inject 3 mL of local anesthetic at the level of the styloid just lateral to the radial artery. After this initial injection, proceed dorsally with subcutaneous injections of the anesthetic along the wrist until the dorsal midline is reached. Approximately 5 mL of local anesthetic is required for this procedure [45].

Ulnar nerve

The ulnar nerve runs into the wrist alongside the ulnar artery, lying just below the flexor carpi ulnaris tendon at the level of the proximal crease. The flexor carpi ulnaris tendon can be localized just proximal to the pisiform bone when the wrist is flexed against resistance. At the palmar crease, the nerve lies deep to the ulnar artery, which makes the volar approach difficult. A lateral approach to the nerve is recommended, which allows access to the nerve without risk of arterial puncture [46]. A 25-gauge needle is inserted in the ulnar side of the wrist at the proximal palmar crease. The needle is advanced in a horizontal plane 1.0 to 1.5 cm underneath the flexor carpi ulnaris. Three to 5 mL of local anesthetic is required for ulnar nerve block. Cutaneous nerve branches of the ulnar nerve wrap around the wrist to supply the dorsum of the hand. These cutaneous nerves may be blocked by injecting 5 to 6 mL of local anesthetic subcutaneously from the lateral border of the flexor carpi ulnaris tendon to the dorsal midline [41].

Median nerve

The median nerve can be blocked at the proximal volar crease, between the flexor carpi radialis tendon and palmaris longus tendon. In 20% of the population, there is no palmaris longus tendon at present. In the absence of this landmark, the median nerve can be found 1 cm in the ulnar direction from the flexor carpi radialis tendon. A 25-gauge needle is inserted vertically through the skin to a depth of approximately 1 cm. At this depth, a "pop" should be appreciated and a paresthesia elicited as the physician penetrates the deep fascia of the flexor retinaculum. During injection, no skin wheel should appear if the deep fascia has been penetrated. It is better to begin the injection too deep and proceed with injection as withdrawing than to inject too superficially. The retinaculum is an effective barrier to anesthetic if it is not penetrated [41].

Hand

Digital nerve

Each digit contains four digital nerves for sensation. The two dorsal nerves run at the 2- and 10-o'clock positions, whereas the palmar nerves lie at the 4- and 8-o'clock positions. Both palmar nerves supply sensation for the volar aspect, whereas dorsal sensation is supplied by the dorsal digital nerves. In addition to the palmar surface, the palmar nerves of the middle three digits supply sensation to the nailbed and dorsum of the fingertip. Because of this distribution, only palmar digital nerves require blockade to provide anesthesia to the area distal to the distal interpharyngeal joint. All four nerves must be blocked in the thumb and fifth finger for adequate anesthesia [41].

There are various approaches that may be used in performing digital blocks. The dorsal approach is preferred over the volar approach because the dorsal skin is thinner and less painful to inject. A small 25- or 27-gauge needle is inserted at the web space distal to the knuckle and just lateral to the bone. A small subcutaneous wheal of 0.5 mL to 1.0 mL of anesthetic is injected at this point. The needle is then advanced lateral to the bone until tenting of the palmar skin is noted. Once tenting is seen, the needle is withdrawn 1 mm and injected with 0.5 mL to 1.5 mL of local anesthetic. The same procedure is repeated on the opposite side of the digit so that all four nerves are blocked [47].

In an effort to cause less pain to the patient, the physician may alter the technique in the following manner. One side of the digit is injected as described in the previous procedure, but instead of withdrawing the needle, it is redirected across the dorsum of the digit to anesthetize the opposite side. The needle is then withdrawn and inserted into the area that was previously anesthetized. The block is then finished as described in the previous paragraph.

When dealing with fingertip injuries on the middle three digits, only blockade of the volar nerve is required for adequate sedation. Although the dorsal approach is less painful, decreased amount of anesthetic make this a useful technique. The needle is inserted over the center of the metacarpal head on the volar side, and local anesthetic is injected while the needle is advanced to the bone. Once at the bone, the needle is withdrawn 3 to 4 mm, then angled to each side of the digit for complete volar nerve block. A total injection of 4 to 5 mL of agent is all that is required for the blockade. When dealing with fingertip injuries in children, a different version of the volar block is effective. The finger of the child is pinched just distal to the proximal finger crease, so that minor skin tenting is formed. A needle is then inserted into the skin, and 0.5 to 1.0 mL of local anesthetic is injected subcutaneously. This single injection will anesthetize both volar digital nerves in children [41].

Most emergency medicine authorities advise against using epinephrine-containing solutions during digital blockade. However, studies and case reports of vasoconstriction are limited. If epinephrine is used and accidentally injected into a digit, phentolamine may be of benefit in reversing the alpha-agonism.

Metacarpal and intrathecal blocks

At least one study has suggested that a digital block provides more rapid and consistent anesthesia than a metacarpal block, but others are mixed [48,49]. The transthecal technique is probably equivalent to the traditional digital block [50]. These techniques are therefore not discussed here.

Bier block (intravenous regional anesthesia)

The Bier block is a form of intravenous regional anesthesia and has been shown in numerous studies to be a safe and effective form of regional anesthesia for upper and lower extremities [51–54]. Its favorable traits are the ability to achieve consistent anesthesia, a bloodless field, and muscle relaxation. There have been no deaths directly linked with its use. The procedure can be used in any patient who is able to cooperate. Contraindications include an allergy to anesthetic, uncontrolled hypertension, severe peripheral vascular disease, and soft tissue damage in the proximal extremity.

Place an intravenous line (IV) in the unaffected extremity in case resuscitation is required. The anesthetic to be used is 0.5% lidocaine without epinephrine. Other anesthetics have no advantage over lidocaine and should not be used. Bupivacaine should never be used because of its risk for severe cardiovascular and neurologic sequelae. The lidocaine can be purchased commercially or made by diluting 1% lidocaine in equal parts with sterile saline. The lidocaine solution should be premixed in a 50-mL syringe. The recommended dose is 3 mg/kg, but a dose of 1.5 mg/kg is nearly as efficacious and should be used as a starting point in the ED [55]. If needed, more lidocaine can always be given up to the recommended dose.

A pneumatic tourniquet is applied over cotton padding proximal to the pathology. A double-cuff pneumatic system is ideal. The tourniquet is inflated and a 20-gauge catheter is placed in a superficial vein, greater than 10 cm distal to the tourniquet. Some studies have shown a higher success rate with more distal catheter placement. After the IV is placed, the cuff is deflated and the extremity is exsanguinated by either elevating it or wrapping it with an elastic bandage. Manual exsanguinations accomplished by wrapping an elastic bandage from the distal to the proximal of the extremity is more painful than elevation, but is faster and more effective. Care must be taken not to dislodge the intravenous catheter. Some authorities do not feel that exsanguination is essential and that simple elevation of the arm is adequate for the procedure. After wrapping the extremity, the arm is elevated and the pneumatic cuff is inflated to 250 mm Hg (or 50 mm Hg above the systolic pressure for children). The extremity is then lowered and the wrap, if used, is removed.

The lidocaine is then slowly injected into the catheter at the predetermined dose. At 3 to 5 minutes, the patient should begin to note paresthesias or warmth in the extremity. It begins distally and then progresses proximally until complete anesthesia is achieved in 10 to 20 minutes. Muscle relaxation follows. If adequate anesthesia is not achieved in 15 minutes, more lidocaine may be infused, but never more than the 3-mg/kg limit. Another option for inadequate anesthesia is to inject 10 to 20 mL of saline solution. Once anesthesia is achieved, the catheter is removed and the site is tightly taped to prevent leakage of the local anesthetic [45].

The double-cuff tourniquet is used to alleviate tourniquet discomfort, which patients may experience after 20 to 30 minutes. The system consists of a proximal and distal cuff, in which the proximal cuff is inflated before infusion of anesthesia. Anesthesia will be obtained under the distal cuff. When the patient complains of pain under the proximal cuff, the distal cuff may be inflated. Do not deflate the proximal cuff until after the distal cuff is fully inflated. Most patients are only able to endure approximately 1 hour of tourniquet time, limiting this block to procedures that can be completed in that amount of time [56].

After the procedure is complete, a careful sequence must be followed to avoid potential lidocaine toxicity. If the procedure takes less than 30 minutes, the lidocaine may not have achieved adequate tissue fixation, and deflation of the cuff may produce a high peak plasma level of lidocaine. Therefore, a full 30 minutes should be complete before deflation of the tourniquet. At this time, the tourniquet is deflated for 5 seconds and reinflated for 1 to 2 minutes. This cycle is repeated three to four times, and the patient is observed for 20 minutes before discharge [45].

Severe complications are rare and include seizures and cardiovascular problems. By cautiously preventing a large intravascular bolus from reaching the systemic circulation by following the deflation procedure, high blood levels of lidocaine may be avoided. Other measures to avoid systemic circulation include waiting 30 minutes before deflation, using double cuff tourniquet rather than blood pressure cuffs, never exceeding the 3-mg/kg dosage, and avoiding placement of the catheter proximal to the tourniquet.

Femoral nerve block

Pain from femoral shaft fractures has been treated with femoral nerve blocks for over 50 years. Hip fractures have also been responsive to pain control with femoral blocks [57]. There is also evidence that patients who have femoral neck fractures prefer femoral blocks to opioid analgesia [58]. Proximity of the femoral vein and artery create high potential for intravascular injection, but careful aspiration of the syringe before injection greatly reduces this risk [59]. A careful neurovascular examination must be performed both before and after the procedure.

The block is performed with the patient in a supine position. Antiseptic technique is used to prepare the skin over the femoral triangle. Palpate the femoral artery 1 to 2 cm distal to the inguinal ligament. Once localized, move 1 to 2 cm laterally and inject a subcutaneous wheal of local anesthetic. In order to sustain landmarks, the nondominant hand is kept on the femoral artery throughout the remainder of the procedure. A 1.25-cm 22-gauge needle is attached to a 20 mL syringe using an extension tube technique. The needle is inserted just laterally to the artery at a 90° angle and is advanced until a paresthesia is produced or the needle pulsates laterally. If a paresthesia is elicited, the needle is assumed to be in close proximity to the nerve, and 10 to 20 mL of local anesthetic is injected. If no paresthesia is elicited, 10 to 20 mL of agent is injected in a fan-like distribution lateral to the artery in an attempt to anesthetize the nerve. Careful aspiration of the needle is required to avoid intravascular injection [41].

3 in 1 block (inguinal perivascular block)

The 3-in-1 block is used to block the femoral, obturator, and lateral femoral cutaneous nerves with a single injection. The nerve sheath that surrounds the femoral nerve travels proximally and becomes continuous with a wider nerve sheath that contains all three nerves. By injecting large amounts of local anesthetic in to the femoral nerve sheath, fluid will track proximally and block all three nerves. The femoral nerve injection site is used, while 20 to 30 mL of local anesthetic is injected. During the injection, the nondominant hand must be used to apply firm pressure distal to the injection site, and continuous pressure must be applied for 5 minutes after the injection. It may take up to 30 minutes for this block to reach its peak efficacy [41].

Ankle blocks

The foot is supplied by five peripheral nerve branches. The superficial peroneal, deep peroneal, and saphenous nerves course anteriorly and supply sensation to the dorsum of the foot. Multiple branches of the superficial peroneal nerve lie close to the surface between the lateral malleolus and extensor hallucis longus tendon. These branches provide sensory supply to most of the dorsum of the foot. The deep peroneal nerve supplies the web space between the first and second toes, and runs into the ankle under the extensor hallucis longus tendon. The saphenous nerve runs parallel with the saphenous vein between the medial malleolus and tibialis anterior tendon. It supplies sensation to the medial foot around the arch. The posterior tibial and sural nerves are posterior and supply sensation to the volar aspect of the foot. The sural nerve lies superficially between the lateral malleolus and Achilles tendon. It supplies the lateral aspect of the foot, both volar and dorsal. The posterior tibial nerve lies deep and posterior to the posterior tibial artery between the medial malleolus and Achilles tendon. It provides sensation to most of the volar surface of the foot and toes [41].

Posterior tibial nerve
The patient is placed in the prone position, with the foot hanging off the end of the bed in slight dorsiflexion. In this position, the posterior tibial artery is located just posterior to the medial malleolus [60]. A 3.75-cm 25-gauge needle is inserted here, just posterior to the artery, and directed at a 45° angle to the mediolateral plane. Advance the needle to a 0.5 to 1.0 cm depth, and then move from side to side in an attempt to produce a paresthesia. Once a paresthesia is induced, aspirate and then inject 3 to 5 mL of local anesthetic. In cases whereby no paresthesia can be elicited, advance the needle further until it contacts the posterior border of the tibia. After contact is made, withdraw the needle 1 mm and inject 5 to 7 mL of local anesthetic while withdrawing the needle another 1 cm [41].

Sural nerve
Place the patient in the same prone position as with the posterior tibial nerve block. The sural nerve lies superficially and is easily blocked using a subcutaneous wheel. The nerve is found 1 cm above the lateral malleolus, between the Achilles tendon and lateral malleolus. At this site, a skin wheel of 3 to 5 mL is produced to block this superficial nerve [54].

Superficial peroneal nerves
Place the patient in a supine position. The superficial nerves are located between the extensor hallucis longus tendon and the lateral malleolus [41]. Blockade of the nerves can be achieved by placing 4 to 10 mL of local anesthetic subcutaneously at this location. An alternative method consists of

placing a wheal of 0.5 to 1.0 mL of local anesthetic midway between the anterior tibial edge and the lateral malleolus [54].

Deep peroneal nerve

With the patient in the supine position, and the foot dorsiflexed, palpate the anterior tibial tendon above the medial malleolus. The extensor hallucis longus tendon is then palpated by having the patient dorsiflex the great toe. The needle is inserted 1 cm above the base of the medial malleolus between these two tendons. A subcutaneous wheal of local anesthetic is deposited, and the needle is then advanced under the extensor hallucis longus tendon (approximately 30° laterally) until it contacts the tibia. This occurs at a depth of less than 1 cm. At this point the needle is withdrawn 1 mm, and 1 mL of local anesthetic is injected [41,54].

Saphenous nerve

The saphenous nerve is located superficially and is blocked by subcutaneously injecting 3 to 5 mL of local anesthetic between the medial malleolus and anterior tibial tendon.

Digital toe blocks

Digital nerve blocks in the foot are more efficacious and comfortable for the patient than attempts with local infiltration. Discomfort with local infiltration is thought to be secondary to the fibrous septa and limited subcutaneous space. In certain instances, these factors cause the block to be ineffective and increase the likelihood of local ischemia.

As with digits of the hand, two volar and two dorsal nerves supply each toe. The volar nerves branch from the posterior tibial and sural nerves, whereas the dorsal nerves are branches of the deep and superficial peroneal nerves. In the toes, the nerves lie close to the bone at the 2-, 4-, 8-, and 10-o'clock positions. As the nerves travel proximally, they parallel the tendons and are further from the bone [41].

There are multiple injection sites that may be considered for digital blocks. The metatarsal approach is performed by inserting the needle dorsally between metatarsal bones and injecting 1 mL of local anesthetic in a subcutaneous wheal. The needle is then slowly advanced until tenting of the volar surface is noted. At that time 2 mL of local anesthetic is deposited as the needle is being withdrawn. Before being removed from the skin, the needle is then redirected laterally and the procedure is repeated. To fully block one digit, this procedure must be performed in two or three adjacent spaces because of sensory overlap of the nerves. Consistent blocks of the digital nerves are difficult to achieve with this technique, because the nerves do not lie in a predictable location.

The recommended and most commonly used approach for a digital block of the toe is the web space block. A 3.75-cm 27-gauge needle is inserted at the lateral edge of the bone just proximal to the base of the toe. A subcutaneous wheal is created by injecting 0.5 to 1.0 mL of local anesthetic. The needle is then advanced until tenting of the volar skin is visualized. While stationary, inject 0.5 to 1.0 mL of local anesthetic. Another 0.5 mL of local anesthetic is then injected while simultaneously withdrawing the needle. The procedure is then repeated on the opposite side of the toe. As discussed with digital blocks of the finger, variations may be used to minimize patient discomfort and multiple needle sticks. In cases whereby only the distal portions of the toe must be anesthetized, the block can be performed further away from the web space. In these situations, it is important to decrease the amount of local anesthetic due to risking vascular compromise in such a small subcutaneous space [41].

Intercostal block

Intercostal nerve blocks provide cutaneous relief over the affected area. They are commonly used in the ED to provide analgesia for broken or contused ribs. In theory, the advantages of eliminating pain with inspiration may decrease hypoventilation, atelectasis, and pneumonia, but there are no good studies that show it to be more effective than oral analgesics in outpatient settings [41]. Intercostal blocks are contraindicated in patients who have flail chest or infection over the site of injection.

There is a small chance of creating a pneumothorax with intercostals blocks. The rate is reported as high as 1.4%, and is increased in patients who have underlying lung disease. The questionable relief and inconsistent duration of the block, along with a small chance for pneumothorax, require thorough counseling of the patient beforehand. A trial of oral analgesics may be indicated first [61].

Successful blocks require a thorough understanding of the involved anatomy. Each thoracic nerve exits the spinal column at the intervertebral foramen. Immediately after exiting the foramen, the posterior cutaneous branch splits off to supply the paraspinal area. The intercostals nerve runs along the subcostal groove with the vein and artery. As the nerve reaches the midaxillary line, it gives off lateral cutaneous branches. Blocking these lateral cutaneous nerves will provide relief to the anterior and posterior lateral chest wall.

Performing the block in the posterior midaxillary line is advantageous because of several factors. In the posterior region, only a thin layer of fascia separates the nerve from the pleura, creating greater potential for pneumothorax. In the posterior midaxillary line, the internal intercostal muscles lie between the nerve and pleura creating a small buffer. Because most rib fractures occur in the anterior or lateral portion of the ribs, most blocks can be performed in the posterior midaxillary line and still provide adequate relief [41].

The patient is placed sitting in an upright position and leaning forward on a Mayo stand. The injured rib is then palpated and followed posteriorly to the posterior midaxillary line [62]. The overlying area is then prepared in a sterile manner. Retract the skin at the inferior border of the rib superiorly with the index finger of the nondominant hand. A 3.75-cm 25-gauge needle on a 10-mL syringe is then inserted by the dominant hand into the skin at the tip of the finger. The needle is directed cephalad at an 80° angle. The needle is then advanced until it contacts the rib. Release skin traction with the dominant hand, which will move the needle perpendicular to the chest wall and to the inferior edge of the rib. At this time, the syringe is switched to the nondominant hand. The palm is rested against the chest wall and the middle finger is used to walk the needle off the inferior edge of the rib. Slowly advance the needle 3 mm, aspirate, and inject 2 to 5 mL of local anesthetic while slowly moving the needle in and out 1 mm. This in and out movement ensures penetration of the compartment between the internal and external intercostals muscles where the nerve lies. The same technique is then repeated on the two ribs above and below the initial injection to ensure blockage of overlapping nerves.

The patient should then be observed for 30 minutes after the procedure for signs and symptoms of a pneumothorax. If the patient is stable after this time, they may be discharged home with return precautions. Symptomatic patients should receive a chest radiograph and treated with the standard of care in instances of pneumothorax [41].

Facial and oral blocks

General recommendations

The best local anesthetic for ED procedures in this area is bupivacaine. The prolonged duration of action makes it superior to lidocaine in these cases. Epinephrine should be used (when not contraindicated) for dental blocks, because of the high vascularity of the oral cavity. One exception to the use of bupivacaine is performance of the maxillary supraperiosteal injection. Lidocaine with epinephrine provides the most prolonged anesthesia for this procedure [63].

Because of the high vascularity involved, a 27-gauge or larger needle should be used to facilitate aspiration and prevent intravascular injection of anesthetic. Needles specifically designed with a thumb ring or finger grip help improve aspiration technique. Multiple techniques may be used to decrease the pain of injection in this sensitive area. Topical anesthetics can be placed on a thoroughly dried area by using a cotton tip applicator. Low concentrations are ineffective, but agents such as 20% benzocaine or 5% to 10% lidocaine are effective. Benzocaine is highly preferred because of its rapid onset of action (30 seconds), brief duration (5–15 minutes), and low systemic absorption. Distraction techniques, such as shaking the lip during injection, can also be used in concordance with topical anesthetics to decrease pain [64].

Supraperiosteal

Supraperiosteal blocks provide anesthesia to a single tooth. Preparation of the oral mucosa is used before injection. The mucous membrane is then pulled in the necessary direction to expose the mucobuccal fold. The needle is inserted into the mucobuccal fold with the bevel facing the bone. Deposit 1 to 2 mL of local anesthetic at the apex of the tooth, close to the periosteum. Complete anesthesia may take 5 to 10 minutes. Because the nerve runs inside the cortex of the bone, this procedure may fail if the local anesthetic is placed too far from the periosteum or the root [58].

Anterior superior alveolar nerve

By performing this block, anesthesia is provided to the maxillary canine, the central and lateral incisors, and one half of the upper lip. General preparation is the same as previously described. The needle is inserted with the bevel facing bone superior to the apex of the canine and directed into the canine fossa. After insertion, 2 mL of local anesthetic are injected [65].

Middle superior alveolar nerve

This nerve provides sensation to the maxillary premolars and part of the first molar. The needle is inserted with the bevel facing bone superior to the apex of the second premolar tooth. Two mL of local anesthetic are injected [57].

Posterior superior alveolar nerve

This block will provide anesthesia to the maxillary molars. In some instances to gain complete anesthesia, the first maxillary molar must be separately anesthetized.

The patient's mouth should be half open and the cheek retracted laterally. The needle is inserted in the mucosal reflection just distal to the distal bucal root of the upper second molar. The needle is advanced along the curvature of the maxillary tuberosity to a depth of 2 to 2.5 cm. At this point, the needle is aspirated, and 2 to 3 mL of local anesthetic is then injected, being careful to avoid injection into the pterygoid plexus [57].

Infraorbital nerve

Infraorbital blockade is extremely useful in repairing cosmetic lacerations that would become distorted with local infiltration. This block provides anesthesia to the intraoral areas previously discussed, as well as the skin of the lower eyelid, nose, and upper lip. The infraorbital foramen is located in line with the pupil and on the inferior border of the infraorbital ridge. The intraoral approach is preferred to the extraoral variation, because it provides a longer duration of anesthesia [66].

The block is performed by holding one finger over the inferior border of the infraorbital rim and inserting the needle in the labial mucosa opposite the apex of the first premolar tooth approximately 0.5 cm from the bucal surface. The needle is advanced superiorly until it is palpated near the foramen at a depth of approximately 1.5 cm. At this point, 2 to 3 mL of local anesthetic is deposited near, but not within, the foramen [58,67].

Inferior alveolar nerve block

The inferior alveolar nerve provides sensation to the ipsilateral mandibular teeth and the lower lip and chin. The bucal mucosa is prepared in the usual fashion, and the physician should position him/herself on the side of the patient opposite of the one being injected. Hold the syringe parallel to the occlusal surfaces of the teeth and angle it so that it overlies the first and second premolars on the opposite side of the mandible. If needed, a 25-gauge needle may be bent to 30° to facilitate this angle. Use the non-dominant hand to palpate the coronoid process of the mandible. At this point, a triangle should be visualized in the mucosa posterior to the molars. The needle is then inserted into this triangle approximately 1 cm above the occlusal surface of the molars. Advance the needle until contact is made with the mandibular bone, which creates the posterior surface of the mandibular sulcus. Ensuring the needle comes in contact with the bone will prevent posterior injection of anesthetic into the parotid gland. If this occurs, the seventh cranial nerve will be anesthetized and will create a temporary Bells palsy. After location is verified, inject 1 to 2 mL of local anesthetic after aspiration. Up to 3 to 4 mL can be used as necessary if the needle is placed suboptimally. After the needle is withdrawn, it is reinserted into the bucal mucosa opposite the second molar, and 0.5 mL of local anesthetic is injected [58,68].

Mental nerve block

The mental nerve is a continuation of the inferior alveolar nerve and innervates the skin and mucosa of the ipsilateral lip, with mild midline crossover. For this reason, both mental nerves must be blocked when midline lip anesthesia is required.

The mental nerve emerges from the mental foramen 1 cm inferior and anterior to the second premolar tooth. In children, the foramen lies between the first and second primary molars. Internal approach to the nerve is generally less painful than an external approach if a topical anesthetic is used. Palpate the mental foramen in the described location; then insert the needle in the lower mucobuccal fold at a 45° angle. At this time, 1 to 3 mL of local anesthetic is injected into the area around the mental foramen [58,69].

Ophthalmic nerve block

The ophthalmic nerve provides sensation to the forehead and scalp as far posteriorly as the lambdoid suture. The nerve consists of lateral and medial branches of the supraorbital, supratrochlear, and infratrochlear nerves. The nerves all emerge for the superior aspect of the orbit. The supraorbital nerve emerges from the supraorbital notch, which is found on the supraorbital rim directly above the pupil. The supratrochlear nerve is located 0.5 to 1.0 cm medial to the foramen, and the infratrochlear nerve is found on the most medial portion of the supraorbital rim.

The block is performed by placing 1 to 3 mL of local anesthetic subcutaneously adjacent to the supraorbital notch. If this initial injection does not provide adequate anesthesia, 5 mL of local anesthesia can be injected subcutaneously along the supraorbital rim the entire length of the eyebrow. Eyelid swelling can be reduced by firmly placing a finger just below the supraorbital rim [58,70].

Procedural sedation and analgesia in wound management

Most wounds in the ED may be adequately anesthetized with local and regional techniques as previously described. Larger, multiple, and more extensive wounds are generally addressed in an operative setting; however, procedural sedation and anesthesia (PSA) does have a limited role in certain clinical scenarios. PSA may be utilized as a primary means of decreasing pain and discomfort during assessment, cleansing, and definitive repair of more painful and extensive wounds. PSA agents may also be given to ease the pain of local anesthetics in areas that are particularly painful to inject (ears, nose, genitalia), or as an adjunct to local anesthetics when they alone cannot completely anesthetize a given wound. Examples of wounds seen in the ED that may not be adequately anesthetized with local or regional anesthetics include burns, deep puncture wounds requiring debridement or packing and diffuse, and superficial abrasions with foreign bodies (such as seen with road rash). PSA as a primary or adjunctive method for analgesia may be appropriate at times, and the practicing emergency physician should be comfortable with several agents that can be used in this role. This section provides a brief overview of agents that may be useful in this setting, but the reader should refer to a more in-depth review of PSA for more specific recommendations on dosages, adverse effects, and medication profiles.

General concepts

Selecting an appropriate agent depends on several factors. Adequate analgesia will be a primary goal in most scenarios, although sedation, anxiolysis, or amnesia may also be necessary because some patients have a significant aversion or fear of injections. Sedation may be required (eg, a terrified and struggling pediatric patient with wounds to the face) to provide motion control during local injections. In these instances, a short period of sedation (enough to inject the wounds) may be all that is necessary. The length of time for the management of a wound should be considered and the proper agent should be chosen that will provide adequate analgesia while allowing timely discharge from the ED if that is a goal.

Intravenous delivery of any PSA agent is the most reliable and effective method. This provides quicker peak levels and allows the provider to more accurately titrate the agent when necessary. Intramuscular (IM) methods provide less reliable absorption rate and peak effects. IM delivery may be occasionally considered when IV access is not available or easily obtainable, or the act of obtaining IV might cause more anxiety and discomfort for a given patient. Ketamine, which is discussed later, is an exception because it can reliably and quickly be delivered IM. Oral and transmucosal (rectal and intranasal) routes can be excellent choices, especially in the pediatric population. Inhaled nitrous oxide is a good analgesic/sedative choice that does not require injection or an IV; however, most EDs do not carry this because of difficulty maintaining the required delivery and scavenging systems. Regardless of the route of administration, proper monitoring of blood pressure, pulse oximetry, and ventilatory status of the patient should be maintained until the patient's mental status and vital signs have returned to their preprocedural state.

Opioid analgesics

Opioids, in general, are a good choice for PSA in wound management. They provide analgesia as well as some level of sedation. They differ in potency and half-lives, but generally all function to elevate pain thresholds and may be used in conjunction with other agents. Respiratory depression, nausea, and hypotension are potential adverse effects, but serious effects may be reversed with opioid antagonists. Care must be taken when using with sedatives, because synergism may occur that worsens the adverse effects such as respiratory depression and hypotension. Patients who have significant pain can be given IM analgesics upon arrival, but monitoring of the respiratory status is required with larger doses because there may be a delay to peak effect using this route.

Morphine

Morphine is a longer acting opioid with peak effect in approximately 15 to 20 minutes and duration of action of approximately 1 to 2 hours when given IV. Onset of action with IM delivery of morphine is more variable with delayed onset (5–20 minutes) and peak onset of approximately 60 minutes. The terminal half-life of morphine is 1.5 to 2 hours and duration of analgesia approximately 3 to 4 hours. Because it is poorly lipid soluable, morphine does not quickly enter the cerebrospinal fluid and is therefore poorly titratable. This makes morphine a poor choice for PSA in the ED. As an adjunct to local anesthesia, it may be used for a patient who has a painful wound early in the ED course, but the operator must allow adequate time to pass before beginning the procedure. This can allow the provider time to prepare for a local or regional block while instituting analgesia and sedation for the procedure. It is a good choice for painful injuries and wounds that should require extended analgesia even after ED wound management.

Fentanyl

Fentanyl is approximately 100 times more potent than morphine but is lipid soluable and therefore reaches peak cerebrospinal fluid concentrations quickly within a few minutes. This makes it desirable as a PSA agent because it is easily titratable. Fentanyl also has a shorter duration of action (30–40 minutes) than morphine, which theoretically allows a more timely discharge of patients. It has much less histamine release than morphine, resulting in less bronchospasm and hypotension than morphine. Nausea, vomiting, and hypotension are possible but rare. A reasonable starting dose for fentanyl is 1 to 2 µg/kg IV, especially if used with a sedative or for an adjunct to local anesthetic. A typical cumulative dose of fentanyl for PSA is approximately 2 to 5 µg/kg, titrating boluses of 1 µg/kg at a time to achieve the desired effect. Chest wall rigidity is a rare complication seen with rapid administration of IV fentanyl in doses much higher than used with PSA (>5 µg/kg bolus) and should not be of concern.

Ketamine

Ketamine is an excellent choice for PSA in painful ED wound management. It is a dissociative anesthetic and provides analgesia with amnesia and sedation. This produces an "awake" patient that is dissociated from external stimuli in a trance-like state, but whose respiratory drive is maintained. It has an outstanding side effect profile and only rarely causes respiratory depression, as with other analgesics or sedatives. Most often this is seen when IV opioids or benzodiazepines are added to ketamine as adjuncts. Most respiratory difficulties are related to positioning and increased airway secretions; therefore, suctioning and repositioning of the airway usually suffice to address airway difficulties. Laryngospasm is an infrequent complication that can usually be managed with bag valve mask ventilation, and severe laryngospasm requiring paralysis and intubation has only rarely been reported [71].

Ketamine may be effectively delivered IM at doses of 2 to 5 mg/kg, depending on the depth of desired sedation and length of sedation, with approximate onset of action within 5 minutes and duration of 20 to 30 minutes. IV administration allows for repeated titration and onset of action of 1 minute with duration of 15 to 20 minutes. Doses range from 0.5 to 2 mg/kg IV, with repeat doses of 0.5 mg/kg infused as needed. Return to baseline consciousness generally occurs in 15 to 20 minutes after the last IV dose, unless larger doses are employed. Oral ketamine at doses of 10 mg/kg may also be employed in patients in whom IV access is not obtained, and seems to allow for better sedation than oral midazolam [72]. Because ketamine is a sialagogue, glycopyrrolate or atropine are often used to decrease secretions, although this has not been definitively proven in clinical trials. Concomitant administration of a benzodiazepine may decrease the incidence of the emergence phenomenon (hallucinations, bizarre movements, agitation) in adults, but has not been shown to be effective in children [73,74].

Ketamine would be a good choice in several clinical scenarios in ED wound management. Repeat boluses of 0.5 mg/kg ketamine IV, or 2 mg/kg

IM may allow for adequate analgesia and a cooperative semialert patient. This state would be ideal for certain painful procedures such as burn/ wound debridement or follow-up wound care (painful packing changes). Ketamine generally provides adequate analgesia and sedation if delivered alone, but low-dose ketamine may be effective with IV opioids for opioid-resistant pain [75]. No definitive human data exist to clarify if opioids provide additional benefit to low-dose ketamine in opioid naïve patients without increasing side effects, but this combination may be useful in performing painful procedures such as burn debridement in the ED.

Sedatives/anxiolytics/amnestics

Sedatives alone do not provide analgesia, which is the primary desired characteristic sought in an agent used for wound management. Sedatives may be employed with analgesics to decrease anxiety or impart amnesia so that the painful manipulation of a wound is not recalled by the patient. When used alone, sedatives usually require a significant depth of sedation for painful procedures. Often the risk of deeper sedation for this purpose is not appropriate because better options exist. In addition, sedated patients may still perceive the pain and purposefully withdraw or move, making wound management difficult.

Low-dose sedatives may be added to opioids for certain painful procedures, although this may increase the incidence of side effects through synergism, and close monitoring is again warranted.

Benzodiazepines

Midazolam is a short acting benzodiazepine with an onset of 2 to 3 minutes and duration of 30 to 60 minutes, depending on the dose. Intravenous doses range from 0.02 to 0.04 mg/kg and may be titrated based on patient response, making midazolam the preferred benzodiazepine in ED PSA. It is often combined with fentanyl to achieve the desired effect, because both possess a quick onset and short duration. Case reports of death from this combination of agents exist, but it carries a level B recommendation in clinical policy consensus despite the concerns for significant respiratory depression [76,77].

Barbiturates

Barbiturates are also sedatives that provide no analgesic effects. Ultra-short-acting agents, such as methohexital, can produce significant and brief sedation for painful procedures. Hypotension and respiratory depression are frequently seen at doses that impart deep sedation in patients (1–2 mg/kg IV of methohexital or thiopental). Barbiturates are not routinely combined with opioids for PSA, and their short duration may be suitable only as an adjunct for local anesthetics or brief painful wound manipulation.

Etomidate

Etomidate produces brief sedation, anxiolysis, and amnesia but without analgesia. Unlike barbiturates, it does not affect hemodynamic stability. Respiratory depression is a dose-related side effect and myoclonus, seen in approximately 10% of patients, may initially prevent motion control until it subsides. Nausea and vomiting occurs occasionally at the usual dosage of etomidate for PSA (0.1–0.15 mg/kg IV) [78]. Evidence for use of etomidate as a PSA agent in the ED in adults and children is mounting, but currently etomidate has a level C recommendation in a clinical policy consensus [79]. Drug characteristics also limit its usefulness in wound management and, like barbiturates, may be primarily suitable as an adjunct for local anesthetics or brief painful wound manipulation.

Propofol

Propofol is also a pure sedative without analgesic properties with brief onset and duration (less than 1 minute onset and several minutes duration). A usual PSA dose for propofol is 0.75 to 1 mg/kg and then 0.5 mg bolus every 1 to 2 minutes, or given as a continuous infusion of 25 to 75 µg/kg/min. Propofol produces amnesia, sedation, and hypnosis, but no analgesic effects. It produces less nausea and vomiting due to its antiemetic effects but has a high incidence of respiratory depression, apnea, and hypotension. Fortunately, most of these effects are brief and, with proper monitoring of the airway and blood pressure, have not been shown to cause significant complications in limited studies [80]. It may be used in combination with fentanyl to provide adequate analgesia in addition to sedation for the management of painful wound manipulation. In pediatric patients, the fentanyl–propofol combination currently carries a level B recommendation, and propofol alone has a level C recommendation in a national consensus clinical policy [79].

Summary

The practicing emergency physician should be comfortable in his or her ability to alleviate pain when managing patients' wounds in the ED. This can be effectively and safely accomplished through a firm understanding of regional and local anesthetic techniques, procedural sedation and analgesia, and the possible side effects and toxicities of any agents that are employed for this purpose.

References

[1] Tetzlaff JE. The pharmacology of local anesthetics. Anesthesiol Clin North America 2000; 18(2):217–33.

[2] Piccinini F, Chiarra A, Villani F. The active form of local anesthetic drugs. Experientia 1972; 28:140–1.

[3] Covino BG. Pharmacology of local anesthetic agents. Br J Anaesth 1986;58:701–16.
[4] Morgan GE, Mikhail MS, Murray MJ, et al. Local anesthetics. In: Morgan GE, Mikhail MS, Murray MJ, editors. Clinical anesthesiology, 4th edition. New York: Lange Medical Books; 2006. p. 233–40.
[5] Strichartz G, Berde C, Miller RD, editors. Miller's anesthesia, 6th edition. Philidelphia: Churchill Livingstone; 2005. p. 593–4.
[6] Ahlstrom KK, Frodel JL. Local anesthetics for facial plastic procedures. Otolaryngol Clin North Am 2002;35(1):29–53.
[7] Rodriguez E, Jordan R. Contemporary trends in pediatric sedation and analgesia. Emerg Med Clin North Am 2002;20(1):199–222.
[8] Markakis DA. Regional anesthesia in pediatrics. Anesthesiol Clin North America 2000; 18(2):355–81.
[9] Bartfield JM, Jandreau SW, Raccio-Robak N. Randomized trial of diphenhydramine versus benzyl alcohol with epinephrine as an alternative to lidocaine local anesthesia. Ann Emerg Med 1998;32(6):650–4.
[10] Xia Y, Chen E, Tibbits DL, et al. Comparison of effects of lidocaine hydrochloride, buffered lidocaine, diphenhydramine, and normal saline after intradermal injection. J Clin Anesth 2002;14(5):339–43.
[11] Dire DJ, Hogan DE. Double-blinded comparison of diphenhydramine versus lidocaine as a local anesthetic. Ann Emerg Med 1993;22(9):1419–22.
[12] Wilder RT. Local anesthetics for the pediatric patient. Pediatr Clin North Am 2000;47(3): 545–58.
[13] Zempsky WT, Karasic RB. EMLA versus TAC for topical anesthesia of extremity wounds in children. Ann Emerg Med 1997;30:163–6.
[14] Blanke W, Wlater, Hallern BV, et al. Sharp wound debridement in local anaesthesia using EMLA cream: 6 years' experience in 1084 patients. Eur J Emerg Med 2003;10(3):229–31.
[15] Bjerring P, Arendt-Nielson L. Depth and duration of skin analgesia to needle insertion after topical application of EMLA cream. Br J Anaesth 1990;64:173–7.
[16] Eichenfield LF, Funk A, Fallon-Friedlander S, et al. A clinical study to evaluate the efficacy of ELA-max (4% liposomal lidocaine) as compared with eutectic mixture of local anesthetics cream for pain reduction of venipuncture in children. Pediatrics 2002;109(6):1093–9.
[17] Bucalo BD, Mirikitani EJ, Moy RL. Comparison of skin anesthetic effect of liposomal lidocaine, EMLA nonliposomal lidocaine, and EMLA using 30-minute application time. Dermatol Surg 1998;24:537–41.
[18] Carter Eric L, Coppola C, Barsanti F. A randomized, double-blinded comparison of two topical anesthetics formulations prior to electrodesiccation of dermatosis papulosa nigra. Dermatol Surg 2006;32:1–6.
[19] Wallace MS, Ridgeway B, Jun E, et al. Topical delivery of lidocaine in healthy volunteers by electroporation, electroincorporation, or iontophoresis: an evaluation of skin anesthesia. Reg Anesth Pain Med 2001;26:229–38.
[20] Kim MK, Kini NM, Troshynski TJ, et al. A randomized clinical trial of dermal anesthesia by iontophoresis for peripheral intravenous catheter placement in children. Ann Emerg Med 1999;33(4):395–9.
[21] Schultz AA, Strout TD, Jordan P, et al. Safety, tolerability, and efficacy of iontophoresis with lidocaine for dermal anesthesia in ED pediatric patients. J Emerg Nurs 2002;28(4): 289–96.
[22] Dailey RH. Fatality secondary to misuse of TAC solution. Ann Emerg Med 1988;17:159–60.
[23] Moppett I, Szypula K, Yeoman P. Comparison of EMLA and lidocaine iontophoresis for cannulation analgesia. Eur J Anaesthesiol 2004;21:210–3.
[24] Jacobsen S. Errors in emergency practice. Emerg Med 1987;19:109.
[25] Blackburn PA, Butler KH, Hughes MJ, et al. Comparison of tetracaine-adrenaline-cocaine (TAC) with topical lidocaine-epinephrine (TLE): efficacy and cost. Am J Emerg Med 1995; 13(3):315–7.

[26] Ernst AA, Marvez-Valls E, Nick TG, et al. LAT (lidocaine-adrenaline-tetracaine) versus TAC (tetracaine-adrenaline-cocaine) for topical anesthesia in face and scalp lacerations. Am J Emerg Med 1995;13(2):151–4.

[27] Schilling CG, Bank DE, Borchert BA, et al. Tetracaine, epinephrine (adrenaline), and cocaine (TAC) versus lidocaine, epinephrine, and tetracaine (LET) for anesthesia of lacerations in children. Ann Emerg Med 1995;25(2):203–8.

[28] Resch K, Schilling C, Borchert BD, et al. Topical anesthesia for pediatric lacerations: a randomized trial of lidocaine-epinephrine-tetracaine solution versus gel. Ann Emerg Med 1998; 32:693–7.

[29] Mattson U, Cassuto J, Jontell M, et al. Digital image analysis of erythema development after experimental thermal injury to human skin: effect of postburn topical local anesthetics (EMLA). Anesth Analg. 1999;88(5):1131–6.

[30] Johnson A, Brofeldt BT, Nellgard P, et al. Local anesthetics improve dermal perfusion after burn injury. J Burn Care Rehabil. 1998;19(1 Pt 1):50–6.

[31] Wilhelmi BJ, Blackwell SJ, Miller JH, et al. Do not use epinephrine in digital blocks: myth or truth? Plast Reconstr Surg 2001;107(2):393–7.

[32] Green D, Walter J, Heden R, et al. The effects of local anesthetics containing epinephrine on the digital blood perfusion. J Am Podiatr Med Assoc 1992;82(2):98–110.

[33] Krunic AL, Wang LC, Soltani K, et al. Digital anesthesia with epinephrine: an old myth revisited. J Am Acad Dermatol 2004;51:755–9.

[34] Panni M, Segal S. New local anesthetics: are they worth the cost? Anesthesiol Clin North Am 2003;21(1):19–35.

[35] Santos AC, DeArmas PI. Systemic toxicity of levobupivacaine, bupivacaine, and ropivacaine during continuous intravenous infusion to nonpregnant and pregnant ewes. Anesthesiology 2001;95(5):1256–64.

[36] Scarfone RJ, Jasani M, Gracely EJ. Pain of local anesthetics: rate of administration and buffering. Ann Emerg Med 1998;31:36–40.

[37] Bartfield JM, Sokaris SJ, Raccio-Robak N. Local anesthesia for lacerations: pain of infiltration inside vs outside the wound. Acad Emerg Med 1998;5(2):100–5.

[38] McKay W, Morris R, Mushlin P. Sodium bicarbonate attenuates pain on skin infiltration with lidocaine, with or without epinephrine. Anesth Analg 1987;66:572–4.

[39] Christoph RA, Buchanan L, Begalla K, et al. Pain reduction in local anesthetic administration through pH buffering. Ann Emerg Med 1988;17:117–20.

[40] Bartfield JM, Gennis P, Barbera J, et al. Buffered versus plain lidocaine as a local anesthetic for simple laceration repair. Ann Emerg Med 1990;19(12):1387–9.

[41] Matsumoto AH, Reifsnyder AC, Hartwell GD, et al. Reducing the discomfort of lidocaine administration through pH buffering. J Vasc Interv Radiol 1994;5:171–5.

[42] Colaric KB, Overton DT, Moore K. Pain reduction in lidocaine administration through buffering and warming. Am J Emerg Med 1998;16:353–6.

[43] Morgan GE, Mikhail MS, Murray MJ, et al. Peripheral nerve blocks. In: Morgan GE, Mikhail MS, Murray MJ, editors. Clinical anesthesiology, 3rd edition. New York: Lange Medical Books; 2002. p. 283–308.

[44] Faccenda KA, Finucane BT. Complications of regional anesthesia: incidence and prevention. Drug Saf 2001;24(6):413–42.

[45] Ducharme J. Wrist blocks. In: Rosen P, Chan TC, Vilke GM, editors. Atlas of emergency procedures. St. Louis (MO): Mosby; 2001. p. 170–3.

[46] Kelly JJ, Spektor M. Nerve blocks of the thorax and extremities. In: Roberts JR, Hedges JR, editors. Clinical procedures in emergency medicine, 4th edition. Philadelphia: Saunders; 2004. p. 567–90.

[47] Taleghani NN, Sternbach G. Digital nerve block. In: Rosen P, Chan TC, Vilke GM, editors. Atlas of emergency procedures. St. Louis (MO): Mosby; 2001. p. 174–5.

[48] Knoop K, Trott A, Syverud S. Comparison of digital versus metacarpal blocks for repair of finger injuries. Ann Emerg Med 1994;23(6):1296–300.

[49] Hung VS, Bodavula VK, Dubin NH. Digital anesthesia: comparison of the efficacy and pain associated with three digital nerve block techniques. J Hand Surg [Br] 2005;30:581–4.

[50] Hill RG Jr, Patterson JW, Parker JC, et al. Comparison of transthecal digital block and traditional digital block for anesthesia of the finger. Ann Emerg Med 1995;25(5):604–7.

[51] Roberts JR. Intravenous regional anesthesia. In: Roberts JR, Hedges JR, editors. Clinical procedures in emergency medicine, 4th edition. Philadelphia: Saunders; 2004. p. 591–5.

[52] Colbern EC. Intravenous regional anesthesia: the perfusion block. Anesth Analg 1966;45(1): 69–72.

[53] Dunbar RW, Mazze RI. Intravenous regional anesthesia: experience with 779 cases. Anesth Analg 1967;46(6):806–13.

[54] Roberts JR. Intravenous regional anesthesia—"Bier block". Am Fam Physician 1978;17(2): 123–6.

[55] Farrell RG, Swanson SL, Walter JR. Safe and effective IV regional anesthesia for use in the emergency department. Ann Emerg Med 1985;14(4):288–92.

[56] Gerancher JC. Regional anesthesia: upper extremity nerve blocks. Anesthesiol Clin North America 2000;18(2):297–317.

[57] Ducharme J. Acute pain and pain control: state of the art. Ann Emerg Med 2000;35(6): 592–603.

[58] McGlone R, Sadhra K, Hamer DW, et al. Femoral nerve block in the initial management of femoral shaft fractures. Arch Emerg Med 1987;4(3):163–8.

[59] Dilger JA. Regional anesthesia: lower extremity nerve blocks. Anesthesiol Clin North America 2000;18(2):319–40.

[60] Taleghani NN, Sternbach G. Foot blocks. In: Rosen P, Chan TC, Vilke GM, editors. Atlas of emergency procedures. St. Louis (MO): Mosby; 2001. p. 176–7.

[61] Shanti CM, Carlin AM, Tyburski JG. Incidence of pneumothorax from intercostal nerve block for analgesia in rib fractures. J Trauma 2001;51(3):536–9.

[62] Barton ED. Intercostal nerve block. In: Rosen P, Chan TC, Vilke GM, editors. Atlas of emergency procedures. St. Louis (MO): Mosby; 2001. p. 34–5.

[63] Yagiela JA. Oral-facial emergencies: anesthesia and pain management. Emerg Med Clin North Am 2000;18(3):449–70.

[64] Amsterdam JT, Kilgore KP. Regional anesthesia of the head and neck. In: Roberts JR, Hedges JR, editors. Clinical procedures in emergency medicine, 4th edition. Philadelphia: Saunders; 2004. p. 552–66.

[65] Amsterdam JT. Internal maxillary-superior alveolar nerve block. In: Rosen P, Chan TC, Vilke GM, editors. Atlas of emergency procedures. St. Louis (MO): Mosby; 2001. p. 162–3.

[66] Lynch MT, Syverud SA, Schwab RA, et al. Comparison of intraoral and percutaneous approaches for infraorbital nerve block. Acad Emerg Med 1994;1(6):514–9.

[67] Taleghani NN, Sternbach G. Facial and oral blocks. Infraorbital nerve block. In: Rosen P, Chan TC, Vilke GM, editors. Atlas of emergency procedures. St. Louis (MO): Mosby; 2001. p. 160–1.

[68] Amsterdam JT. Mandibular and inferior alveolar nerve block. In: Rosen P, Chan TC, Vilke GM, editors. Atlas of emergency procedures. St. Louis (MO): Mosby; 2001. p. 164–5.

[69] Amsterdam JT. Mental nerve block. In: Rosen P, Chan TC, Vilke GM, editors. Atlas of emergency procedures. St. Louis (MO): Mosby; 2001. p. 166–7.

[70] Taleghani NN, Sternbach G. Facial and oral blocks: supraorbital nerve block. In: Rosen P, Chan TC, Vilke GM, editors. Atlas of emergency procedures. St. Louis (MO): Mosby; 2001. p. 158–9.

[71] Green SM, Rothrock SG, Lynch EL, et al. Intramuscular ketamine for pediatric sedation in the emergency department: safety profile in 1,022 cases. Ann Emerg Med 1998;31(6):688–97.

[72] Younge PA, Kendall JM. Sedation for children requiring wound repair: a randomised controlled double blind comparison of oral midazolam and oral ketamine. Emerg Med J 2001; 18(1):30–3.

[73] Chudnofsky CR, Weber JE, Stoyanoff PJ, et al. A combination of midazolam and ketamine for procedureal sedation and analgesia in adult emergency department patients. Acad Emerg Med 2000;7(3):228–35.

[74] Sherwin TS, Green SM, Khan A, et al. Does adjunctive midazolam reduce recovery agitation after ketamine sedation for pediatric procedures? Ann Emerg Med 2000;35(3):229–38.

[75] Weinbroum AA. A single small dose of postoperative ketamine provides rapid and sustained improvement in morphine analgesia in the presence of morphine-resistant pain. Anesth Analg 2003;96:789–95.

[76] Mace SE, Barata IA, Cravero JP, et al. Clinical policy: evidence-based approach to pharmacologic agents used in pediatric sedation and analgesia in the emergency department. Ann Emerg Med ;44(4):342–77.

[77] Miner JR, Heegaard W, Plummer D. End-tidal carbon dioxide monitoring during procedural sedation. Acad Emerg Med 2002;9(4):275–80.

[78] Ruth WJ, Burton JH, Bock AJ. Intravenous etomidate for procedural sedation in emergency department patients. Acad Emerg Med 2001;8(1):13–8.

[79] Godwin SA, Caro DA, Wolf SJ, et al. Clinical policy: procedural sedation and analgesia in the emergency department. Ann Emerg Med 2005;45(2):177–96.

[80] Green SM, Krauss B. Propofol in emergency medicine: pushing the sedation frontier. Ann Emerg Med 2003;42(6):792–7.

ELSEVIER
SAUNDERS

Emerg Med Clin N Am
25 (2007) 73–81

EMERGENCY
MEDICINE
CLINICS OF
NORTH AMERICA

Closure Techniques

Jeremy D. Lloyd, MD[a],*, Melvin J. Marque III, MD[a],
Robert F. Kacprowicz, MD[b]

[a]Department of Emergency Medicine, Wilford Hall Medical Center, 959 MSGS/MCED,
2200 Bergquist Drive, Suite 1, Lackland Air Force Base, TX 78236, USA
[b]US Air Force Pararescue School, Det 1, 342 TRS, Building 437,
Kirtland Air Force Base, NM 87117, USA

Emergency physicians (EPs) encounter many traumatic wounds requiring closure in an emergency department (ED). The decision to close a wound and the technique used are influenced by many factors, including location, depth, and contamination of wound; age of patient; and resources or time available. Most wounds can be managed adequately with simple, interrupted sutures. Prudent EPs, however, are familiar with many alternative techniques that may serve them better in times of need and the limitations associated with each of the alternatives.

Sutures

The most common method of wound closure in an ED is the use of sutures. Sutures are a time-honored method of wound closure and offer several advantages, including familiarity, lowest rate of dehiscence, and greatest tensile strength [1]. Despite advantages of some of the newer techniques, sutures remain the standard approach to laceration management and remain the technique of choice for closure of complicated wounds, wounds in areas of high skin tension, and deeper wounds requiring multiple layers of closure [2].

Suture selection

Nonabsorbable sutures, such as nylon, long have been the standard material for use in closure of skin wounds, with absorbable suture reserved for use in closure of deep tissue layers. Recent literature calls this practice into question and provides evidence that absorbable suture may be appropriate for skin closure.

* Corresponding author.
E-mail address: jeremy.lloyd@lackland.af.mil (J.D. Lloyd).

Patients frequently request the use of "dissolving" suture for closure of superficial wounds, primarily because of the discomfort and time involved in returning for removal of nonabsorbable suture. Classic teaching assumes the use of absorbable suture for skin closure results in significantly more scarring than similar wounds closed with nonabsorbable suture, and, as a result, the practice of closing skin with absorbable suture is discouraged.

Suture integrity of absorbable sutures varies widely, from as short as 7 days for rapid-absorbing surgical gut to up to 60 days for polydioaxanone and polyglyconate (Maxon, US Surgical, Norwalk, Connecticut) [1]. Only the shortest duration sutures should be considered for use in closure of the skin. Ethicon recently introduced coated irradiated polyglactin 910 (Vicryl Rapide), which has integrity similar to rapid-absorbing gut but reportedly less tissue reactivity, making it an attractive choice for skin closure [3].

Several studies addressing the use of absorbable suture have appeared in the recent literature. Parrell and Becker [4] randomly assigned patients who had surgical facial wounds to closure with 5-0 coated polypropolene (Prolene, Eithicon) or 5-0 coated irradiated polyglactin 910 (Vicryl Rapide, Ethicon) and followed the patients for 6 months, at which time scars were compared. No significant difference between scars was found.

Karounis and colleagues [5] studied the long-term outcomes with the use of surgical gut versus nylon sutures in pediatric lacerations sutured in an ED. Wounds were followed up at 4 to 5 months by a blinded plastic surgeon using the visual analog scale, and no significant difference was found in cosmetic result. In fact, a trend toward improved outcome with gut was seen.

Holger and colleagues [6] similarly studied 9- to 12-month outcomes after closure of facial wounds with either rapid-absorbing gut, octylcyanoacrylate (OCA), or nylon suture. No significant difference in cosmetic outcome was seen between any of the groups.

Finally, Al-Qattan [7] studied the use of irradiated polyglactin 910 (Vicryl Rapide) versus standard polyglactin 910 (Vicryl) in the closure of elective pediatric hand surgeries and found improved cosmetic outcomes and fewer wound complications with the use of irradiated polyglactin 910.

Taken together, these studies provide significant evidence that absorbable suture may be appropriate for skin closure in EDs. The smallest available size of irradiated polyglactin 910 (Vicryl Rapide), however, is 5-0, which may make it somewhat less attractive than rapid-absorbing gut for the closure of facial wounds.

Techniques

For the vast majority of simple wounds encountered in an ED, simple interrupted sutures are sufficient. In some cases, more involved closure may be necessary. Recent literature provides guidance for decision making in more complicated cases.

Deep sutures clearly are indicated for closure of lacerations, which are deep enough to penetrate into muscle, with closure of the fascia indicated to prevent dead space. Elimination of dead space in the wound is essential to prevent hematoma formation and accumulation of exudate [1]. Once the fascial layer is closed, placement of subcutaneous sutures with apposition of the skin edges before skin closure is believed to result in improved cosmetic outcome [1]. The use of absorbable suture is mandatory for this indication, and choice of material should be based on the use of security and minimal tissue reactivity. Polyglactin (Vicryl, US Surgical, Norwalk, Connecticut) and polyglycolic acid (Dexon) are reasonable choices for deep sutures, as the use of synthetic suture seems to decrease the rate of infection [8]. Placement of stitches in fat should be avoided, as they provide no significant benefit to wound healing [9].

Additional caveats to the placement of deep sutures include avoidance of deep suture placement in wounds that seem to be contaminated, as they seem to increase the rate of infection. Mehta and colleagues [10] showed that placement of subcutaneous sutures in contaminated wounds, despite thorough irrigation, increased the rate of infection in the rat model. In contrast, however, placement of subcutaneous sutures in a similar model of noncontaminated wounds showed no significant increase in wound inflammation or infection [11].

In uncomplicated wounds of the face, however, placement of dermal sutures is not shown to affect the clinical outcome at 90 days. Singer and colleagues [12] studied the 90-day outcome of nongaping facial wounds closed with dermal sutures compared with the outcome of wounds closed with a single layer closure and found the cosmetic outcomes and scar width to be similar. Application of these results in wounds other than simple, nongaping wounds should be viewed with caution, however, and multilayer closure used if any doubt exists.

In wounds involving areas of high skin tension, use of occasionally overlooked techniques may provide improved cosmetic outcome. The use of the horizontal mattress stitch is a useful adjunct in cases where the distance between wound edges is large to spread the tension over a longer area with each stitch or in areas of higher skin tension, such as across joints. The horizontal mattress suture also is useful particularly in those who have thin, fragile skin, such as the elderly [13].

Finally, the use of the half-buried horizontal mattress stitch, or corner stitch, is a useful technique in the closure of wounds with V-shaped flaps, such as those suffered as a result of blunt trauma. The use of the corner stitch provides fewer suture marks and good corner apposition and is believed to provide better blood flow to the skin flap [13]. This was confirmed by Kandel and Bennet [14], who showed increased blood flow to the flap by laser Doppler imaging compared with alternate techniques. The rate of tip necrosis was not significantly different among groups; however, only three cases of tip necrosis were seen in this study, making conclusions about flap necrosis rates difficult to make [14]. Regardless, the corner stitch seems to result in a more meticulous and pleasing closure.

To place the corner stitch, the suture is placed transcutaneously across from the wound flap and exits subcutaneously from the wound edge. The corner flap then is elevated with forceps and the suture is placed horizontally through the dermis of the flap. Once the horizontal portion is placed, the suture then is passed into the opposing subcutaneous wound edge and brought out through the skin, with the knot placed between the transcutaneous suture ends.

The use of sutures to close traumatic wounds in EDs remains an important tool for practicing EPs. Recent literature provides significant guidance for the best cosmetic outcome for patients while minimizing stress and discomfort. Use of absorbable suture for cutaneous wound closure is an important technique, particularly in children. Underused techniques of wound closure, including multilayer closure and use of adjunctive suturing techniques, continue to be important to EPs.

Cyanoacrylates

Cyanoacrylates are chemicals that form an adhesive bond when contact is made with moisture. Short-chain cyanoacrylates are used in commercial, nonmedical products, such as glue, but their toxicity has prevented their use as tissue adhesives. Butyl cyanoacrylates are intermediate-length cyanoacrylates that are less toxic and maintain a stronger bond than the shorter-chain molecules. They have not been approved for use in the United States by the Food and Drug Administration (FDA); however, they have been used for many years in a host of countries for laceration repair and other procedures [15–17]. 2-OCA is FDA approved for use in the United States and marketed as Dermabond (Ethicon, Sommerville, New Jersey) topical skin adhesive. 2-OCA has a longer 8-carbon chain, which offers greater flexibility, a stronger bond, and slower degradation than the butylcyanoacrylates [18].

Several studies of 2-OCA show it to be equivalent or superior to conventional suture techniques. When compared prospectively to sutures in the repair of pediatric facial lacerations, long-term cosmetic outcomes were equivalent [16]. A large, randomized clinical trial, including 814 patients from multiple clinical settings, compared 2-OCA to standard suture closure. Cosmetic outcome, infection rate, and rate of dehiscence were equivalent. Time to wound closure with 2-OCA was faster than standard suture closure (2.9 minutes versus 5.3 minutes, $P < .0001$) [18]. Most studies comparing the two methods of wound closure parallel these results.

There are several advantages to 2-OCA over standard sutures. The application of tissue adhesives is relatively painless and easy to perform, no foreign material is introduced into the wound, and no suture removal is required. There also is evidence that cyanoacrylates possess inherent antimicrobial properties [19,20]; however, the use of skin adhesives should not preclude standard wound irrigation and preparation.

2-OCA has a higher direct cost compared with sutures, but an overall reduction in cost might be achieved with tissue adhesives. When considering factors, such as equipment, medication cost, follow-up visits, procedure time, patient and parent preference, and loss of parental income, 2-OCA has an advantage over standard suture. A Canadian study compared the cost to the health care system when using tissue adhesives versus absorbable and nonabsorbable sutures. The reduction in cost (in Canadian dollars) per patient was $49.60 for switching to tissue adhesive and $37.90 for absorbable sutures compared with nonabsorbable sutures. Additionally, 90% of parents chose tissue adhesives as their primary choice for wound closure [21].

2-OCA is a sterile, liquid, topical agent colored with violet die. It is packaged in a single-use ampule with an inner glass container that has an applicator tip. When the inner glass ampule is crushed, the polymerization process begins and 2-OCA flows freely only for a few minutes. It is indicated for use on skin lacerations with easily approximated skin edges or in deeper lacerations in conjunction with deep dermal sutures. 2-OCA should not be used alone in areas of high tension or areas of repetitive movement (ie, joints). It should be used with caution in the vicinity of the eye. When using it in this area, patients should be positioned so that runoff is directed away from the eye and protect the eye with wet gauze. A high viscosity version of 2-OCA now is available, which should minimize the likelihood of runoff.

Follow standard wound preparation before closure with tissue adhesives. After irrigation, dry the area with sterile gauze. Keep the wound in a horizontal position to prevent inadvertent runoff, and use immediately after the ampule is crushed. Approximate wound edges with gloved fingers or sterile forceps and apply the liquid slowly in multiple thin layers (at least 2–4 coats). Wait approximately 30 seconds between layers. When closure is complete, allow the adhesive to dry completely (approximately 5 minutes) before applying a dressing. Bandages or dressings are not necessary as the adhesive provides an adequate barrier; however, they may prevent a young or noncompliant patient from picking at the wound. Full apposition strength is achieved in 2.5 minutes after the top layer is applied. Antibiotic ointment or other topical preparations should not be used as they can weaken the polymerized film and lead to dehiscence. Instruct patients not to pick or scrub the area. The adhesive sloughs off naturally in 5 to 10 days and no follow-up is needed unless otherwise indicated. If the closure is suboptimal or there is inadvertent adherence of undesired surfaces, antibiotic ointment or petroleum jelly can facilitate removal of the adhesive.

Adhesive tapes

Skin closure tapes allow for rapid closure of wounds that have well-approximated margins with little discomfort to patients. Their use for primary laceration repair is limited, however, by several factors. Although they are less reactive than sutures and staples, they lack the tensile strength of other wound closure modalities [22]. They require the use of adhesive adjuncts, such as tincture of benzoin, which increases the local inflammatory reaction and rate of infection [23]. They have a high rate of dehiscence and are not adequate for primary closure of wounds under tension [24]. As a result of these factors, adhesive tapes have little usefulness for primary wound closure in an ED.

Staples

Stapling devices have been used for decades in closure of surgical incisions and have proved an efficient alternative to sutures. They also have gained acceptance as alternatives to sutures for traumatic wounds. Multiple studies have shown equivalent outcomes when comparing staples to sutures in cosmetic results, cost-effectiveness, and complications. The greatest advantage to staples is the speed of closure. They also are shown to have a lower rate of infection and less foreign-body reaction [24].

The current automatic staplers are indicated for use on wounds located on extremities, trunk, and scalp, with the exception of the face, neck, hands, and feet. Providers benefit from the speed of closure when caring for intoxicated or agitated patients or multiple trauma victims. Avoid use of metal staples in scalp wounds, however, if CT or MRI of the head is anticipated, as the staples produce undesired artifact on the images or may be dislodged because of the powerful magnetic forces. Particularly deep wounds may require use of absorbable sutures to reduce tension and close dead space before the placement of the skin staples.

One person can perform the technique of closing wounds with staples; however, two people are preferable. The wound should be prepared in the standard fashion and any necessary deep sutures should be placed to relieve tension. The skin edges then are everted with forceps or pinched together between the thumb and forefinger. The staple is placed across the wound and the trigger of the staple gun is squeezed to advance the staple and secure it into the skin. Care must be taken to avoid placing the staple too deep in the skin, resulting in tissue necrosis. The crossbar is 1 mm above the skin surface when placed properly.

Removal of the staples requires a special instrument. The jaws of the device are used to grab the crossbar of the staple and bend the points out of the skin for removal. It is more painful than suture removal, but overall patient satisfaction is similar. The timing of staple removal is the same as with sutures. Consider discharging patients who have a staple removal device if they are to follow-up in their primary care clinic, as not all clinics have the devices readily available.

Recent advances in absorbable staples may make many limitations of the standard metal staples obsolete. The relatively new devices aim to provide convenience and cosmetic results of a subcuticular closure with the speed and ease of use of metal staples. Studies thus far are limited to animal models and surgical incisions. A recent study compared absorbable staples, metal staples, and absorbable braided sutures for closing contaminated wounds on an animal model. The rate of infection at 7 days was the primary outcome, whereas speed of closure and dehiscence also were measured. The results showed a lower rate of infection compared with vicryl sutures and metal staples with speed of closure comparable to the metal staples with no dehiscence [25]. If these promising results are reproducible in randomized controlled trials in an ED setting, then this may be a viable option for EP physicians.

Hair apposition technique

The hair apposition technique (HAT) is a novel method for closing selected scalp wounds using the patient's existing hair. It involves bringing strands of hair together from both sides of the wound, making a single twist, and securing it with a drop of glue. There are several advantages compared with standard suturing. First, it requires no injection of anesthetic, thus minimizing pain associated with closure. There are no special tools required except for the tissue adhesive. A nurse can perform the technique, freeing physicians for more critical tasks. Also, there are no sutures to remove, which requires a follow-up visit by patients.

Selected scalp wounds should be less than 10 cm in length with scalp hair greater than 3 cm long. Severely contused tissue and actively bleeding wounds that do not stop with pressure should be excluded. This also probably is not the best choice for contaminated wounds.

In 2002, Hock and colleagues [26] reported the first randomized controlled trial using HAT. Of the 189 patients enrolled in the study, half received the HAT procedure and the other half received standard suturing. The results of the HAT group showed less scarring (6.3% versus 20.4%) and fewer overall complications (7.3% versus 21.5%). They also reported significantly lower pain scores (median 2 versus 4) and shorter procedure times (median 5 versus 15 minutes). A follow-up study in 2005 also has shown HAT to be more cost effective than standard suturing. These results were attributed to lower complication rates, decreased duration of the procedure, fewer equipment needs, and no need for return visit for suture removal [27].

Summary

There are many techniques available for the closure of traumatic wounds in EDs. Each method has its own unique benefits and limitations that must be considered in each case individually. The best technique provides durability, simplicity, excellent cosmetic outcome, and overall patient satisfaction. Unfortunately, at this time no single method is superior for all situations.

EPs must be familiar with multiple techniques to provide the best outcomes for their patients.

References

[1] Hollander JE, Singer AJ. Laceration management. Ann Emerg Med 1999;34:356–67.
[2] Schremmer RD. New concepts in wound management. Clinical Pediatric Emergency Medicine 2004;5(4):239–45.
[3] Dunn DL. Ethicon wound closure manual. Sommerville (NJ): Ethicon Inc; 2004.
[4] Parrell GJ, Becker GD. Comparison of absorbable with nonabsorbable sutures in closure of facial skin wounds. Arch Facial Plast Surg 2003;5(6):488–90.
[5] Karounis H, Gouin S, Eisman H, et al. A randomized, controlled trial comparing long-term cosmetic outcomes of traumatic pediatric lacerations repaired with absorbable plain gut versus nonabsorbable nylon sutures. Acad Emerg Med 2004;11(7):730–5.
[6] Holger JS, Wandersee SC, Hale DB. Cosmetic outcomes of facial lacerations repaired with tissue-adhesive, absorbable and nonabsorbable sutures. Am J Emerg Med 2004;22(4):254–7.
[7] Al-Qattan MM. Vicryl Rapide versus Vicryl suture in skin closure of the hand in children: a randomized prospective study. J Hand Surg [BR] 2005;30(1):90–1.
[8] Sharp WV, Belden TA, King PH, et al. Suture resistance to infection. Surgery 1982;91:61–3.
[9] Milewski PJ, Thompson H. Is a fat stitch necessary? Br J Surg 1980;67:393–4.
[10] Mehta PH, Dunn KA, Bradfield JF, et al. Contaminated wounds: infection rates with subcutaneous sutures. Ann Emerg Med 1996;27:43–8.
[11] Austin PE, Dunn KA, Eily-Cofield K, et al. Subcuticular sutures and the rate of inflammation in noncontaminated wounds. Ann Emerg Med 1995;25:328–30.
[12] Singer AJ, Gulla J, Hein M, et al. Single layer versus double-layer closure of facial lacerations: a randomized controlled trial. Plast Reconstr Surg 2005;116:363–8.
[13] Zuber TJ. The mattress sutures: vertical, horizontal, and corner stitch. Am Fam Physician 2002;66:2231–6.
[14] Kandel EF, Bennet RG. The effect of stitch type on flat tip blood flow. J Am Acad Dermatol 2001;44:265–72.
[15] Osmond MH, Wuinn JV, Sutcliffe T, et al. A randomized, clinical trial comparing butylcyanoacrylate with octylcyanoacrylate in the management of selected pediatric facial lacerations. Acad Emerg Med 1999;6(3):171–7.
[16] Quinn JV, Drzewiecki A, Li MM, et al. A randomized, controlled trial comparing a tissue adhesive with suturing in the repair of pediatric facial lacerations. Ann Emerg Med 1993; 22(7):1130–5.
[17] Keng TM, Bucknall TE. A clinical trial of tissue adhesive (histoacryl) in skin closure of groin wounds. Med J Malaysia 1989;44(2):122–8.
[18] Singer AJ, Quinn JV, Clark RE, et al. Closure of lacerations and incisions with octylcyanoacrylate: a multicenter randomized controlled trial. Surgery 2002;131(3):270–6.
[19] Quinn JV, Osmond MH, Yurack JA, et al. N-2-butylcyanoacrylate: risk of bacterial contamination with an appraisal of its antimicrobial effects. J Emerg Med 1995;13(4):581–5.
[20] Quinn J, Maw J, Ramotar K, et al. Octylcyanoacrylate tissue adhesive versus suture wound repair in a contaminated wound model. Surgery 1997;122(1):69–72.
[21] Osmond MH, Klassen TP, Quinn JV. Economic comparison of a tissue adhesive and suturing in the repair of pediatric facial lacerations. J Pediatr 1995;126(6):892–5.
[22] Rodeheaver GT, Halverson JM, Edlich RF. Mechanical performance of wound closure tapes. Ann Emerg Med 1983;12(4):203–7.
[23] Panek PH, Prusak MP, Bolt D, et al. Potentiation of wound infection by adhesive adjuncts. Am Surg 1972;38(6):343–5.
[24] Capellan O, Hollander JE. Management of lacerations in the emergency department. Emerg Med Clin North Am 2003;21:205–31.

[25] Pineros-Fernandez A, Salopek L, Rodheaver PF, et al. A revolutionary advance in skin clo-sure compared to current methods. J Long Term Eff Med Implants 2006;16(1):19–27.

[26] Hock MO, Ooi SB, Saw SM, et al. A randomized controlled trial comparing the hair apposition technique with tissue glue to standard suturing in scalp lacerations (HAT study). Ann Emerg Med 2002;40:19–26.

[27] Ong ME, Coyle D, Lim SH, et al. Cost-effectiveness of hair apposition technique compared with standard suturing in scalp lacerations. Ann Emerg Med 2005;46:237–42.

ELSEVIER
SAUNDERS

Emerg Med Clin N Am
25 (2007) 83–99

EMERGENCY
MEDICINE
CLINICS OF
NORTH AMERICA

Advanced Laceration Management

Daniel J. Brown, MD[a],[*], Jon E. Jaffe, MD[b], Jody K. Henson, MD[c]

[a]SAUSHEC Emergency Medicine, Brooke Army Medical Center, MCHE-EM,
3851 Roger Brooke Dr., Fort Sam Houston, San Antonio, TX 78234-6200, USA
[b]Department of Emergency Medicine, Texas A&M Health Science
Center-College of Medicine, Scott and White Hospital,
2401 South 31st Street, Temple, TX 76508, USA
[c]Texas A&M Health Science Center, Scott and White Hospital, 2401 South 31st Street,
Temple, TX 76508, USA

Many lacerations seen in the emergency department setting require specific management based on anatomic location. Lacerations of the fingertip, ear, nose, lip, tongue, and eyelid can be complex and require advanced management techniques. Many can be treated primarily by emergency clinicians; however, it is important for the clinician to know when consultation is appropriate for treatment by a specialist. Current literature recommendations are presented for initial management, methods of repair, technical tips to facilitate repair, appropriate consultation, and postoperative care for these complex lacerations.

Fingertip

Fingertip lacerations in adults

Fingertip lacerations in adults are commonly seen in the emergency department. Management focuses on loss of tissue or pulp, fracture of the distal phalanx, and damage to the nailbed. Proper management preserves maximum finger length, sensation, and proper regrowth of the fingernail to avoid pain, deformity, and functional impairment.

After a wrist, metacarpal, or digital block and a digital tourniquet for a bloodless field, simple lacerations of the palmar surface without extension

* Corresponding author.
E-mail address: daniel.brown1@lackland.af.mil (D.J. Brown).

0733-8627/07/$ - see front matter © 2007 Elsevier Inc. All rights reserved.
doi:10.1016/j.emc.2006.11.001

to bone and without visualization of ligament injury may be primarily repaired with single- or multifilament absorbable or nonabsorbable suture. If flexor or extensor tendons are partially or completely disrupted, consultation to the hand surgeon is indicated for repair. If phalangeal bone is exposed, it is trimmed back just below skin level with a rongeur.

Fingertip amputations require microsurgical expertise and should be referred to a hand surgeon for digital artery anastomosis and replantation. When comparing replantation to flap repair/amputation closure, microsurgical replantation has several benefits, including less finger shortening, longitudinal nail curvature, absence of proximal interphalangeal (PIP) flexion contracture, better functional outcome, and higher patient satisfaction [1,2]. Near-normal nail regeneration occurs in fingertip amputations that are proximal to the lunula after replantation by a specialist [3]. Some non-microsurgical replantations have been successful [4]; however, the literature is inconclusive. No anatomic boundary has been consistent in predicting successful composite grafting, and some studies required multiple surgeries for nonmicrosurgical replantation to be successful [5,6]. Multiple flap-repair techniques have been published, but these techniques require mobilizing and advancing tissue near digital arteries and nerves and can have severe complications if not performed by a specialist [7]. One technique that is neurovascularly safe and appropriate in the emergency department setting is the thenar-flap graft described herein.

Dorsal fingertip injuries are often complicated by fingernail and nailbed injuries. It was previously thought that any subungual hematoma comprising 25% or more of the visible nail had to removed for nailbed inspection, but a recent systematic review concluded that a subungual hematoma with no other significant fingertip injury may be treatment by trephining alone with good cosmetic and functional results [8]. Additional finger tip injury, including displacement of a distal phalangeal fracture, is highly suspicious for nailbed laceration [9]. The nailplate must be removed to assess and repair nailbed lacerations because future fingernail growth is determined primarily by the accuracy of nailbed repair [10]. This is not emergent, but a delay of more than 2 weeks impairs regrowth [9]. There is a direct correlation between final outcome in nail regrowth and degree of crush injury [10].

The nailplate is separated from the sterile matrix with a fine scissor or scalpel directly under the distal nailplate attachment (Fig. 1). The nail may then be removed with traction and examined for attached remnants of the bed, which must be removed and replaced for complete restoration of the nailbed. After thorough debridement and irrigation of the wound, primary repair of the nailbed is performed with 6-0 or 7-0 absorbable suture.

After nailbed repair, the nailplate or substitute material may be replaced over the germinal and sterile matrix. No statistically significant correlation has been found between nail replacement and improving nail regrowth [10]. It does preserve the contours of the nailfold, prevents adhesions between the fold and the repaired nailbed, and decreases pain. Carefully fitted

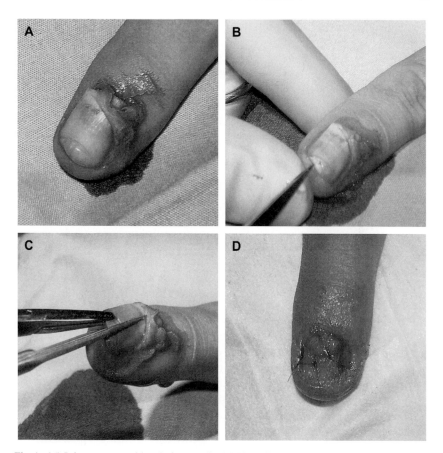

Fig. 1. (*A*) Injury to eponychium before repair. (*B*) The nailplate is separated from the sterile matrix with a fine scissor directly under the distal nailplate attachment. (*C*) Removing eponychium tissue with scissor and removing nailplate with forceps traction. (*D*) After nailbed repair.

nonadherent material, such as polyurethane sponge or paraffin-gauze, has proven to be effective. Dove and colleagues [11] compared nailplate replacement with gauze and found that nail replacement caused less pain and was more adherent than gauze dressings. In addition, 75% of the nailplates remained in place after the initial dressing at 7 days. Nails that spontaneously separate are usually shed at 14 to 21 days [11]. Many other materials have been suggested for nailbed cover, including acrylic nails [12], a nasogastric catheter splint [13], a silicone sheet, or aluminum suture package material [7].

The original nailplate or substitute material should be placed under the eponychium and may be held in place by bilateral single paronychium nonabsorbable sutures [7,9,11]. The sutures securing the nailplate or substitute material should be removed after 3 weeks, at which time the nail will be adherent or spontaneously slough and allow for new nail growth. Another method of anchoring the nailplate to the nailbed is with octyl-2-cyanoacy-late adhesive. No prospective trials have been reported using this tissue adhesive for nailbed repair; however, Hallock [14] published a prospective review demonstrating the common use of octyl-2-cyanoacylate as a nailplate adhesive. One of the most promising uses of octyl-2-cyanoacylate in finger-nail injuries is for a split or torn nail that can be easily pieced together and glued in the appropriate position, securing the nail properly to the nailbed. The finger is then placed in a short volar or hairpin splint isolating the PIP but allowing motion if the distal interphalangeal (DIP) for 4 weeks. Oral an-tibiotics should be given in all cases of nailbed laceration with underlying distal phalangeal fracture because this is an open fracture [9].

Fingertip lacerations in preschool children

The treatment of fingertip injuries in preschool children is common for the emergency specialist. Of hand injuries in children, the fingertip is the most commonly injured area for children 2 years of age and under [15]. Most of the literature endorses meticulous repair of the fingertip, especially the nail, but there is little literature to support this statement. Although for-mal nail bed reconstruction in children has been advocated for hematomas larger than 25%, no notable difference in outcome was found regardless of hematoma size, presence of fracture, or injury mechanism [16]. Other tech-niques, such as reimplantation of the nail, though widely done, have not been supported with good evidence [17].

With the widespread use of sedation techniques, formal operative repair is rarely necessary. Regarding the use of a microscope for the nail bed repair of the preschool child, the literature is inconclusive but suggests that it is not necessary.

What is rarely mentioned in the emergency literature is the technique for dressing the wound after surgery. An active toddler can destroy a poor dress-ing in less than an hour. Green [18] has stated "In no other field of surgery does the postoperative management of the patient play so critical role as it does in hand surgery." A recent study of dressings in children found that frequent dressing changes are not needed if the initial dressing is well applied [19].

After nonadhesive petrolatum gauze is applied to the margins of the wound, gauze should be used. This should be followed by careful applica-tion of splints in function. An outer dressing such as Coban can then be ap-plied extending to the mid forearm. Major repairs of the hand would be extended to the axilla. A well applied dressing can be maintained for several weeks, although it is not necessary with the fingertip injury.

Grafting

Frequently, the fingertip injury causes loss of skin at the tip or the palmar surface. If there is subcutaneous tissue covering the bone, then the wound can be closed with autografting. Although many times this type of wound is closed with a "VY" or left to heal spontaneously, autografting may provide rapid return of function and an excellent outcome.

The donor skin can be obtained from the ipsilateral hypothenar eminence. After gently scraping away the fat with the end of a scalpel from the subcutaneous side, the graft can be sutured in place over the defect. It should be slightly larger than the defect and will contract over time as it takes. The donor site can then be sutured (Fig. 2) [20–22].

Simplified pinning

Frequently in fingertip injuries, there is a fracture of the distal phalanx. Although a small distal chip requires no intervention, a more substantial fragment might need a pin to prevent nonunion [23]. Kirschner wires are rarely available in the emergency department. Before closure of the skin, in a well anesthetized finger, a 22-gauge hypodermic needle can be easily used to bridge the fracture fragments. The hub end should be partially filled with petrolatum or antibiotic ointment and capped (Fig. 3). This can be easily removed after a reasonable union is established.

Ear

As in many facial injuries and lacerations, a precise, delicate repair of complex ear lacerations is necessary to achieve a cosmetically appealing result and to prevent the need for future cosmetic surgical intervention.

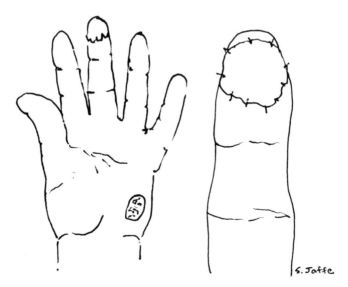

Fig. 2. Hypothenar-flap graft.

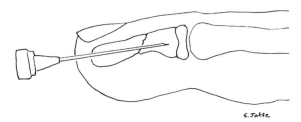

S. Jaffe

Fig. 3. Pinning of distal phalangeal fractures.

Because one ear has a symmetric counterpart that is easily comparable to the observer, repair of the injured ear to best duplicate its counterpart is crucial.

The external ear (auricle or pinna) consists of the prominent outer rim (the helix) and the inner, parallel rim (the antihelix). The helix terminates in a crux immediately above the external auditory meatus, and the antihelix terminates into superior and anterior crura, which create the triangular fossa. The deep furrow between the helix and antihelix is known as the scapha. The cavity surrounded by the antihelix, which leads to the meatus, is known as the concha [24]. These cartilaginous folds assist in the acquisition and amplification of sound and create shadows and curves that must be diligently recreated in wound repair. The auricle is composed of elastic cartilage covered by a firmly attached perichondrium and by delicate, tightly adhering skin with little subcutaneous tissue in between. A potential space exists in the space between the cartilage and the perichondrium that can allow the accumulation of blood after an injury. The lobule of the ear is an exception to the cartilaginous structure of the ear because it contains subcutaneous fat and lacks cartilage.

Knowledge of the physiology of the ear cartilage is essential to prevent disfiguring complications from disruption of its normal state. Cartilage is an avascular tissue. Its nutrients and thus its metabolic support are supplied by the surrounding periosteum. If deprived of the nutrients, protection, and immune mediators provided by this surrounding tissue, the cartilage is prone to infection, erosive chondritis, and subsequent necrosis. It is thus of paramount importance in repair of the auricle to adequately cover exposed cartilage [25].

Goals of repairing lacerations to the ear include cosmesis, appropriate and expedient coverage of cartilage to avoid the aforementioned complications, and avoidance of a large wound hematoma or abscess. The formation of a wound hematoma or a wound abscess prevents adherence of the nutrient-rich perichondrium to the cartilage and can result in destruction of the cartilaginous structure of the ear and abnormal cartilage production, which leads to the development of a fibrotic, calcified mass referred to as the "cauliflower ear" deformity [25–27]. This deformity is often not amenable to reconstructive repair; thus, care should be taken to avoid its formation [28].

Initial wound care of through-and-through ear lacerations consists of appropriate irrigation, taking care not to irrigate with such force as to further dissect the cartilage form its adherent tissue. The innervation of the ear is supplied by the greater auricular nerve (a branch off the cervical plexus) and the auriculotemporal nerve (a branch of V3). Anesthesia for repair can thus be obtained using the great auricular nerve block [29]. The great auricular nerve ascends upward on the facial surface of the sternoclei-domastoid. The nerve divides into end branches 6.5 cm down from the lower external ear canal; therefore, anesthetizing in the mid-sternocleidomastoid area 6.5 cm distally to the meatus should result in an insensate area of the lower portion of the ear. The remainder of the ear can be anesthetized using a V3 block [29]. Infiltration should be 2.5 cm anterior to the tragus in the sigmoid notch (the area between the condyle and the coronoid process of the mandible.) A cotton plug should be inserted into the ear canal to avoid discomfort to the patient during irrigation and to prevent an occlusive clot in the external canal. Jagged or devitalized cartilage and skin should be trimmed. Up to 5 mm of cartilage can be debrided without risk of significant deformity or asymmetry [30]. Tissue debridement should be kept to a mini-mum because it is important in the coverage and thus in the viability of the underlying damaged cartilage. Overzealous skin debridement may result in the need to overstretch the skin and may disrupt the natural contour of the underlying cartilage. The first step in suturing the defect should be the reapproximation of the cartilage. If reapproximation of the cartilage can be performed with approximation of the overlying tissue, then suturing the cartilage is not critical; however, if a defect will remain, then suturing the cartilage is necessary. 4-0 or 5-0 absorbable sutures are recommended and should initially be placed at critical grooves and folds in the cartilage. The stitch through the cartilage should include the anterior and posterior perichondrium to ensure maximum stability of the suture, to prevent tearing through the delicate cartilage, and to ensure nutrient supply to the damaged cartilage. The posterior skin, followed by the anterior skin, should be repaired using 5-0 or 6-0 nonabsorbable interrupted sutures [31]. In wounds in which significant cartilage and tissue loss preclude an adequate and cosmetic closure, appropriate consultation is recommended.

A pressure dressing must be applied to the ear after repair to prevent bleeding, hematoma formation, and the resulting deformity. Moist or petrolatum-coated cotton should be placed in the fissures and folds of the ear until the cotton is level with the helix. Cotton gauze can then be placed behind the ear and cut to fit the shape of the pinna. This padding prevents pain and pressure necrosis caused by the ear pressing against the skull. Gauze can then be placed on the anterior portion of the ear. The entire as-sembly should be secured in place with a circumferential head bandage. Do not include the other ear in the bandage to avoid causing pressure necrosis of the unaffected ear [31]. An alternative, more aggressive dressing uses dental cotton rolls secured with suture passed through the cartilage [30].

Nose

The nose is composed of a bony and cartilaginous skeleton. The cartilaginous, protruding tip of the nose is mainly responsible for the great variation in the size and shape of the nose and is often vulnerable to injury. It is one of the most commonly injured structures in assault victims [26]. It, even more so than the ears, is a focal point of the face, and thus cosmesis of repair is of utmost importance.

The cartilage of the nose is divided into right and left halves by the septal cartilage. The alar cartilage provides the form and support for the tip of the nose. The major alar cartilage of each side of the nose is divided into the medial and lateral crus. The cartilages are connected by aponeurotic tissue. The remainder of the nasal ala is formed by alar fibrous-fatty tissue [24]. The ala is covered by delicate, thin skin. The epithelium of the outer nose transitions into the sebaceous gland and the hair-filled mucous membrane of the inner nose at the transition zone just inside the ala of each nostril.

Nasal lacerations can vary from simple skin lacerations to more complex lacerations involving the cartilaginous framework and nasal mucous membrane. In any injury, the nasal septum must first be visualized to inspect for a septal hematoma. The nasal cartilage, like the cartilage in the external ear, depends on its surrounding perichondrium and supporting tissue for its metabolic needs. An untreated septal hematoma physically separates the cartilage from its perichondrium and thus deprives the nasal cartilage of its nutrients. This results in destruction of the septal cartilage, which can result in septal perforation or an unsightly saddle nose deformity [26]. A septal hematoma should be drained and packed to prevent reaccumulation. Visualization despite significant bleeding can be facilitated using intranasal vasoactive agents.

Repair of nasal lacerations involves accurate reapproximation of each tissue layer. Simple superficial lacerations may by closed using 5-0 to 6-0 monofilament nonabsorbable sutures. In full-thickness lacerations that involve cartilage, debridement of tissue and cartilage should be kept to a minimum. Unlike the ear, where 5 mm of cartilage may be removed in debridement, even a small amount of nasal cartilage removed can produce a significant defect and resultant asymmetry of the healed wound. Likewise, the nasal skin should be minimally debrided because it is inflexible, tears easily, and has minimal redundancy.

Anesthesia of the nose can be attained by performing a dorsal nasal nerve block [29]. Injection and infiltration directly into the laceration not only is extremely painful but can disrupt landmarks and dissect the perichondrial tissue planes; therefore, a nerve block is preferred. A dorsal nerve block is performed by infiltrating 1 to 2 ml of anesthetic per side at the junction of the nasal bones and the nasal cartilage approximately 6 to 10 mm from the midline of the nose. This block provides anesthesia for the cartilaginous dorsum and tip of the nose [29].

A three-layered approach to the full thickness nasal laceration should be used, beginning with the intranasal mucosa (preferably with dissolvable suture), followed by cartilage (if necessary) and finally the external skin [24]. Secondary to the naturally curved form of the ala, disruptions in the nasal cartilage can frequently be approximated and thus repaired by repair of the overlying skin. For cartilage lacerations that cause significant deformity and asymmetry between the nostrils, 4-0 or 5-0 absorbable sutures can be used to gently reapproximate the cartilage. Care should be taken to exactly align the alar edges. The overlying nasal skin can be repaired using 5-0 or 6-0 simple interrupted suture. A subcuticular suture may be used to provide greater strength in the thin, easily friable tissue [32]. Precise alignment of the free rim of the nostril is the most cosmetically important aspect of the repair. Misalignment of the free rim can produce unsightly notching of the alar edge. In lacerations involving the inner nasal mucosa, care must be taken to repair the mucosa to avoid contraction and subsequent retraction of the nasal margin.

Lip

The lips are mobile muscular folds. The external surface of the lip has three distinct regions: the skin, the vermilion, and the oral mucosa. The vermilion is a noncornified layer of stratified epithelium. Its epithelial cells contain a compound called eleidin, which makes it translucent. The translucency allows the underlying vascular papillae to give the lips their pink color [24]. The skin meets the vermilion at the vermilion border, which is further separated into the red line and the white line. These borders and distinctions become of utmost importance during a cosmetic repair. The vermilion joins the mucous membrane at the "wet–dry" border. The labial mucosa meets the alveolar mucosa vestibular fold, which meets the gingival proper.

The primary muscle of the upper and lower lip is the orbicularis oris. It is located between the skin and the oral mucosa. Its integrity is essential for many necessary functions, including speech, facial expressions, and retaining oral secretions.

There are two main classifications of lip injuries: lacerations and avulsions. Lacerations can frequently be managed in the emergency department. Larger avulsions may require surgical intervention. Large lacerations through the lip frequently produce a V-type deformity. These should be repaired using a three-layered technique. Anesthesia of the lower lip can best be attained by performing a mental nerve block on the side of injury [29]. This block allows for anesthetic without disruption of the delicate borders of the lip. To perform the block, infiltrate anesthetic into the buccal sulcus near the base of the second lower bicuspid. The upper lid is best anesthetized using an infraorbital nerve block [29]. This is performed by infiltrating 1 to 2 ml of anesthetic into the infraorbital foramen by inserting the needle just laterally to the alar base of the nose and directing upward and laterally. After anesthetizing, irrigation, and inspection for foreign objects (eg, tooth fragments and dental devices), focus must be placed on alignment of the aforementioned borders.

If the vermilion border is involved in the laceration, the first stitch in repair should exactly reapproximate the red-line and the white-line of the border using 6-0, nonabsorbable suture. Even a discordance of 1 mm can be cosmetically displeasing [32]. After the approximation of the vermilion border, the repair can proceed using an "inside-out" technique. The wet–dry junction can first be approximated, after which the remainder of the mucosal defect can be closed with 5-0 absorbable suture. The approximation of the orbicularis oris muscle can then be performed with 5-0 absorbable suture, using a simple interrupted or horizontal mattress technique [30,32]. Finally, the skin can then be repaired using 6-0 nonabsorbable suture or tissue adhesive [26].

Intraoral lacerations continue to be a subject of controversy. Because the oral mucosa is highly vascular and heals quickly, repair has been recommended mainly in the following situations: (1) if the laceration is longer than 2 cm, (2) if the laceration creates a flap of tissue that falls between the occlusive surfaces of the teeth, or (3) if the wound is gaping and likely to trap food particles [33]. If a buccal laceration involves Stenson's duct, an oral surgery consult may be appropriate to facilitate cannulation and thus ensure patency of the duct.

Lacerations at the vestibular fold and at the border of the gingival and the intraoral mucosa present an additional challenge. Deep lacerations in the vestibular fold can be repaired with absorbable sutures, and we propose the use of a small drain to facilitate wound closure and prevent fluid accumulation and possible subsequent infection in the space created by the contaminated laceration. Avulsions of the tissue overlying the mandibular or maxillary ridge can be difficult because of the thin tissue and the lack of underlying anchoring tissue. If possible, the gingival flap can be sutured using 5-0 absorbable suture to neighboring tissue. If this proves impossible, sutures can be brought circumferentially around teeth to anchor the repair (Figs. 4 and 5) [30,33]. Approximation and avoiding overlapping of tissue in these repairs is especially necessary in elderly edentulous patients to best facilitate denture comfort and ease of fitting.

Tongue

Tongue lacerations can create difficult decisions for emergency physicians. Proper tongue laceration management is important to prevent infection, prevent aspiration, facilitate swallowing, and preserve articulation

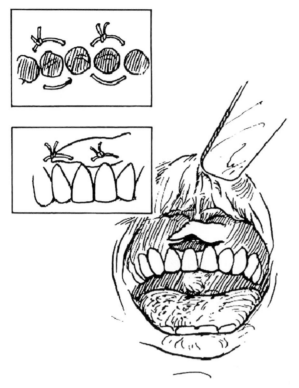

Fig. 4. Avulsion of gingival mucosal tissue. The technique to close this injury is shown. The sutures are brought around the teeth and through the avulsed tissue flap (*insets*). (*From* Trott A. Special anatomic sites. In: Weimer R, Cochran A, editors. Wounds and lacerations: emergency care and closure. St. Louis (MO): Mosby-Year Book; 1991. p. 172; with permission.)

[34,35]. Some lacerations can create airway complications, especially when the lingual arteries are severed, and profuse hemorrhage requires the emergency physician to establish a definitive airway through nasotracheal intubation or cricothyroidotomy/tracheostomy [36]. Oral intubation may complicate laceration repair but may take priority over tongue repair in emergent oral trauma situations.

Most tongue lacerations can be managed by emergency physicians. These include common small lacerations from seizures and falls. Simple lacerations less than 1 cm that are linear, superficial, in the central portion of the tongue, and do not gape open heal well without intervention and therefore do not need repair. These also have a low risk of infection [31,33].

Oral-maxillofacial and dental texts present conflicting recommendations as to which lacerations need repair. Lamell and colleagues [35] used the anecdotal recommendations in the texts to develop a protocol to study outcomes of tongue laceration management in children. Three selection criteria were established to determine need for primary repair by suturing: (1)

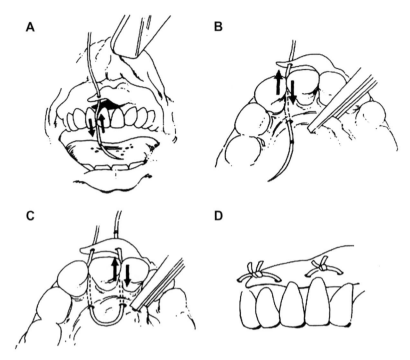

Fig. 5. The technique of flossing the suture material through the teeth in cases in which the needle cannot be passed between the teeth because of tight interproximal contacts. (*A*) Pass needle through facial tissue, then floss through teeth. (*B*) Pass needle through palatal tissue. (*C*) Pass needle through palatal tissue again and floss through teeth. (*D*) Tie suture on facial aspect. (*From* Armstrong BD. Lacerations of the mouth. Emerg Med Clin North Am 2000;18(3): 471–80; with permission.)

wounds gaping (margins not approximated) when the tongue was at rest position, irrespective of wound location on the tongue; (2) lateral border wounds; and (3) wounds with active hemorrhage. Most of the patients studied had lacerations due to falls at home. The most common laceration found was located on the anterior-dorsum of the tongue and averaged 13 mm in length, and the majority were not gaping at rest and were closed with 4-0 chromic gut. The authors found no significant relationship between choice of management (suture versus not) when evaluated for quality of outcome or post-trauma morbidity. Similarly, no significant relationship was found in the quality of outcome with regard to length, width, or depth of wound. They concluded that suturing tongue lacerations does not improve outcome or reduce morbidity. None of the patients received antibiotics, and none of the patients experienced a post-trauma infection. All lacerations that bisect the tongue require primary suture repair [31]. Partial amputations have been successfully replanted, but this requires microsurgical technique for microvascular repair and should be referred to oral-maxillofacial surgery or otolaryngology for repair under general anesthesia [36]. Hemorrhage must be controlled, and suturing lacerations is an effective method; however, hemostasis may be achieved conservatively with simple pressure, cold, or inactivity [31].

Suturing in the oral cavity can be difficult, but many adjuncts can be used to facilitate repair. A Denhardt-Dingman side mouth gag [31] and bite blocks [33] may be used to keep the mouth open. To protrude the tongue for repair, manually holding the tongue with gauze sponges is often adequate. Once the patient is anesthetized, towel clamps or a 0-silk single suture may be passed through the tongue to maintain protrusion (Fig. 6) [33].

Local anesthesia may be performed topically by covering the area with 4% lidocaine–soaked gauze for 5 minutes or local infiltration of 1% lidocaine with buffered epinephrine. For large lacerations, a lingual nerve block may be performed [35].

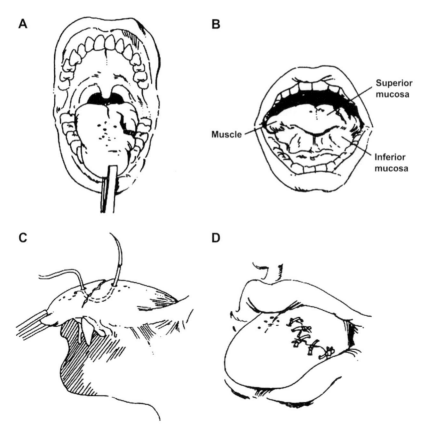

Fig. 6. The closure of a tongue laceration. (A) Towel clamp to hold tongue. (B) Layers of the tongue. (C) Stitch should include half the thickness of the tongue. (D) Tongue with sutured laceration. (From Armstrong BD. Lacerations of the mouth. Emerg Med Clin North Am 2000;18(3):471–80; with permission.)

Suture of the tongue should be performed with an absorbable suture, such as chromic gut. Nylon has sharp ends and therefore should be avoided. The size should be 4-0 or 5-0 [33]. The sutures are placed with wide margins and deep penetration to close all layers with a single stitch and are finished with four square knots. Sutures should be placed on the superior, inferior, and lateral borders as required. Tongue sutures often untie, but that should not prompt the physician to over-tie [33]. The use of a closed hemostat tip may be helpful to prevent over-tying knots. Sutures are rapidly absorbed or fall out in approximately 1 week and therefore do not need removal [33]. All patients who have tongue lacerations regardless of management technique should be instructed to gently swish and spit with a mild antiseptic mouthwash after discharge [37].

Eyelid

Simple upper and lower eyelid lacerations can be managed by the emergency physician. Proper laceration management in the emergency department can prevent cornea or conjunctival irritation or abrasion from irregular scaring or cut suture ends. Knowing periorbital anatomy is the key to recognizing which lacerations need to be referred to an ophthalmologist or to a facial plastic surgeon for repair.

Time to primary closure from 12 to 36 hours is acceptable, and the same delay is acceptable when referring to consultants for primary closure. In the case of canalicular injuries, iced saline gauze applied in the interim can decrease edema and allow for better visualization for microsurgery by the consultant [38].

It is essential that the emergency physician recognize eyelid lacerations that require referral to an ophthalmologist for management. Lacerations that require microsurgical technique to place layered closure through the tarsal plate or microintubation of the canaliculus system should be left to the expertise of ophthalmologists [31,38]. This includes lacerations to upper or lower lid margins or lacerations involving the lacrimal sac or duct. High suspicion for canalicular injuries should be maintained in any laceration medial to the puncta. When in doubt, the integrity of the canalicular system can be assessed by instilling fluorescein into the eye and assessing for dye in the wound [37]. Complete lacerations of the lid margin require exact realignment to avoid entropion or ectropion that may cause corneal or conjunctival irritation. In addition, traumatic lacerations of the upper eyelid with exposure of orbital fat indicates a breach of the orbital septum and requires exploration by an ophthalmologist to rule out underlying levator palpebrae superioris muscle damage [38]. Another sign of levator palpebrae muscle disruption is ptosis in the presence of a horizontal upper lid laceration and requires repair by the consultant [31]. Lid trauma with tissue avulsions should be left to an ophthalmologist.

Many lid lacerations can be treated conservatively without suture repair. Wounds that are good candidates for healing by secondary intension include lacerations that comprise less than 25% of the lid, are superficial, and do not have exposed bone or cartilage [39]. When suture management is indicated in the emergency department setting, 6-0 or 7-0 soft suture is recommended. Multiple studies have shown benefit in using absorbable sutures, such as chromic gut, and using buried mattress sutures to improve postoperative care in juxtamarginal lacerations [40,41]. This technique prevents the complication of suture end abrasion to the globe itself [42,43] and everts the margins of repaired tissue, allowing for better cosmesis by avoiding contraction during healing [39]. Another technique to avoid postoperative corneal abrasions in juxtamarginal laceration repair is to cut the ends long and incorporate the ends into remaining sutures as the wound is closed from proximal to distal away from the lid margin [38,44].

Other superficial cutaneous lacerations that do not include the lid margin or the area immediately near the margin can be closed with any 6-0 or 7-0 soft suture material (absorbable or not). Close attention must be made to avoid vertical tension on the wound site or surrounding tissues during closure because this increases lid retraction, ectropion, or lagophthalmos [39]. Postoperative care includes liberal application of topical antibiotic ointment to the wound, avoiding sun and water exposure, and limiting make-up application for 2 to 3 weeks [38].

Summary

The majority of lacerations to the face and fingertip can be managed by the emergency clinician. Fingertip lacerations can often be left to heal by secondary intention. Complete amputations should be referred to a hand surgeon. Nailbed lacerations should be repaired, and the nail or other splinting material should be replaced for protection. Needle pinning may be useful to splint simple distal phalangeal fractures. A thenar autograft may be performed when reimplantation of a complete amputation is not possible. Ear lacerations require careful irrigation and prompt repair to avoid dissection of the perichondrium, followed by a pressure dressing to prevent bleeding. Septal hematomas of the nose must be drained and packed to avoid destruction of the septal cartilage. Nasal lacerations require careful approximation of the cartilage and limiting debridement of overlying skin. Lip repair is initiated with the approximation of the vermilion border. Most tongue lacerations heal without primary repair, and infection is uncommon. Through-and-through tongue lacerations and lateral wounds often need repair. Upper and lower eyelid repair can be performed by primarily approximating the tarsal plate. Lid margin lacerations and wounds involving the canalicular system require referral to a specialist.

References

[1] Hattori Y, Doi K, Ikeda K, et al. A retrospective study of functional outcomes after successful replantation versus amputation closure for single fingertip amputations. J Hand Surg [Am] 2006;31(5):811–8.

[2] Dubert T, Houimli S, Valenti P, et al. Very distal finger amputations: replantation or "reposition-flap" repair? J Hand Surg [Br] 1997;22(3):353–8.

[3] Nishi G, Shibata Y, Tago K, et al. Nail regeneration in digits replanted after amputation through the distal phalanx. J Hand Surg [Am] 1996;21(2):229–33.

[4] Hirase Y. Salvage of fingertip amputated at nail level: new surgical principles and treatments. Ann Plast Surg 1997;38(2):151–7.

[5] Lin TS, Jeng SF, Chiang YC. Fingertip replantation using the subdermal pocket procedure. Plast Reconstr Surg 2004;113(1):247–53.

[6] Muneuchi G, Kurokawa M, Igawa K, et al. Nonmicrosurgical replantation using a subcutaneous pocket for salvage of the amputated fingertip. J Hand Surg [Am] 2005;30(3): 562–5.

[7] Stevenson TR. Fingertip and nailbed injuries. Orthop Clin North Am 1992;23(1):149–59.

[8] Batrick N, Hashemi K, Freij R. Treatment of uncomplicated subungual haematoma. Emerg Med J 2003;20(1):65.

[9] Melone CP Jr, Grad JB. Primary care of fingernail injuries. Emerg Med Clin North Am 1985; 3(2):255–61.

[10] O'Shaughnessy M, McCann J, O'Connor TP, et al. Nail re-growth in fingertip injuries. Ir Med J 1990;83(4):136–7.

[11] Dove AF, Sloan JP, Moulder TJ, et al. Dressings of the nailbed following nail avulsion. J Hand Surg [Br] 1988;13(4):408–10.

[12] Purcell EM, Hussain M, McCann J. Fashionable splint for nailbed lacerations: the acrylic nail. Plast Reconstr Surg 2003;112(1):337–8.

[13] Bayraktar A, Ozcan M. A nasogastric catheter splint for a nailbed. Ann Plast Surg 2006; 57(1):120.

[14] Hallock GG. Expanded applications for octyl-2-cyanoacrylate as a tissue adhesive. Ann Plast Surg 2001;46(2):185–9.

[15] Salazard B, Launay F, Desouches C, et al. Fingertip injuries in children: 81 cases with at least one year follow-up. Rev Chir Orthop Reparatrice Appar Mot 2004;90(7):621–7 [in French].

[16] Roser SE, Gellman H. Comparison of nail bed repair versus nail trephination for subungual hematomas in children. J Hand Surgery [Am] 1999;24:1166–70.

[17] Boyd R, Libetta C. Towards evidence based emergency medicine: best BETs from the Manchester Royal Infirmary. Reimplantation of the nail root in fingertip crush injuries in children. Emerg Med J 2002;19(2):141.

[18] Green D. General principles. In: Green DP, editor. Operative hand surgery. New York: Livingstone; 1913. p. 15–9.

[19] Cooney WP 3rd, Dobyns JH. Pediatric hand dressing: technical report. J Hand Surg [Am] 2005;30(5):1009–13.

[20] Hutchinson J, Tough JS, Wyburn GM. Regeneration of sensation in grafted skin. Br J Plast Surg 1949;2:82.

[21] Patton H. Split-skin grafts from the hypothenar area for fingertip avulsions. Plast Reconstr Surg 1969;43:426–9.

[22] Schenck RR, Cheema TA. Hypothenar skin grafts for fingertip reconstruction. J Hand Surgery [Am] 1984;9A:750–3.

[23] Rea L. Non-union in a fracture of the shaft of the distal phalanx. Hand 1982;14(1):85–8.

[24] Edlich R, Kenney J. Soft tissue injuries of the face. In: Champion H, editor. Rob & Smiths operative surgery: trauma surgery part 1. London: Butterworths; 1989. p. 133–46.

[25] Belleza WG. Otolaryngologic emergencies in the outpatient setting. Med Clin North Am 2006;90(2):329–53.

[26] Hollander J, Singer A. Emergency wound management. In: Tintinalli JE, editor. Emergency medicine: a comprehensive study guide. New York: McGraw-Hill; 2004. p. 287–305.

[27] Rubin A. Facial trauma. Clinics of Family Practice 2000;2(3):565–80.

[28] Hirsch BE. Infections of the external ear. Am J Otolaryngol 1992;13(3):145–55.

[29] Zide B. How to block and tackle the face. J Plast Reconstr Surg 1998;101(3):840–51.

[30] Trott A. Wounds and lacerations: emergency care and closure. 2nd edition. Mosby Inc.; 1997. p. 192–204.

[31] Lammers RL, Trott AT. Methods of wound closure. In: Roberts JR, Hedges J, editors. Clinical procedures in emergency medicine. 4th edition. Philadelphia: Saunders; 2004. p. 682–6.

[32] Lammers R. Principles of wound management. In: Roberts JR, Hedges J, editors. Clinical procedures in emergency medicine. 4th edition. Philidelphia: Saunders; 2004. p. 640–4.

[33] Armstrong BD. Lacerations of the mouth. Emerg Med Clin North Am 2000;18(3):471–80.

[34] Wells MD, Edwards AL, Luce EA. Intraoral reconstructive techniques. Clin Plast Surg 1995; 22(1):91–108.

[35] Lamell CW, Fraone G, Casamassimo PS, et al. Presenting characteristics and treatment outcomes for tongue lacerations. Pediatr Dent 1999;21(1):34–8.

[36] Buntic RF, Buncke HJ. Successful replantation of an amputated tongue. Plast Reconstr Surg 1998;101(6):1604–7.

[37] McKay MP. Facial trauma. In: Marx JA, Hockberger RS, Walls RM, editors. Rosen's emergency medicine: concepts and clinical practice. 6th edition. St. Louis (MO): Mosby, Inc.; 2006. p. 382–98.

[38] Chang EL, Rubin PA. Management of complex eyelid lacerations. Int Ophthalmol Clin 2002;42(3):187–201.

[39] Chandler DB, Gausas RE. Lower eyelid reconstruction. Otolaryngol Clin North Am 2005; 38(5):1033–42.

[40] Custer PL, Vick V. Repair of marginal eyelid defects with 7-0 chromic sutures. Ophthal Plast Reconstr Surg 2006;22(4):256–8.

[41] Tyers AG, Mokete B, Self J. Comparison of standard eyelid margin closure using silk with a modified repair using 7/0 vicryl and a buried knot. Orbit 2005;24(2):103–8.

[42] Burroughs JR, Soparkar CN, Patrinely JR. The buried vertical mattress: a simplified technique for eyelid margin repair. Ophthal Plast Reconstr Surg 2003;19(4):323–4.

[43] Devoto MH, Kersten RC, Teske SA, et al. Simplified technique for eyelid margin repair. Arch Ophthalmol 1997;115(4):566–7.

[44] Ali SN, Budny PG. "Minding the ends": a simple technique for repair of lower eyelid lacerations. Emerg Med J 2004;21(2):263.

ELSEVIER
SAUNDERS

Emerg Med Clin N Am
25 (2007) 101–121

EMERGENCY
MEDICINE
CLINICS OF
NORTH AMERICA

Emergency Management of Difficult Wounds: Part I

Vincent Ball, MD,
MAJ Bradley N. Younggren, MD, FACEP*

*Department of Emergency Medicine, Madigan Army Medical Center,
Building 9040 Fitzsimmons Drive, Tacoma, WA 98431, USA*

Emergency physicians treat millions of wounds annually in the United States. In 2004 approximately 6.4 million open wounds were seen in United States emergency departments, representing approximately 5.8% of all visits [1]. This article covers difficult traumatic wounds that emergency physicians encounter on a daily basis, including mammalian bites, puncture and high-pressure wounds, and crush injuries, with special emphasis given to individuals at high risk for infectious complications. Information is provided on epidemiology, pathophysiology, management, and treatment of various wounds. The authors highlight available guidelines, provide the best evidence available, and provide recommendations when data are limited.

Mammalian bite wounds

Approximately 2 million bites per year in the United States are treated by physicians. The true incidence is uncertain because reporting is not mandatory in all areas and not all bite victims seek treatment. It is generally agreed that dog bites are the most common type of mammalian bites. Numerous sources cite that approximately 1% of all emergency department visits in the United States are because of bites. No recent evidence exists as to the overall incidence of bite injuries. A retrospective analysis done by Merchant and colleagues [2] of International Classification of Disease, Ninth Revision, codes covering three pediatric emergency departments in the northeast United States from 1995 to 2001 summarized that human bites, the least common of mammalian bite wounds, composed 0.04% of total visits. Regardless of the prevalence of bite wounds, they are sources of polymicrobial

---

* Corresponding author.
E-mail address: bradley.n.younggren@us.army.mil (M.B.N. Younggren).

0733-8627/07/$ - see front matter © 2007 Elsevier Inc. All rights reserved.
doi:10.1016/j.emc.2007.01.003

infection with potential for disastrous infectious and cosmetic outcomes if not treated properly.

Dog bites

In 2001 an estimated 368,245 people were treated for dog bite–related injuries [3]. This figure represents an estimated 80% to 90% of all bite wounds [4]. In data obtained from 1979 to 1996 United States Humane Society, NEXIS database, and death certificates, pit bulls and Rottweilers were implicated most often in fatal bite injuries [5]. Most pediatric bite victims (82%) are familiar with the biting dog [6]. Fatal bites typically involve small children who have bites to the neck resulting in exsanguination. The larger-breed dogs are capable of exerting forces in excess of 450 psi [3]. In 2001 the injury rate was highest for children 5 to 9 years of age and decreased in incidence with increasing age. Among victims less than 14 years of age, the rate for males (293.2 per 100,000) was higher than that for females (216.7 per 100,000). After the age of 15, the gender difference was not significant. The incidence of dog bites increases in the summer, with a peak of 11.1% of bites occurring in July. A minority of dog-bite injuries in 2001, 4.5%, were work related. Dog-bite injuries occur most commonly to the upper extremity (45.3%), followed by the lower extremity (25.8%) and head and neck area (22.8%) [2]. Bite wounds to the hand are at risk for tenosynovitis, abscess formation, osteomyelitis, and septic arthritis. Wounds to the face can be disfiguring and provide significant cosmetic concerns.

Dog-bite injuries may present as punctures, abrasions, tears, or avulsions. Larger breeds of dogs can generate pressures in excess of 450 psi [7], which is sufficient to penetrate a human skull [8]. The force and relative bluntness of the teeth also increases the possibility of a crush injury with devitalized tissue rather than a laceration or puncture injury.

Cat bites

Cat bites are the second most common type of mammalian bites, representing an estimated 5% to 15% of bites with an estimated annual incidence of 400,000 [3]. Because of their finer, sharper teeth and weaker biting forces, cat bites generally present as puncture wounds. Similar to dog bites, the distribution of cat bite wounds is more commonly on the upper extremity. Some 60% to 67% of bites occur on the upper extremity, with 15% to 20% occurring on the head and neck, 10% to 13% on the lower extremity, and up to 5% on the trunk (Fig. 1) [9–11].

Microbiology

There have been few recent studies isolating pathogens from dog and cat bites. Although earlier studies emphasized aerobic pathogenic organisms,

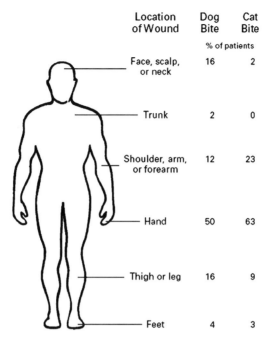

Location of Wound	Dog Bite	Cat Bite
	% of patients	
Face, scalp, or neck	16	2
Trunk	2	0
Shoulder, arm, or forearm	12	23
Hand	50	63
Thigh or leg	16	9
Feet	4	3

Fig. 1. Distribution of wound infections in 50 dog bites and 57 cat bites. (*From* Talan DA, Citron DN, Abrahamian FM, et al. Bacteriologic analysis of infected dog and cat bites. Emergency Medicine Animal Bite Infection Study Group. N Engl J Med 1999;340(2):86; with permission © Copyright 1999 Massachusetts Medical Society. All rights reserved.)

especially *Pasteurella* sp, *Streptococcus* sp, and *Staphylococcus* sp, recent studies emphasize the multitude of aerobic and anaerobic pathogenic species not previously associated with bite wounds [6,8]. In the previous *Emergency Medicine Clinics of North America* article discussing management of dog and bite wounds, Dire [9] summarized the relevant bacteriologic studies up until 1992. More recently Brook [7] studied wounds cultured from 17 dog bites and 4 cat bites in pediatric patients and isolated aerobic bacteria only in 5 of 21 wounds, anaerobic bacteria only in 2 of 21 wounds (10%), and both aerobic and anaerobic isolates in 14 of 21 wounds (66%).

Talan and colleagues [11], as part of a 12-center collaborative, studied infected bite wounds in 50 dog-bite and 57 cat-bite victims isolating an average of five bacteria per culture (range 0–16). Combined aerobes and anaerobes were isolated in 56% of the wounds with aerobes alone from 36% and anaerobes alone in 1%. *Pasteurella canis* was the most frequent isolate from dog bites (50%) and *Pasteurella multocida* subspecies *multocida* and *septica* were the most common isolates of cat bites (75%). Seven percent of the clinically infected wounds had no growth [10]. The incidence of *Pasterurella* species in dog bites found by Talan and colleagues (50%) is greater than previously described (Table 1) [11].

Table 1
Isolates from 50 dog bites and 57 cat bites

	Dog bites (%)	Cat bites (%)
Aerobes		
Pasteurella	50	75
Pasteurella canis	26	2
Pasteurella multocida	12	54
Streptococcus	46	46
Staphylococcus	46	35
Neisseria	16	19
Corynebacterium	12	28
Moraxella	10	35
Enterococcus	10	12
Bacillus	8	11
Pseudomonas	6	5
Capnocytophaga	2	7
Eikenella corrodens	2	2
Anaerobes		
Bacteroides	30	28
Porphyromonas	28	30
Propionibacterium	20	18
Fusobacterium nucleatum	16	25
Peptostreptococcus	16	5
Prevotella	28	19
Prevotella heparinolytica	14	9
Prevotella melaninogenica	2	2

Data from Talan DA, Citron DM, Abrahamian FM, et al. Bacteriologic analysis of infected dog and cat bites. N Engl J Med 1999;340:85–92.

The consensus in the literature of the microbiologic analysis of dog and cat bites is that *Pasteurella, Staphylococcus,* and *Streptococcus* species are the most prevalent aerobic pathogens and polymicrobial infections are the norm [3,6,10]. The use of postexposure antibiotic prophylaxis remains controversial among practitioners. Overall, dog-bite wound infection rates approximate those of non-bite lacerations at 3% to 20% [6,10,12] and represent the lowest risk for infection among mammalian bite wounds. Some bites, however, are at higher risk for infection, including those on the hand, of which an estimated 28% to 47.6% become infected [6,13]. Facial dog bites carry an estimated 4% chance of becoming infected [6]. Puncture wounds are more likely to become infected, as demonstrated by cat bite infection rates. Cats, because of their narrower, sharper teeth, are able to deliver inoculum deeper through a smaller-diameter wound, resulting in an infection rate estimated at 60% to 80% [6,10].

Insufficient studies exist analyzing the efficacy of antibiotic prophylaxis in dog and cat bites that present within 24 hours and do not appear infected. A recent Cochrane Database review on the subject revealed eight studies comprising 674 patients who had mammalian bites, of which none showed a statistically significant reduction in the rate of infection with prophylactic antibiotics after uncomplicated bites by dogs or cats [14]. A study by Brakenbury [15] in 1989 in a series of 185 patients found a significant benefit in prescribing amoxicillin/clavulanate after animal bites presenting 9 to 24 hours after injury. Despite the scarcity of data the general consensus and the authors' recommendations are to prescribe antibiotics for all cat bites and for high-risk dog bites, such as those that present greater than 9 hours after bite, appear as a deep puncture, occur on the hand or over a joint, and occur in high-risk patients (extremes of age, asplenic, immunocompromised). Five to 7 days of antibiotics that cover *Staphylococcus*, *Streptococcus*, and *Pasteurella* species is recommended. In penicillin-allergic children, clindamycin and trimethoprim-sulfamethoxazole are recommended. In adults who are allergic to penicillin a combination of clindamycin and a fluoroquinolone is sufficient. Table 2 provides empiric recommendations. Wounds that are obviously infected may benefit from an initial parenteral or oral dose in the emergency department, although no evidence supports this practice [16].

Systemic infection from dog and cat bites is rare in otherwise healthy individuals, but one organism commonly found in dog and cat oral flora is linked with septicemia. *Capnocytophaga* species are frequently found in animal bites but rarely result in clinical infection, presumably because of slow growth, low virulence, and susceptibility to antibiotics used for prophylaxis. In one review of 103 cases, 94 of which were septicemia, 33% of the infections occurred in asplenic patients, 24% in alcoholics, and 5% in patients with immunosuppression. Forty-one percent of systemic infections, however, occurred in patients who had no predisposing factors [17]. The route to infection was an animal bite in 54% of cases, an animal scratch in 8.5%, and animal exposure alone in 27%. The remaining 10.5% had no

Table 2
Recommendations for empiric antibiotic prophylaxis

Bite source	Cause of infection	Primary treatment[a]	Alternative treatment[a]
Dog	*Pasteurella sp.* *Staphylococcus aureus* *Bacteroides sp.* *Fusobacterium* *Capnocytophaga*	Amoxicillin/clavulanate 875/125 mg po bid or 500/125 mg po tid	Clindamycin 300 mg po qid + FQ (adults) Clindamycin + TMP-SMX (children)
Cat	*Pasteurella sp.* *Staphylococcus aureus*	Amoxicillin/Clavulanate 875/125 mg po bid or 500/125 mg po tid	Cefuroxime axetil 0.5 gm po q12h or doxycycline 100 mg po bid

Abbreviations: FQ, fluoroquinolones (FQ contraindicated in children and pregnant women); TMP-SMX, trimethoprim-sulfamethoxazole (contraindicated during pregnancy).

[a] Duration of all regimens 5–7 days.

Data from Talan DA, Citron DM, Abrahamian FM, et al. Bacteriologic analysis of infected dog and cat bites. N Engl J Med 1999;340:85–92; and Broder KR, Cortese MM, Iskander JK. Preventing tetanus, diphtheria, and pertusis among adolescents: use of tetanus toxoid, reduced diphtheria toxoid and acellular pertussis vaccine. MMWR Morb Mortal Wkly Rep 2006; 55(RR-03):1–34.

identifiable source. Dogs accounted for 91% of cases, whereas cats accounted for 8% of cases [15]. Rarer presentations include septicemia with concurrent meningitis, infective endocarditis, arthritis, and localized eye infection. Recently a case of a mycotic abdominal aneurysm secondary to *Capnocytophaga canimorsus* has been reported. The patient was presumably infected when he allowed his dog to lick a scratch on his forearm [18]. *C canimorsus* is susceptible to the recommended empiric antibiotics.

Management

Management of bite victims includes initial assessment, local wound care, antibiotics described above, and recognition and management of systemic illness. Initial evaluation of all bite victims should be approached as a trauma victim. Local protocols vary for trauma team activation and resuscitation, but appropriate consultants should be notified as necessary. After ensuring initial stabilization and hemostasis, the practitioner should elicit a history of the incident identifying the vaccination status of the animal and victim, and rabies and tetanus prophylaxis should be administered as necessary (Table 3) [19]. The local health department should be notified per department and locality protocol. A history of allergies, current medications, and medical conditions that would preclude proper wound healing, such as diabetes, immunosuppression, peripheral vascular disease, smoking, splenectomy, and alcoholism, should be obtained.

All bites and scratches should be thoroughly washed with soap and water as described by Rondeau and McManus in this issue. Use of a virucidal agent, such as povidone-iodine solution, early after rabid animal bites has

Table 3
Tetanus prophylaxis recommendations

	Clean, minor wound		All other wounds[a]
Tetanus history	Tdap or Td[b]	TIG	Tdap or Td
Unknown or ≤3 immunizations	Yes	No	Yes
Primary 3 series Completed			
Last <5 years ago	No	No	No
Last >5 and <10 years ago	No	No	No
Last >10 years ago	Yes	No	No

Abbreviations: Td, tetanus diptheria; Tdap, tetanus-diptheria-acellular-pertussis; TIG, tetanus immune globulin; TT, tetanus toxoid.

[a] Such as, but not limited to, wounds contaminated with dirt, feces, soil; puncture wounds; avulsions; and wounds resulting from crushing, burns, and frostbite.

[b] Tdap is preferred to Td for adolescents (11–18 years) who have never received Tdap. Td is preferred to TT for adolescents who received Tdap previously or if not available. If TT and TIG are both used, Tetanus Toxoid Adsorbed rather than Tetanus Toxoid for Booster Use Only (fluid vaccine) should be used.

Data from Human rabies prevention—United States, 1999. Recommendations of the Advisory Committee on Immunization Practices (ACIP). MMWR Morb Mortal Wkly Rep 1999;48(RR-1):1–21.

been shown to decrease the risk for rabies infection [20]. A thorough examination under proper lighting conditions should be conducted. Devitalized tissue and debris should be removed from the wound and special care should be taken if wounds are overlying vascular structures, joints, or bone. Radiographs of the injured area may be indicated to detect foreign bodies, abscess, fracture, and joint involvement. Skull imaging may be necessary for victims who have scalp bites in which the extent of wound involvement is not readily apparent by physical examination [7]. A search for signs of localized and systemic infection should be identified, such as erythema, fluctuance, purulent drainage, lymphangitis, and fever, with the understanding that immunocompromised patients may not exhibit these classic findings.

No specific guidelines exist recommending the culture of bite wounds; however, it is prudent to culture all clinically infected wounds. Although data are limited, bite wounds are almost always managed by delayed primary or secondary closure. As long as the wound is closed before the proliferative phase of healing the results are indistinguishable from those of primary healing [21]. Specifics of closure techniques are provided by Lloyd and Marque in this issue.

Human bites

Human bites are the third most common type of mammalian bite in the United States, accounting for 3.6% to 23% of bite wounds, but perhaps the most potentially disastrous because of the abundant pathogenic oral flora found in humans [3]. It is estimated that 10% to 17.7% of all bite wounds become infected with a higher rate found among clenched-fist injuries, also known as fight bites. In addition to the risk for infection associated with human bite injuries, human bites pose a potential for the transmission of systemic infections. Studies have found that the incidence of human bites is more common among males with the peak incidence from 10 to 34 years of age [22]. Approximately 60% of reported bites occur in the upper extremity, whereas 15% occur in the head and neck region, commonly on the ears, nose, or lips [3].

Human bite wounds occur from one of two mechanisms: occlusion and clenched fist. Occlusional bites occur when the teeth are sunk into the skin, as occurs with a dog or cat bite. Clenched-fist injuries occur when a closed fist impacts another individual's teeth leaving an injury over the dorsal aspect of the third, fourth, or fifth metacarpophalangeal (MCP) joints, most classically over the third MCP. Occlusional injuries can result from aggressive play among children in day care, accidents during sporting events, rough sexual play, child abuse, domestic violence, or seizure-related activity. Occlusional bites can occur anywhere on the body but when they occur on the hand they must be viewed similar to clenched-fist injuries because of their risk for infection. In a study of 434 human bites and 803 lacerations in individuals institutionalized because of developmental disabilities, 17.7% of bite wounds became infected versus 13.4% of lacerations. Bites occurring anywhere on the hand were twice as likely to become infected, however [23]. The area over the MCP joints is more prone to injury because of the relative lack of soft tissue covering the ligaments, joints, and bone.

The human oral flora is extremely diverse. In a recent study of infected human bite wounds conducted by Talan and Abrahamian [24] as part of the Emergency Medicine Human Bite Infection Study Group, a 12-center collaborative effort that studied 50 patients who had infected human bites, the median number of isolates per wound was four (three aerobes and one anaerobe). Aerobic species were isolated alone in 44% of wounds, anaerobes alone were isolated in 2%, and both aerobes and anaerobes were isolated in 54% of wounds. The most common aerobic isolates were *Streptococcus*, *Staphylococcus*, and *Eikenella* species. The most common anaerobic pathogens were *Prevotella* and *Fusobacterium* species (Table 4).

Management

History should elicit the mechanism of injury, timing, and risk factors for systemic disease transmission. Patients who have a fight bite may hesitate to

Table 4
Common pathogenic bacteria isolated from infected human bite wounds in 50 patients

	% of wounds with organism
Aerobes	
Streptococcus sp	84
S anginosus	52
Staphylococcus sp	54
Staphylococcus aureus	30
Staphylococcus epidermidis	22
Eikenella corrodens	30
Enterococcus	6
Neisseria	8
Haemophilus	22
H parainfluenza	12
Corynobacterium	12
Candida	8
Anaerobes	
Fusobacterium	34
Prevotella	36
P melaninogenica	22
P intermedia	14
Veillonella	24
Eubacterium	16
Peptostreptococcus	22
Campylobacter	16
Eubacterium	16
Actinomyces	8

Data from Talan DA, Abrahamian FM. Clinical presentation and bacteriologic analysis of infected human bites in patients presenting to emergency departments. Clin Infect Dis 2003;37:1481–9.

reveal the actual mechanism for fear of legal repercussions. Any wound occurring over the MCP joints should alert the physician for this type of mechanism. Wounds over joints or vascular structures should be examined throughout the complete range of motion to identify retracted injuries. All bite marks in a young child should raise suspicion of abuse. The normal distance between the maxillary canine teeth in adults is 2.5 to 4.0 cm. Any human bite marks with an intercanine distance greater than 3.0 cm were likely inflicted by an adult. Suspicious wounds should be photographed next to a ruler, a thorough skin examination should be done, and appropriate consultations should be made [25]. A thorough neurovascular examination should be documented, including two-point discrimination. Physical examination of bite wounds should be done with appropriate lighting after the wound has been copiously irrigated.

Radiographs are recommended to exclude foreign bodies or abscesses and to identify fractures and assess joint spaces. Because of the increased risk for infection for hand wounds, consultation with a hand surgeon should be made for all but superficial hand wounds for possible admission and exploration. Antibiotic prophylaxis is warranted if the wound is believed to be at higher risk for infection (eg, significant contamination; involvement of bone, tendon, or joint space; bites on the hand; puncture wounds; or bites occurring in high-risk patients) [26]. Antibiotics should cover *Streptococcus* species, *Staphylococcus* species, and *Eikenella*, and provide broad anaerobic coverage. Because of the increasing number of β-lactam–producing species, amoxicillin/clavulanate is recommended for 5 days. In penicillin-allergic patients, clindamycin plus either ciprofloxacin or trimethoprim-sulfamethoxazole is appropriate. Borrom discusses appropriate antimicrobials in detail in this issue. The decision to close the wound primarily is multifactorial. As a rule, human bite wounds are at increased risk for infection and may be closed by delayed primary or secondary closure without worsened cosmetic outcome [20]. Lloyd and Marque discuss the closure techniques in detail in this issue. The patient should be re-examined in 48 to 72 hours in the emergency department or by the primary care provider.

In all cases involving bite wounds, patients should be counseled that they may have retained foreign bodies, even if not identified radiographically or by physical examination. Additionally, patients should be told that they will have a scar and that they should use adequate sun block and limit sun exposure to the affected area for 1 year.

Plantar puncture injury

Plantar puncture wounds are a common injury encountered by emergency medicine practitioners. Few trials exist and most studies have small sample sizes, which gives rise to controversy in management. The typical mechanism involves stepping on a nail, glass, or other sharp object. The incidence of plantar puncture wounds among pediatric patients has been estimated at 0.82% of pediatric emergency department visits with 7% of lower extremity trauma presentations involving a puncture wound of the foot [27]. Infection rates are estimated from 2.2% to 10.8% and complications include retained foreign body, cellulitis, abscess, osteomyelitis, and septic arthritis [28–30]. Proper emergency department management includes wound care, identification of foreign body, and preventing complications.

A focused history should include time of injury, footwear worn during injury, source of puncture, tetanus status, and underlying medical conditions that would preclude adequate healing. Wounds with delayed presentation are more prone to infection and complications. A study by Schwab [30] involving 63 patients identified a higher complication rate associated with presence of symptoms 48 hours postinjury. The wearing of tennis shoes at the time of injury predisposes to infection with *Pseudomonas aeruginosa* [26,27,31]. The peripheral neuropathy associated with diabetes mellitus and peripheral vascular disease also predispose to infection.

Physical examination of plantar puncture wounds should include assessing for signs of infection and the neurovascular status of the distal extremity. The location of the puncture may have an impact on risk for complications. In a study involving 70 patients (36 inpatients and 34 outpatients) an injury to the forefoot, defined as the area overlying the metatarsal necks extending distally, was more commonly associated with complications, including osteomyelitis and pyarthrosis. Of the 36 inpatients, 35 had injury of the forefoot. The authors attribute their finding to the small amount of soft tissue overlying the forefoot and the fact that the metatarsal heads are a primary weight-bearing area of the foot. The midfoot has abundant soft tissue and is not a primary weight-bearing area unless the lateral foot is punctured. Although the hindfoot has the greatest amount of soft tissue, it is a major area of weight-bearing and thus is prone to deep puncture injuries [27].

All wounds should be cleaned appropriately and tetanus status updated as necessary. Puncture wounds are considered contaminated wounds. Devitalized tissue should be removed and the wound should be inspected for foreign bodies. Determining the depth of the wound and bone involvement may prove difficult. No study has shown a benefit to extensive exploration of puncture wounds. After appropriate local or regional anesthesia, gentle probing with a blunt instrument, such as a nasal forceps or hemostat, to determine the depth, presence of a foreign body, and bone, tendon, or joint involvement is appropriate [26]. No evidence exists to indicate when imaging is necessary but it should be considered in all but superficial involvement without signs of infection. Imaging should also be considered in unexplained foot cellulitis or cellulitis unresponsive to antibiotics [32]. Radiographs may identify radiopaque objects, abscess, or gas and air in the soft tissue. Bony changes in osteomyelitis may not be evident for 7 to 12 days [33]. Ultrasound or CT is preferred in identifying radiolucent foreign bodies. The sensitivity in ultrasound of identifying foreign bodies is operator dependent and is complicated by the fascial planes, tendons, and muscles in the foot. If surgical exploration is expected, CT aids in preoperative planning. Blankenship discusses imaging techniques in detail elsewhere in this issue. Local wound culture may be necessary in systemically ill patients or those not responsive to antibiotics.

Antibiotics

No widely recognized guidelines exist indicating when antibiotics are necessary for plantar puncture wounds [34]. A prospective case series by Schwab and Powers [30] treated 63 patients (aged 18 to 59 years) who presented within 24 hours with surface cleansing alone and all patients were kept non–weight-bearing for 24 hours. On follow-up at 48 hours, 1 week, 1 month, and 6 months, only presence of symptoms 48 hours postinjury was associated with risk for complication (five infections and two retained foreign bodies). The authors found no predictive symptoms of complications at initial presentation. Multiple factors are involved in the decision to prescribe antibiotics: time to presentation, footwear, health status of individual, and availability of close follow-up. Fluoroquinolones, such as ciprofloxacin, provide adequate coverage of *P aeruginosa*, which should be considered if tennis shoes were worn at time of injury [26,27,30]. Alternatively, ceftazidime or cefepime are recommended parenterally if admission is indicated [18]. Patients who are systemically ill, are suspected of having osteomyelitis, or require surgical exploration necessitate admission. Analgesia may be necessary in addition to local wound care, antibiotics, and tetanus update. Consultation with the orthopedic or podiatric service is made as necessary. Discharged patients should be counseled of the possibility of retained foreign bodies despite negative imaging and educated about the warning signs of infection. Non–weight-bearing and crutches may be indicated on a case-by-case basis.

High-pressure injection injury

High-pressure injuries are uncommon but have potentially devastating consequences that represent a surgical emergency. Failure to identify what appears to be an innocuous injury may result in significant functional loss and possible amputation. Optimal outcome depends on the practitioner recognizing the injury and arranging definitive care by a specialist.

This type of injury occurs when equipment capable of generating sufficient pressure injects its contents into the human body. Commercial high-pressure guns reach pressures from 2000 to 12,000 psi. A pressure of only 100 psi can break intact skin; a pressure of 5100 psi can breach clothing and intact skin [35,36]. Various products are delivered through high-pressure guns, including water, hydraulic oil, molten metal, paint, thinner, and solvents [37].

In recent reviews the populations at risk are industrial painters, farmers, and autoworkers. The typical patient is a man (99.1% of reported cases) with injury to the nondominant hand of a single wound, most commonly to the index finger [35,38]. Injection injuries have been reported less commonly in the forearm and foot [39]. Injury occurs commonly while attempting to clean the nozzle. Prognosis depends on various factors summarized in Box 1.

The toxicity of the injected material depends on its viscosity and chemical composition. Paint solvents and diesel fuel are highly viscous and spread farther on injection than paint, grease, or oil. Lipid-soluble materials produce greater tissue destruction and a greater inflammatory response. Paint solvents have resulted in amputation rates as high as 80% versus a 20% risk for amputation with grease [40]. Paint, although less viscous, may contain 40 raw materials, including solvent, pigment, and transport vehicles, all of which may directly damage tissue. Oil-based paint may result in a higher amputation rate than latex. No cases of water or air injection have resulted in amputation, although they have been associated with long-term functional deficit [37]. Additionally, injection material may be contaminated with bacteria, which may lead to additional inflammation and secondary infection.

The material injected travels until it meets resistance. The angle of entry, velocity, and resistance determine the spread of injectant. Penetration of the digital tendon sheaths is more likely if injury occurs along joint creases where the tendon sheaths are weakest, whereas proximal spread of material to the wrist is more likely if injury occurs over the thumb and little finger because of the radial and ulnar bursae. Injection velocities greater than 7000 psi are associated with an increased risk for amputation. Injection into the fingers is three times more likely to result in amputation compared with injection into the palm because of the fingers' limited distensibility [37].

Initial emergency department examination may be underwhelming (Figs. 2 and 3). If presentation is immediate the patient may have minimal pain and physical examination findings. Over time the wound may have significant edema, discoloration, pain, and possibly ischemia. The practitioner should elicit the timing of injury, type of material injected, and pressure of equipment used. Physical examination should document the

---

Box 1. Factors determining the severity of a high-pressure injection injury

Viscosity and chemical composition of material
Amount and velocity of injection
Anatomy and distensibility of the injection site
Interval between injury and treatment

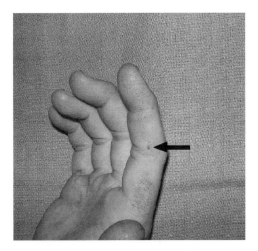

Fig. 2. High-pressure injection injury.

neurovascular status of the extremity with emphasis on recognizing pain out of proportion to findings in the digits and forearm, which may indicate compartment syndrome. Immediate consultation should be made with the hand surgeon in all cases. Radiographs should be obtained to identify proximal spread of material if radiopaque, to identify subcutaneous emphysema,

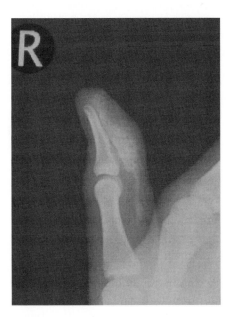

Fig. 3. Radiograph of thumb that has been injected with paint. Note proximal dispersion. (*From* Hogan CJ. High-pressure injection injuries to the upper extremity: a review of the literature. J Orthop Trauma 2006;20:503–11; with permission.)

and for preoperative planning. Broad-spectrum antibiotics should be administered parenterally. Cultures are typically obtained during initial surgical debridement and are likely unobtainable in the emergency department. Standard preoperative laboratory tests should be obtained, tetanus status updated, and analgesia administered as needed. Digital block should not be used for anesthesia as it would increase the pressure within the digit and increase ischemia. Controversy exists as to the indications for steroids. Several case reports report favorable clinical response and animal studies suggest that steroids may be beneficial for injection injuries of organic solvents by reducing inflammation [37]. Any decision to administer steroids should be made in consultation with the hand surgeon.

All patients who have high-pressure injection injuries should be admitted for surgical debridement or discharged from the emergency department with close follow-up only after being examined by the consultant.

Crush injuries

In recent years physicians have seen an increase in the number of crush injuries. Larger population densities coupled with impoverished conditions result in large groups of people living in close proximity in buildings with poor structural integrity. Modern warfare and large-scale natural disasters, such as earthquakes or tsunamis, can be the inciting event. Collapsing structures result in a large number of people being trapped by rubble, and thus we have seen an increase in the number of crush injuries from these events. Crush injury–related renal failure and wound infection are complications that can be treated with the appropriate resources and training.

In recent times there have been several devastating earthquakes that resulted in large numbers of crush injuries. In 1976 a 7.8 Richter scale earthquake in Tangshan, China resulted in 350,300 injuries and 242,769 deaths, with approximately 20% of those deaths coming from crush syndrome [41]. Other recent examples include the earthquake in Bam, Iran in 2005 that resulted in more than 26,000 deaths and 124 crush syndrome cases with 96 of these cases requiring dialysis. These are just a few examples of natural disasters with large-scale mortality and crush syndromes resulting in secondary wound management and dialysis issues [42].

Pathophysiology

Crush syndrome was first described in the literature by Bywaters and Beall [43] in 1941. Their observations came from taking care of soldiers who were crushed during bombing raids in London during the Blitz. It was recognized during this time period that myoglobin deposition in the kidneys was responsible for renal failure. Since that time, numerous observations have been made regarding crush syndrome demonstrating involvement of many organ systems (Box 2).

Box 2. Complications secondary to crush syndrome

Limb injury; maim or amputation
Acute renal failure
Acute respiratory distress
Disseminated intravascular coagulation
Bleeding and hypovolemic shock
Cardiac failure
Arrhythmias
Electrolyte disturbances
Psychologic trauma

Data from Sever MS, Vanholder R, Norbert L. Medical progress: management of crush-related injuries after disasters. N Engl J Med 2006;345:1052–63.

Following the initial insult to muscle provides a framework to understand the various processes occurring during crush syndrome. After a muscle cell is crushed or stretched, potassium and myoglobin are released from the damaged cell. Also, damaged cells absorb water, calcium, and sodium from the extracellular space through leaky sarcolemmas [44].

A large efflux of potassium from these cells can result in hyperkalemia and the secondary cardiotoxicity that results from it. The myoglobin is released from the cells along with urate and phosphate, which precipitates in the distal convoluted tubules and forms casts leading to obstruction. Metabolic acidosis and hypovolemia potentiate this problem in the renal tubules [43]. Acidemia causes myoglobin to form a gel, which leads to decreased urine output and acute renal failure [40]. Oligemia, hyperkalemia, hypocalcemia, and uremia progress to death in 3 to 7 days if untreated.

In addition to the renal disaster there are other medical issues in patients involved in significant crush injuries. There is the risk for infection and subsequent sepsis from the initial crush injury and also from fasciotomy sites. Patients are also susceptible to acute respiratory distress syndrome following such a systemic insult. Additionally, if crush injuries result in bony abnormalities fat embolism syndrome must be considered in the differential diagnosis.

Prehospital care

Prehospital care is paramount in patients involved in significant crush injuries. The rate of complications, such as renal failure and compartment syndrome, is inversely proportional to the elapsed time from injury to prehospital medical care [45]. Additionally, following the Marmara earthquake in Turkey in 1999, it was demonstrated that time under the rubble was positively correlated with the need for amputation [46].

As in other instances, primary management of airway, breathing, and circulatory issues must be addressed before transport. These cases are unique because, as opposed to the relatively short transport time for most intercity EMS transport, many of these patients are managed by prehospital providers for extended periods of time while awaiting extrication. Normal saline should be administered to these patients because of the risk for worsening preexisting hyperkalemia and inability to accurately monitor urine output in these patients. The eventual goal is to maintain urine output at 1 to 2 mL/kg/h. Hemorrhage must be controlled, and some would argue for the early administration of antibiotics in these patients.

Hospital management

These patients arrive with multiple issues that need to be addressed. Specifically, primary trauma can result in issues regarding hemorrhage, pneumothoraces, and unstable fractures that need to be managed concurrently. Some patients require fasciotomies, whereas some have already received such therapy in the prehospital environment.

Fluids

Fluids are a key component to resuscitation in an effort to maintain peripheral organ perfusion and, specifically, preserve renal function. Initially normal saline can be used, but eventually potassium- and glucose-containing solutions are needed. Many suggest alternating between normal saline and a glucose solution in an effort to keep as many electrolytes in balance as possible. Large amounts of fluid can be required, sometimes upwards of 12 L in the first 48 hours [43]. A reasonable goal is to maintain urine output at 200 to 300 mL/h [40]. Central venous pressure (CVP) monitoring is a good way to have continuous data regarding intravascular volume. One can also tailor fluid resuscitation using this monitor. One suggestion is to give continuous small boluses until there is a sustained increase in CVP. For example, one approach might be to continue with boluses until there is a sustained increase of 3 mm Hg in the CVP after 15 minutes [43]. In general, fluid input must take into account losses from third spacing, bleeding, and urine output.

Alkalinization

Alkalinizing the urine of patients undergoing rhabdomyolysis secondary to crush syndrome has been a proven technique for some time. Urinary alkalinization increases the solubility of myoglobin and minimizes the formation of gel that causes tubule obstruction and subsequent oliguria. For comparison, 7.5% of myoglobin is precipitated at a urine pH of 8.5 versus 46% at a pH of 5.0 [40]. There are numerous suggested regimens in the literature to achieve urinary alkalinization. One such model is to add 50 mmol bicarbonate to the initial fluid boluses with a goal of keeping urine pH greater than 6.5 [47].

Mannitol

Although somewhat controversial, many authors suggest that the use of the osmotic diuretic mannitol as an adjunctive therapy in crush injury patients improves outcomes. The suggested dose is 1 to 2 g/kg of 20% solution administered over a 4-hour period. It is believed that this creates a forced diuresis thereby increasing urine output and helping to wash out tubular myoglobin. Mannitol also has the potential benefit of reducing intracompartmental pressures (which could potentially decrease the need for fasciotomies) and protecting the kidneys from oxidative injury by acting as a free radical scavenger [48]. As an intravascular volume expander, it must be monitored closely and should not be given until urine output is established in the patient [47]. Electrolytes, osmolarity, urine output, and CVP must be monitored closely while administering mannitol.

Renal disaster

Despite physicians' best efforts, some patients succumb to renal disaster. Patients who have complete failure of their kidneys will die if dialysis is not available. It is evident from disasters in the last 10 years that an organized approach to crush patients following disasters has saved lives. One of the main ways this has been successful is through the use of mobile dialysis units. This process is labor-intensive, but it is required and should be anticipated in all disasters in which there are crush injury patients. One can expect crush syndrome patients requiring dialysis to continue this therapy for 13 to 18 days [49].

Compartment syndrome

Compartment syndrome results when injured muscle cells increase in size with intracellular fluid uptake while total space remains constant. This swelling results in increases in intracompartmental pressures. As pressure increases, blood flow to the damaged tissue decreases resulting in tissue ischemia and eventual necrosis. It is classically taught that increased pressures resulting in tissue ischemia for more than 6 to 8 hours result in permanent damage.

The treatment for compartment syndrome is fasciotomy. This procedure allows the swelling muscle to expand outside of its compartment, thereby preserving afferent blood flow. Fasciotomy continues to be a controversial subject in the realm of crush syndrome management [50]. Some authors argue that this is a lifesaving intervention that also decreases the risk for complications related to crush syndrome [51]. Other studies have not shown such profound benefits with fasciotomy [52]. The benefits of fasciotomy must be compared with the outcomes related to localized wound infection, sepsis, subsequent amputations, and increased mortality.

Additional treatment modalities

In general, surgical amputation is not a recommended course of action in patients who have crush syndrome and should be considered a last resort in all patients. Sometimes this is the only method available for patient extraction, however. Even consensus statements recommend this only as a last resort because many severely crushed limbs can return to near or full function [53]. There is some evidence that exposing crush injuries to subatmospheric pressures lowers serum myoglobin levels. Further research involving human subjects is needed to quantify when this therapy should be initiated in patients. Additionally, hyperbaric oxygen (HBO) could be an effective adjunctive therapy for crush injury patients. A recent review of nine studies concluded that there might be some beneficial effects to HBO and that further studies are warranted [54].

Infections and wound management

Wound management and infection are concerns for the provider when patients make it out of the acute phase in which concern about renal disaster predominates. These patients who have crushed extremities have varying severity of wounds, but the one common feature is that they are all dirty wounds. Both endogenous and exogenous bacteria are introduced into an open wound site following these types of injuries. This, combined with the loss of the protective skin barrier, makes these patients susceptible to infection, sepsis, and risk for death. Also, a main site of infection risk is the fasciotomy site following a few days of hospitalization.

There is one study that attempted to quantify the type and severity of wound infection in crush syndrome patients. Kazancioglu and colleagues [55] retrospectively reviewed the bacterial characteristics of crush syndrome patients following the Marmara earthquake. This earthquake occurred on August 17, 1999 in northwestern Turkey and caused 17,480 deaths and 43,953 injuries. The conclusion of the study was that infections were still a major factor in crush syndrome–related deaths. Microbial growth was detected in 95% of the patients studied. Nonfermenting Gram-negative bacilli (67%), Gram-positive cocci (17%), Enterobacteriaceae (12%), and yeast-like fungi (4%) were isolated in these samples. *Acinetobacter* (36%) and *P aeruginosa* (21%) were the major bacterial isolates and were found to be resistant to carbapenems but sensitive to quinolone therapy. In total, 9 (22%) patients died of sepsis despite physicians' best efforts. Perhaps one of the most important observations from this article was that after a few days of hospitalization most infections occurred at the site of previous fasciotomies. The use of fasciotomies, especially in the prehospital environment, remains controversial and this study demonstrates the increased infection and mortality complicated by this surgical procedure [55,56].

References

[1] McCaig LF, Nawar EW. National Hospital Ambulatory Medical Care Survey: 2004 emergency department summary. Advance data from vital and health statistics. No. 372. National Center for Health Statistics; 2006.

[2] Merchant RC, Fuerch F. Comparison of the epidemiology of human bites evaluated at three US pediatric emergency departments. Pediatr Emerg Care 2005;21:833–8.

[3] Gilchrist J, Gotsch K, Annest JL, et al. Nonfatal dog bite, related injuries treated in hospital emergency departments, United States 2001. MMWR Morb Mortal Wkly Rep 2003;52: 605–10.

[4] Griegro RD, Rosen T, Orengo IF, et al. Dog, cat, and human bites: a review. J Am Acad Dermatol 1995;33:1019–29.

[5] Lockwood R. Dog-bite–related fatalities—United States, 1995–1996. MMWR Morb Mortal Wkly Rep 1997;46:463–7.

[6] Schalamon J. Analysis of dog bites in children who are younger than 17 years [abstract]. Pediatrics 2006;117:374–9.

[7] Brook I. Microbiology and management of human and animal bite wound infections. Prim Care Clin Office Pract 2003;30:25–39.

[8] Ianelli A. Penetrating brain injuries from a dog bite in an infant [abstract]. Pediatr Neurosurg 2005;41:41–5.

[9] Dire DJ. Emergency management of dog and cat bite wounds. Emerg Med Clin North Am 1992;10:719–36.

[10] Dire DJ. Cat bite wounds: risk factors for infection [abstract]. Ann Emerg Med 1991;20: 973–9.

[11] Talan DA, Citron DM, Abrahamain FM, et al. Bacteriologic analysis of infected dog and cat bites. N Engl J Med 1999;340:85–92.

[12] Presutti RJ. Prevention and treatment of dog bites. Am Fam Physician 2001;63:1567–70.

[13] Broder J, Jerrard D. Low risk of infection in selected human bites treated without antibiotics. Am J Emerg Med 2004;22:10–3.

[14] Turner TWS. Do mammalian bites require antibiotic prophylaxis. Ann Emerg Med 2004;44: 274–6.

[15] Brakenbury PH. A comparative double blind study of amoxicillin/clavulanate vs placebo in the prevention of infection after animal bites [abstract]. Arch Emerg Med 1989;6:251–6.

[16] Gilbert DN. The Sanford guide to antimicrobial therapy. 36th edition. Sperryville (VA): Antimicrobial Therapy, Inc.; 2006.

[17] Lion C. Capnocytophagia canimorsus infections in human: review of the literature and case reports [abstract]. Eur J Epidemiol 1996;12:521–33.

[18] Tierney DM, Straus LP, Sanchez JL. Capnocytophagia canimorsus mycotic abdominal aortic aneurysm: why the mailman is afraid of dogs. J Clin Microbiol 2006;44:649–51.

[19] Broder KR, Cortese MM, Iskander JK. Preventing tetanus, diphtheria, and pertussis among adolescents: use of tetanus toxoid, reduced diphtheria toxoid and acellular pertussis vaccine. MMWR Morb Mortal Wkly Rep 2006;55(RR-03):1–34.

[20] Human rabies prevention—United States, 1999. Recommendations of the Advisory Committee on Immunization Practices (ACIP). MMWR Morb Mortal Wkly Rep 1999; 48(RR-1):1–21.

[21] Lammers RL. Principles of wound management. In: Roberts, editor. Clinical procedures in emergency medicine. 4th edition. Philadelphia: Saunders; 2004. p. 638.

[22] Perron AD, Miller MD. Orthopedic pitfalls in the ED: fight bite. Am J Emerg Med 2002;20: 114–7.

[23] Lindsay D. Natural course of the human bite wound: incidence of infection and complications in 434 bites and 803 lacerations in the same group of patients. J Trauma 1987;27: 45–8.

[24] Talan DA, Abrahamian FM. Clinical presentation and bacteriologic analysis of infected human bites in patients presenting to emergency departments. Clin Infect Dis 2003;37:1481–9.

[25] Kos LK, Shwayder T. Cutaneous manifestations of child abuse. Pediatr Dermatol 2006;23: 311–20.

[26] American College of Emergency Physicians. Clinical policy for the initial approach to patients presenting with penetrating extremity trauma. Ann Emerg Med 1999;33:612–36.

[27] Chudnofsky CR. Special wounds: nail bed, plantar puncture, and cartilage. Emerg Med Clin North Am 1992;10:801–22.

[28] Patzakis MJ. Wound site as a predictor of complications following deep nail punctures to the foot. West J Med 1989;150:545–7.

[29] Weber EJ. Plantar puncture wounds: a survey to determine the incidence of infection [abstract]. J Accid Emerg Med 1996;13:274–7.

[30] Schwab RA, Powers RD. Conservative therapy of plantar puncture wounds [abstract]. J Emerg Med 1995;13:291–5.

[31] Fisher MC. Sneakers as a source of Pseudomonas aeruginosa in children with osteomyelitis following puncture wounds. J Pediatr 1985;106:607–9.

[32] Wartella J. The foot. In: Schwartz DT, editor. Emergency radiology. New York: McGraw-Hill, Health Professions Division; 2000. p. 154.

[33] Schwartz DT. Fundamentals of skeletal radiology. In: Schwartz DT, editor. Emergency radiology. New York: McGraw-Hill, Health Professions Division; 2000. p. 22.

[34] Harrison M. Antibiotics after puncture wounds to the foot. Best evidence topic report. Emerg Med J 2002;19:49.

[35] Neal NC, Burke FD. High-pressure injection injuries. Injury 1991;22:467–70.

[36] Hart RG, Gillian DS. Prevention of high-pressure injection injuries to the hand. Am J Emerg Med 2006;24:73–6.

[37] Burke F, Brady O. Veterinary and industrial high pressure injection injuries: need swift diagnosis and decompression. BMJ 1996;312:1436.

[38] Hogan CJ. High-pressure injection injuries to the upper extremity: a review of the literature. J Orthop Trauma 2006;20:503–11.

[39] Shea MP. High pressure water injection injuries of the foot: a report of two cases [abstract]. Foot Ankle 1993;14:104–6.

[40] Smith GD. High pressure injection injuries. Trauma 2005;7:95–103.

[41] Gonzalez D. Crush syndrome. Crit Care Med 2005;33(1):S34–41.

[42] Sever MS, Vanholder R, Norbert L. Medical progress: management of crush-related injuries after disasters. N Engl J Med 2006;354(10):1052–63.

[43] Bywaters EGL, Beall D. Crush injuries and renal function. Br Med J 1941;1:427–32.

[44] Smith J, Greaves I. Crush injury and crush syndrome: a review. J Trauma 2003;54: S226–30.

[45] Nagi TM, Kambiz K, Shahriar JM, et al. Musculoskeletal injuries associated with earthquake. A report of injuries of Iran's December 26, 2003 Ban earthquake casualties managed in tertiary referral centers. Injury 2005;26:27–32.

[46] Sever MS, Erek E, Vanholder R, et al. Lessons learned from the Marmara disaster: time period under the rubble. Crit Care Med 2002;30(11):2443–9.

[47] Better OS. Rescue and salvage of casualties suffering from the crush syndrome after mass disasters. Mil Med 1999;164:366–9.

[48] Malinoski DJ, Slater MS, Mullins RJ. Crush injury and rhabdomyolysis. Crit Care Clin 2004;20:171–92.

[49] Sever MS, Ereik E, Vanholder R, et al. Renal replacement therapies in the aftermath of the catastrophic Marmara earthquake. Kidney Int 2002;62:2264–71.

[50] Lin YM, Lee TS. Fasciotomy in crush syndrome patients: debates continue. Emerg Med J 2005;22:78.

[51] Duman H, Kulahci Y, Sengezer M. Fasciotomy in crush injury resulting from prolonged pressure in an earthquake in Turkey. Emerg Med J 2003;20:251–2.

[52] Demirkiran O, Dikmen Y, Utku T, et al. Crush syndrome patients after the Marmara earthquake. Emerg Med J 2003;20:247–50.

[53] Greaves I, Porter KM. Consensus statement on crush injury and crush syndrome. Accid Emerg Nurs 2004;12:47–52.

[54] Garcia-Covarrubias L, McSwain NE, Van Meter K, et al. Adjuvant hyperbaric oxygen ther-
     apy in the management of crush injury and traumatic ischemia: an evidence-based approach.
     Am Surg 2005;71(2):144–51.
[55] Kazancioglu R, Cagatay A, Calangu S, et al. The characteristics of infections in crush syn-
     drome. Clin Microbiol Infect 2002;8:202–6.
[56] Anaya DA, McMahon K, Nathens AB, et al. Predictors of mortality and limb loss in necro-
     tizing soft tissue infections. Arch Surg 2005;140:151–7.

ELSEVIER
SAUNDERS

Emerg Med Clin N Am
25 (2007) 123–134

EMERGENCY
MEDICINE
CLINICS OF
NORTH AMERICA

Emergency Management of Difficult Wounds: Part II

MAJ Bradley N. Younggren, MD, FACEP*,
MAJ Mark Denny, MD, FACEP

*Department of Emergency Medicine, Madigan Army Medical Center, Building 9040,
Fitzsimmons Drive, Tacoma, WA 98431, USA*

Necrotizing fasciitis

Necrotizing fasciitis (NF) is a significant and growing concern among clinicians because of its rapid progression and lethality. Wound management in this instance can mean the difference between life and death, and a delay in care can be detrimental. This puts enormous pressure on emergency physicians not only to be attuned to suspecting the diagnosis but also to understanding the proper emergency department (ED) management.

Even with increased knowledge in the diagnosis and management of this disease process, mortality still is between 24% and 34% percent [1]. Additionally, NF creates a large burden in hospital manpower and resources. It is readily apparent that the costs of treating patients who have NF are high. The economic burden is disproportionate to other types of medical care [2]. As such, emergency physicians must be facile at the diagnosis and management of this dangerous disease.

Predisposing factors

It is fairly difficult to find a specific subset of patients that is predisposed to NF. One study looking specifically at group B streptococcus, NF, and toxic shock syndrome found extremes of age and underlying medical conditions, especially diabetes mellitus, to be significant predisposing factors for this illness [3]. Other studies have found many other comorbid conditions to be predisposing factors. Immunosupression, chronic disease, chronic steroid use, age greater than 60 years old, intravenous drug use, peripheral vascular disease, renal failure, malignancy, and obesity are comorbid

* Corresponding author.
E-mail address: bradley.n.younggren@us.army.mil (M.B.N. Younggren).

conditions that can predispose someone to NF [4,5]. Potential predisposing factors or injuries that could increase the risk for NF do exist. The literature suggests that trauma, soft-tissue infections, surgery, intravenous drug use, childbirth, burns, and muscle injuries all are reported etiologic factors believed to contribute to the development of NF [6].

Clinical features

There are some features that can help guide emergency physicians toward the diagnosis of NF, but nothing is pathognomonic for NF. The superficial skin layers can appear normal until later in the disease, which makes it a more difficult diagnosis to make. Classically it was believed that patients present with fever, diaphoresis, and tachycardia. One case series supported the finding of tachycardia while discovering many patients who presented afebrile to an ED [6].

Pain is a critical part of the history and examination in patients who have NF. Pain may appear out of proportion to a physician's examination. Pain may be present in areas where there is no obvious evidence of infection. Alternatively, the site of infection may appear painless or of decreased sensation.

The skin can appear erythematous, perhaps tense with discolored wound drainage. Patients can have a variety of skin manifestations that include draining infections, ulcers, frank necrosis, and subcutaneous air.

Diagnosis

Laboratory studies

In general it is believed that laboratory studies are not helpful at differentiating between NF and other types of soft-tissue infections. Leukocytosis, anemia, hypocalcaemia, hyponatremia, and hypoprotenemia all may be seen, but there is limited sensitivity and specificity of these findings [7]. Hypoalbumenia, acidosis, hyperglycemia, elevated creatinine, and elevated blood urea nitrogen also are seen in NF [6]. Yet others have found hyperkalemia and elevated alanine aminotransferse levels in addition to the laboratory studies discussed previously [8]. There is evidence that patients who have prolonged prothrombin times have an increased mortality. A case series of black tar heroin-associated NF demonstrated most patients to have a leukocytosis and elevated lactate level [6].

Some believe that admission white blood cell counts of greater than 15,400 cells/mL or a serum sodium less than 135 mmol/L are the two best laboratory studies to help identify cases of NF [9]. In short, there are many laboratory abnormalities that potentially can suggest NF; nothing, however, is sensitive or specific enough to really help identify this dangerous disease.

Diagnostic imaging

Typically, plane radiographs are ordered for initial evaluation of an infected extremity or region. The common belief is that this helps identify signs of severe infection, such as subcutaneous air or periosteal elevation. Although part of a complete evaluation, there is no evidence to suggest a lack of radiographic findings should preclude an emergency physician from pursuing the diagnosis of NF further. CT is an effective imaging modality to help identify the extent of disease progression. Asymmetric fascial thickening and the presence of small amounts of gas can be identified on CT scan [10]. This is used more and more to help surgeons identify the extent of NF and how far surgical débridement might have to occur.

In addition to plane film and CT technology, ultrasound is becoming more and more useful in EDs for a variety of conditions. The speed at which an emergency physician can arrive at a potential diagnosis makes this an increasingly popular modality. Early findings related to NF include thickened, distorted fascia. Swelling of the subcutaneous tissues and muscle or early evidence of frank muscle necrosis also may be found [11]. In one retrospective case series, ultrasound did miss some evidence of subcutaneous inflammation. In this series, however, ultrasound demonstrated changes in the subcutaneous fat (28 of 32 patients), investing fascia (18 of 32 patients), and muscle (15 of 32 patients) [12]. This early study suggests that future work must be done to determine if ultrasound is an effective modality at identifying NF in a short period of time.

Microbiology

In general, most of these infections are polymicrobial in nature with potential bacterial synergy and, thus, require broad-spectrum antibiotic therapy [13]. Species of *Staphylococcus*, *Streptococcus* (group A and otherwise), *Clostridium*, *Pseudomonas*, *Klebsiella*, *Serratia*, *Peptococus*, and *Bacteroides* are some examples of microbes implicated in NF [14].

Management

In a general sense, the most important point regarding treatment of NF is early recognition and aggressive management coupled with early consultation. This is truly a surgical emergency where time is a critical factor in determining patients' morbidity and mortality. There are several predictors that have been identified that foretell mortality and limb loss. This is helpful for emergency physicians to identify a subset of patients who likely will have a worse outcome. In particular, independent predictors of mortality are a white blood cell count greater than $30,000 \times 10^3/\mu L$, creatinine greater than 2 mg/kL, and heart disease at hospital admission. Also, infection with clostridium is an independent predictor of limb loss and mortality [15].

Resuscitation

On recognition of NF, an aggressive medical resuscitation must begin in an ED. Redundant, secure intravenous access must be obtained. Based on new guidelines regarding the management of sepsis in the ED, aggressive early fluid resuscitation and antibiotic therapy must be initiated. As such, consider early placement of a central venous pressure monitor to monitor fluid resuscitation continuously. A Foley catheter should be placed to monitor urine output appropriately. Early fluid resuscitation also is critical because these patients have immense third spacing and insensible losses that only are magnified by the surgical débridement process.

Antibiotics

There are many antibiotic regimens recommended for adjuvant therapy of NF. As discussed previously, this tends to be a polymicrobial infection; therefore, start with broad-spectrum coverage in these patients. Usually double or triple antibiotic therapy is necessary until Gram's stain and culture results can help focus therapy [15]. A reasonable first-line regimen might be ampicillin-sulbactam, gentamicin, and clindamycin [16].

Penicillin continues to be effective for gram-positive coverage. If there is concern for group A streptococcal involvement, the addition of clindamycin is helpful for inhibiting M protein and exotoxin production and providing anaerobic coverage [17]. Additionally, metronidazole can be used for anaerobic coverage in NF. Gram-negative anaerobes are covered by ampicillin or gentamicin. For broader coverage to include pseudomonas, imipenem or miropenem can be considered. Finally, vancomycin can be used if there is a propensity for methicillin-resistant *Staphylococcus aureus* (MRSA) [14].

Surgical débridement

The mainstay of therapy for NF is surgical débridement and all other treatments are adjuncts to this definitive treatment. Early recognition of the need for aggressive surgical debridement is the key to decreasing the morbidity and mortality associated with this disease process. Typically, surgical technique describes persistent débridement until viable tissue is reached. The majority of these patients require re-exploration and eventual skin grafting once the infection has been treated appropriately.

Hyperbaric oxygen

The use of hyperbaric oxygen therapy (HBO) for the treatment of NF is another modality to consider when managing these patients. This treatment first was introduced after Brummelkamp's [18] 1961 research demonstrating that hyperbaric oxygen inhibited anaerobic infection growth. The overlying theory is that increased oxygen can be delivered to infected, ischemic tissue, thereby increasing its viability (tissue preservation) and ability to fight infection. The evidence is mixed, however, and the topic remains controversial. Some trials have found trends toward increased survival and decreased trips to the operating room for débridement [19]. Alternatively, other studies have demonstrated no benefit to HBO in the treatment of these patients [20].

From a physiologic standpoint, the use of HBO makes sense in the treatment of NF. The evidence, however, is inconsistent and seems to have little downside but requires additional randomized clinical trials for further clarification [21].

Intravenous immunoglobulin

Intravenous immunoglobulin (IVIG) is a potential adjunctive therapy to those described previously. Currently, there are not any quality studies to promote or refute the use of IVIG in NF. In theory, streptococcal exotoxin behaves like a superantigen. Superantigens quickly can result in a large production of inflammatory cytokines. IVIG is shown to inhibit superantigen elicited T-cell activation. Thus, there perhaps is a role for IVIG in the treatment of patients who have suspected or confirmed streptococcal-induced NF. The current recommended dose is 1000 mg per kg with up to repeat doses of 500 mg per kg on days 2 and 3 if the patient remains on pressor agents [22].

Summary

NF is a disease much feared by patients and physicians. With the media hype regarding "flesh-eating bacteria," this fear has been only magnified. NF can present in a variety of clinical presentations, with a variety of physical examination and laboratory findings. It is imperative for emergency physicians to have a low index of suspicion for NF and initiate early treatment of and surgical consultation for these patients.

Methicillin-resistant *Staphylococcus aureus*

Part of the decision about wound management involves determining the need for prophylactic antibiotics. Several specific situations involve specific antibiotics that cover organisms unique to a situation. An example of this is antipseudomonal coverage for the through-the-shoe plantar puncture wound. One such unique situation, which may have an impact on wound management in the near future, is the evolution of community-associated MRSA (CA-MRSA). The effect of CA-MRSA on wound management has not been studied extensively and should be an area of future research. Moran and colleagues [23] report the prevalence of MRSA among ED patients presenting with acute, purulent skin and soft-tissue infections, including abscess (81%), infected wounds (11%), and cellulitis with purulent exudates (8%). MRSA was isolated from 53% of the infected wounds and 98% of the MRSA isolates genetically were CA-MRSA. This data indicate that CA-MRSA is a real player in wounds that become infected, so this organism and how ED physicians should combat it are reviewed briefly.

Background

The first case of MRSA presenting in the community occurred in the 1980s. This phenomenon was believed to be a temporary transmission of nosocomial strains into the community and occurred in people who had certain risk factors, such as hospitalization, surgery, dialysis, or residence in a long-term care facility within 1 year; presence of invasive medical devices (tracheostomy tube, gastrostomy tube, or Foley catheter); isolation of MRSA 2 or more days after hospitalization; or previous isolation of MRSA [24]. CA-MRSA, however, has microbiologic characteristics that make it genetically and phenotypically different from hospital-associated MRSA (HA-MRSA), although this distinction is not clean and continues to evolve [25]. The definition of CA-MRSA seems to be in flux. Initially, anyone who developed a MRSA infection without the risk factors (discussed previously) and within 48 to 72 hours of hospital admission was considered to have CA-MRSA. Now that there is an understanding that CA-MRSA is unique genetically, many have come to call an organism CA-MRSA based not on the risk factors but on the genetics. So, paradoxically, CA-MRSA is emerging as a significant cause of nosocomial infection, and, in one study, more than one third of MRSA bacteremia was caused by a genetically identified community strain [26].

Methicillin resistance is conferred by a penicillin-binding protein 2a, which is encoded in a mecA gene within a mobile genetic element called a staphylococcal chromosomal cassette mec (SCCmec). CA-MRSA seems to be mostly SCCmec type IV, whereas HA-MRSA are types I, II, and III. SCCmec type IV (CA-MRSA) strains are more susceptible to other antibiotics, giving physicians more antibiotic choices than available previously for HA-MRSA. Unfortunately, the CA-MRSA strains tend to be more virulent, in part because they frequently are found to carry a gene for Panton-Valentin leukocidin, a toxin that damages cell membranes by creating lytic pores and may play a role in invasive CA-MRSA [27–29].

The past decade has seen the emergence of CA-MRSA, and several articles during this period describe outbreaks in certain populations, including children, day-care attendees, prisoners, intravenous drug users, athletes, military trainees, Native Americans, and men who have sex with men [30–46]. Moreover, it may be that in certain communities, MRSA is the "normal" pathogen in soft-tissue and skin infections. In fact, 51% of positive cultures were MRSA in one ED-based study, with CA-MRSA accounting for 76% to 99% of these [47], and 59% of cultures were MRSA (98% CA-MRSA) in another ED study involving 11 geographically separated areas [23]. Arguably, these data make CA-MRSA the most common cause of purulent (ie, cultureable) skin and soft-tissue infections in ED patients. The incidence in simple cellulitis is unknown, because purulence is not available for culture in this disease process.

Emergency physicians must recognize the importance of this new infectious threat, but at this time there are no data to support a change in basic laceration management or prophylactic antibiotic use. Wound preparation with foreign body removal, débridement when needed, irrigation, and appropriate patient selection are the best methods for preventing wound infection. One of the first decision points regarding treatment of lacerations is the decision to primarily close the wound. Delayed primary closure (DPC) is a seldom-used technique in emergency medicine but is reasonable in heavily contaminated wounds and certain high-risk populations (immuno-compromised, elderly, diabetic, and so forth). Again, there are no data regarding DPC in the prevention of wound infections caused by CA-MRSA, and at this time, the authors recommend the decision for DPC be made independent of this organism's prevalence in a community. As the pathogens that cause soft-tissue and skin infections evolve and antibiotic resistance patterns change, wound management decisions may need to be readdressed.

For patients presenting to an ED with an infected wound, cultures should be taken in every case to isolate the organism and treat according to suscep-tibilities. This is true even if CA-MRSA already has been established as the primary organism responsible for these infections in the community. This is important to monitor for resistance pattern changes in this virulent organ-ism. The choice of empiric antibiotics for infected wounds is discussed briefly in the next section; however, the authors want to emphasize the im-portance of adequate drainage. Abscesses must be incised and drained with loculations broken up and packing placed. Sutures should be removed from infected wounds and a search for retained foreign body completed. In most cases, antibiotics probably are not necessary if the drainage is done well and foreign bodies removed. In the authors' experience, failure of appropriate incision and drainage (I&D) often is the result of poor pain management or patient cooperation during the procedure; they strongly recommend se-dation in the ED or consultation with a surgeon for operative intervention in cases where patient pain and cooperation limit adequate I&D.

Antimicrobial therapy

For some patients, empiric antimicrobial therapy may be used in addition to I&D. Factors that may influence the decision to use antibiotics include signs and symptoms of systemic spread, associated comorbidities or immu-nosuppression, extremes of age, wound location, return visit or lack of response to I&D alone, and the severity and rapidity of progression or the presence of associated cellulitis [25].

The choice of empiric antibiotics for infected wounds is not straightfor-ward. Before CA-MRSA, a β-lactam antibiotic, such as cephalexin, was first choice and provided adequate coverage. This still is a reasonable option for first-line therapy for patients who have mild illness and no significant comorbidities, especially if the local prevalence of CA-MRSA is low. Some experts suggest that a prevalence greater than 10% to 15% warrants a change in empiric therapy, although there are no data to support this rec-ommendation [25,48]. Unfortunately, the mecA gene confers resistance to β-lactam antibiotics, such as cephalexin. In communities where CA-MRSA is found to be the primary organism, a β-lactam may be inadequate. Vanco-mycin is the drug of choice for serious infections caused by HA-MRSA or CA-MRSA and those patients deemed ill enough to need hospital admission. Options for outpatient treatment of CA-MRSA include trimethoprim-sulfa-methoxazole (TMP-SMX), clindamycin, doxycycline, linezolid, and rifam-pin, but there are problems with each of these antimicrobials.

Although not approved by the Food and Drug Administration (FDA) for the treatment of staphylococcal infection, TMP-SMX has been shown to be active against staphylococcal and, specifically, MRSA infections [23,47,49,50]. Furthermore, most CA-MRSA isolates are susceptible to this drug. The problem with TMP-SMX is lack of efficacy in treating group A streptococcus (GAS), which is another common cause of soft-tissue and skin infections. So, depending on the prevalence of local isolates, empiric therapy may involve using a β-lactam agent or clindamycin to cover GAS, plus TMP-SMX for CA-MRSA. Once the isolate and susceptibilities are obtained from culture, the antibiotic should be tailored, which addresses the importance of follow-up within 48 to 72 hours for these patients.

Clindamycin is FDA approved for staphylococcal infections and another possibility that would cover CA-MRSA and GAS. Isolates from recent ED studies demonstrate 94% to 98% susceptibility [23,47,50]. The issue with clindamycin is that some CA-MRSA isolates have an inducible resistance. The Centers for Disease Control and Prevention and the National Commit-tee for Clinical Laboratory Standards recommend that if clindamycin is used empirically, laboratories should complete D-zone testing to identify inducible clindamycin resistance in MRSA isolates.

Doxycycline also is used in the treatment of MRSA with good suscepti-bilities in ED patients (82%–92%) and clinical cure rates (83%), but the data are not sufficient to support use in the treatment of invasive infections [23,47,50,51]. Susceptibility to doxycycline is tested in commercially avail-able kits using tetracycline (similar to methacillin resistance tested as a lack of oxacillin susceptibility in these kits).

Linezolid is a bacteriostatic antistaphylococcal agent with excellent tissue distribution, which can be given orally or parenterally. It is shown to have equivalent or better cure rates then vancomycin [52–54]. This drug should be reserved for serious infections caused by MRSA and consultation with an infectious disease specialist is recommended before initiation of this costly medication.

Rifampin should not be used as a single agent because resistance develops rapidly [55]. Use with other antimicrobials that are active against MRSA may help eradicate MRSA carriage [56]. At this time, however, there are no data to support the routine treatment to eradicate colonization from an ED.

Unfortunately, no simple algorithm exists for the choice of empiric anti-biotics in the new era of CA-MRSA. It is important to check susceptibilities of the isolate and have awareness of the local susceptibility patterns. Local public health departments and hospital antibiograms are sources of this information. In areas of high prevalence, initial therapy should consist of TMP-SMX or clindamycin. The addition of a β-lactam, such as cephalexin, is reasonable depending on the incidence of GAS in the local community. Follow-up within 48 to 72 hours is key to check susceptibilities and tailor antibiotics.

Special considerations

Patients who are diabetic, are morbidly obese, have renal failure, are at the extremes of age, or have altered immune response (chemotherapeutics, HIV, congenital deficiencies, and so forth) are at higher risk for developing wound infections. The type of wound, mechanism of injury, level of contamination, anatomic area, and time of injury are important details to obtain during evaluations of patients who have wounds; however, emergency physicians must take individual characteristics into account and realize that the same wound might be managed differently in at-risk individuals.

Although an in-depth discussion of the pathogenesis of this increased risk of infection is beyond the scope of this article, some of the multifactorial reasons for the predisposition to infection that elderly patients display are outlined briefly. Common living environments, such as long-term care facilities, foster the transmission of infections. Functional impairment, such as incontinence and immobility, also increase the risk of cellulitis and predispose to skin breakdown and sores, creating openings for organisms. The malnutrition prevalent in the elderly also limits the immune response and worsens wound healing. The elderly have decreased physiologic reserves, such as impaired arterial and venous circulation, which also compromise wound healing. Moreover, the integument differs in that there is a much thinner epidermis with loss of subcutaneous fat and elastin fibers and a more permeable dermis [57]. Finally, many elderly have comorbid illnesses (cancer, diabetes, emphysema, and so forth), are on medications that have immunosuppressive effects, or have indwelling devices that compromise host defenses. The incidence of wound infection in hospitalized elderly patients over 85 years of age is 2 times that of persons 18 to 24 years of age [58].

One technique to help avoid the development of wound infections in these special patient populations is DPC. Although emergency physicians use this technique in heavily contaminated wounds, old wounds, and many bite wounds, many fail to consider the use of DPC in at-risk groups. Although the authors could not find any randomized, controlled trials comparing this technique to standard wound management in these populations, they recommend emergency physicians consider DPC in these high-risk patients. Using prophylactic antibiotics in these patients also is not well studied. The authors' opinion is that if one is considering the use of prophylactic antibiotics because a patient is in a high-risk group, then DPC should be considered strongly before the use of antibiotics.

Summary

Difficult wounds constitute a significant amount of the morbidity and mortality emergency physicians face on a daily basis. There are specific traumatic and atraumatic wounds that are difficult to manage and have a high risk of complications. Emergency physicians must be able to identify these high-risk wounds and patients and take steps to mitigate further morbidity and mortality.

References

[1] Anaya DA, McMahon K, Nathens AB, et al. Predictors of mortality and limb loss in necrotizing soft tissue infections. Arch Surg 2005;140:151–7.

[2] Widjaja AB, Tran A, Cleland H, et al. The hospital costs of treating necrotizing fasciitis. ANZ J Surg 2005;75(12):1059–64.

[3] Crum NF, Wallace MR. Group B streptococcal necrotizing fasciitis and toxic shock-like syndrome: a case report an review of the literature. Scand J Infect Dis 2003;35:878–81.

[4] Elliot DC, Kufera JA, Meyers RAM. Necrotizing soft tissue infections: risk factors for mortality and strategies for management. Ann Surg 1996;224:672–83.

[5] Hasham S, Matteucci P, Stanley PRW, et al. Necrotising fasciitis. BMJ 2005;330:830–3.

[6] Longernan S, Rodrigues RM, Schaulis M, et al. A case series of patients with black heroin-associated necrotizing fasciitis. J Emerg Med 2004;26(1):47–50.

[7] Schneier JI. Rapid infectious killers. Emerg Med Clin North Am 2004;22:1099–114.

[8] Ogivie Christain M, Miclau T. Necrotizing soft tissue infections of the extremities and back. Clin Orthop Relat Res 2006;447:179–86.

[9] Wall DB, Klein SR, Black S, et al. A simple model to help distinguish necrotizing fasciitis from nonnecrotizing soft tissue infection. J Am Coll Surg 2000;191:227–31.

[10] Wysoki MG, Santora TA, Shah RM, et al. Necrotizing fasciitis. CT characteristics. Radiology 1997;203(2):859–63.

[11] Chau CLF, Griffith JF. Musculoskeletal infections: ultrasound appearances. Clin Radiol 2005;60:149–59.

[12] Parenti GC, Marri C, Calandra G, et al. Necrotizing fasciitis of soft tissues: role of diagnostic imagine and review of the literature. Radiol Med 2000;99:334–9.

[13] Tahaz L, Erdemir F, Kibar Y, et al. Fournier's gangrene: report of thirty-three cases and a review of the literature. Int J Urol 2006;13:960–7.

[14] Kihiczak GG, Schwartz RA, Kapila R. Necrotizing fasciitis: a deadly infection. J Eur Acad Dermatol Venereol 2006;20:365–9.

[15] Elliot D, Kufera JA, Myers RA. The microbiology of necrotizing soft tissue infections. Am J Surg 2000;179:361–6.

[16] Singer AJ, Hollander JE. Lacerations and acute wounds: an evidence based guide. Philadelphia: FA Davis Co.; 2003. p. 197–9.

[17] Stevens DL. Streptococcal toxic shock syndrome: spectrum of disease, pathogenesis, and new concept sin treatment. Emerg Infect Dis 1995;1:69–78.

[18] Brummelkamp WH, Hogendyk J, Boerema I. Treatment of anaerobic infections by drenching the tissue with oxygen under high atmospheric pressure. Surgery 1961;49: 299–302.

[19] Escobar SJ, Slade JB, Hunt TK, et al. Adjuvant hyperbaric oxygen therapy (HBO2) for treatment of necrotizing fasciitis reduced mortality and amputation rate. Undersea Hyperb Med 2005;32(6):37–43.

[20] Mindrup SR, Kealey GP, Fallon B. Hyperbaric oxygen for the treatment of Fournier's Gangrene. J Urol 2005;173:1975–7.

[21] Jallali N, Withey S, Butler PE. Hyperbaric oxygen as an adjuvant therapy in the management of necrotizing fasciitis. Am J Surg 2005;189;462–6.

[22] Darabi IK, Abdel-Wahab O, Dzik W. Current usage of intravenous immune globulin and the rationale behind it: the Massachusetts General Hospital data and a review of the literature. Transfusion 2006;46:741–53.

[23] Moran GJ, Krishnadasan A, Gorwitz RJ, et al. Methicillin-resistant *Staphylococcus aureus* infections among patients in the emergency department. N Engl J Med 2006;355(7):666–74.

[24] Fridkin SK, Hageman JC, Morrison M, et al. Methicillin-resistant *Staphylococcus aureus* in three communities. N Engl J Med 2005;352:1436–44.

[25] Gorwitz RJ, Jernigan DB, Powers JH, et-al, and Participants in the CDC-Convened Experts' Meeting on Management of MRSA in the Community. Strategies for clinical management of MRSA in the community: summary of an Experts' Meeting Convened by the Centers for Disease Control and Prevention 2006. Available at: http://www.cdc.gov/ncidod/dhqp/ar_mrsa_ca.html. Accessed September 9, 2006.

[26] Seybold U, Kourbatova EV, Johnson JG, et al. Emergence of community-associated methicillin-resistant *Staphylococcus aureus* USA300 genotype as a major cause of health care-associated blood stream infections. Clin Infect Dis 2006;42:647–56.

[27] Baba T, Takeuchi F, Kuroda M, et al. Genome and virulence determinants of high virulence community-acquired methicillin-resistant *Staphylococcus aureus*. Lancet 2002;359: 1819–27.

[28] Naimi TS, LeDell KH, Como-Sabetti K, et al. Comparison of community- and health care-associated methicillin-resistant *Staphylococcus aureus* infection. JAMA 2003;290:2976–84.

[29] Kollef MH, Micek ST. Methicillin-resistant *Staphylococcus aureus*: a new community-acquired pathogen? Curr Opin Infect Dis 2006;19(2):161–8.

[30] Herold BC, Immergluck LC, Maranan MC, et al. Community-acquired methicillin-resistant *Staphylococcus aureus* in children with no identified predisposing risk. JAMA 1998;279: 593–8.

[31] Frank AL, Marcinak JF, Mangat PD, et al. Increase in community-acquired methicillin-resistant *Staphylococcus aureus* in children. Clin Infect Dis 1999;29:935–6.

[32] Centers for Disease Control and Prevention. Outbreaks of community-associated methicillin-resistant *Staphylococcus aureus* skin infections—Los Angeles County, California 2002–2003. MMWR Morb Mortal Wkly Rep 2003;52(5):88.

[33] Baggett HC, Hennessy TW, Leman R, et al. An outbreak of community-onset methicillin-resistant *Staphylococcus aureus* skin infections in southwestern Alaska. Infect Control Hosp Epidemiol 2003;24(6):397–402.

[34] Centers for Disease Control and Prevention. Methicillin-resistant *Staphylococcus aureus* skin or soft tissue infections in a state prison—Mississippi 2000. MMWR Morb Mortal Wkly Rep 2001;50(42):919–22.

[35] Centers for Disease Control and Prevention. Methicillin-resistant *Staphylococcus aureus* infections in correctional facilities—Georgia, California, and Texas, 2001–2003. MMWR Morb Mortal Wkly Rep 2003;52(41):992–6.

[36] Wootton SH, Arnold K, Hill HA, et al. Intervention to reduce the incidence of methicillin-resistant *Staphylococcus aureus* skin infections in a correctional facility in Georgia. Infect Control Hosp Epidemiol 2004;25(5):402–7.

[37] Begier EM, Frenette K, Barrett NL, et al. A high-morbidity outbreak of methicillin-resistant *Staphylococcus aureus* among players on a college football team, facilitated by cosmetic body shaving and turf burns. Clin Infect Dis 2004;39(10):1446–53.

[38] Centers for Disease Control and Prevention. Methicillin-resistant *Staphylococcus aureus* infections among competitive sports participants—Colorado, Indiana, Pennsylvania, and Los Angeles County, 2000–2003. MMWR Morb Mortal Wkly Rep 2003;52(33): 793–5.

[39] Kazakova SV, Hageman JC, Matava M, et al. A clone of methicillin-resistant *Staphylococcus aureus* among professional football players. N Engl J Med 2005;352:468–75.

[40] Nguyen DM, Mascola L, Brancoft E. Recurring methicillin-resistant *Staphylococcus aureus* infections in a football team. Emerg Infect Dis 2005;11(4):526–32.

[41] Lindenmayer JM, Schoenfeld S, O'Grady R, et al. Methicillin-resistant *Staphylococcus aureus* in a high school wrestling team and the surrounding community. Arch Intern Med 1998;158(8):895–9.

[42] Zinderman CE, Conner B, Malakooti MA, et al. Community-acquired methicillin-resistant *Staphylococcus aureus* among military recruits. Emerg Infect Dis 2004;10:941–4.

[43] Adcock PM, Pastor P, Medley F, et al. Methicillin-resistant *Staphylococcus aureus* in two child care centers. J Infect Dis 1998;178(2):577–80.

[44] Shahin R, Johnson IL, Jamieson F, et al. Methicillin-resistant *Staphylococcus aureus* carriage in a child care center following a case of disease. Toronto Child Care Center Study Group. Arch Pediatr Adolesc Med 1999;153(8):864–8.

[45] Lee NE, Taylor MM, Bancroft E, et al. Risk factors for community-associated methicillin-resistant *Staphylococcus aureus* skin infections among HIV-positive men who have sex with men. Clin Infect Dis 2005;40(10):1529–34.

[46] Groom AV, Wolsey DH, Naimi TS, et al. Community-acquired methicillin-resistant *Staphylococcus aureus* in a rural American Indian community. JAMA 2001;286(10):1201–5.

[47] Frazee BW, Lynn J, Charlebois ED, et al. High prevalence of methicillin-resistant *Staphylococcus aureus* in emergency department skin and soft tissue infections. Ann Emerg Med 2005; 45(3):311–20.

[48] Martinez-Aguilar G, Hammerman WA, Mason EO, et al. Clindamycin treatment of invasive infections caused by community-acquired, methicillin-resistant and methicillin-susceptible *Staphylococcus aureus* in children. Pediatr Infect Dis J 2003;22(7):593–8.

[49] Markowitz N, Quinn EL, Saravolatz LD. Trimethoprim-sulfamethoxazole compared with vancomycin for the treatment of *Staphylococcus aureus* infection. Ann Intern Med 1992; 117:390–8.

[50] Moran GJ, Amii RN, Abrahamian FM, et al. Methicillin-resistant *Staphylococcus aureus* in community-acquired skin infections. Emerg Infect Dis 2005;11(6):928–30.

[51] Ruhe JJ, Monson T, Bradsher RW, et al. Use of long-acting tetracyclines for methicillin-resistant *Staphylococcus aureus* infections: case series and review of the literature. Clin Infect Dis 2005;40(10):1429–34.

[52] Stevens DL, Herr D, Lampiris H, et al. Linezolid versus vancomycin for the treatment methicillin-resistant *Staphylococcus aureus* infections. Clin Infect Dis 2002;34:1481–90.

[53] Weigelt J, Itani K, Stevens D, et al. Linezolid versus vancomycin in treatment of complicated skin and soft tissue infections. Antimicrob Agents Chemother 2005;49:2260–6.

[54] Sharpe JN, Shively EK, Polk HC Jr. Clinical and economic outcomes or oral linezolid versus intravenous vancomycin in the treatment of MRSA-complicated, lower-extremity skin and soft-tissue infections caused by methicillin-resistant *Staphylococcus aureus*. Am J Surg 2005; 189:425–8.

[55] Strausbaugh LJ, Jacobson C, Sewell DL, et al. Antimicrobial therapy for methicillin-resistant *Staphylococcus aureus* colonization in residents and staff of a Veterans Affairs nursing home care unit. Infect Control Hosp Epidemiol 1992;13(3):151–9.

[56] Yu VL, Goetz A, Wagener M, et al. *Staphylococcus aureus* nasal carriage and infection in patients on hemodialysis. Efficacy of antibiotic prophylaxis. N Engl J Med 1986;315(2):91–6.

[57] Plewa MC. Altered host response and special infections in the elderly. Emerg Med Clin North Am 1990;8(2):193–206.

[58] Haley RW, Hooton TM, Culver DH, et al. Nosocomial infections in U.S. hospitals 1975–1976: estimated frequency by selected characteristics of patients. Am J Med 1981;70:947–59.

ELSEVIER
SAUNDERS

Emerg Med Clin N Am
25 (2007) 135–146

EMERGENCY
MEDICINE
CLINICS OF
NORTH AMERICA

Management of Burn Wounds in the Emergency Department

Rubén Gómez, MD, PhD,
COL Leopoldo C. Cancio, MD*

*US Army Institute of Surgical Research, 3600 Rawley E. Chambers Avenue,
Fort Sam Houston, San Antonio, TX 78234-6315, USA*

In the United States, more than 1 million patients per year sustain burn injuries [1]. Of these, approximately 700,000 seek care in an emergency department, and approximately 45,000 are hospitalized. One half of these admissions are received by the approximately 125 specialized burn centers; the other one half are admitted to other hospitals. Thus, only approximately 4.5% of burn patients actually are hospitalized. The majority of patients who have burns are seen by emergency medicine providers. Accordingly, this article provides guidance for the triage of burn victims and an approach to the treatment of patients who have major burns in the first several hours after injury. There are some general remarks with respect to special injuries, such as electrical and chemical injuries. Finally, outpatient treatment of patients who have minor burns is described.

Pathophysiology of the burn wound

To understand burn wounds better, some basic facts about the skin should be reviewed [2,3]. The skin is a laminar structure. The outer layer or epidermis arises from the stratum germinativum. As cells from this layer migrate upward, they differentiate into keratinocytes that finally desquamate. The dermal layer contains epidermal appendages: hair follicles, sweat glands, and sebaceous glands. Blood vessels, nerve endings, immunocytes, fibroblasts, and elastin and collagen fibers also reside in the dermis. The subcutaneous layer is deep to the dermis. With these anatomic landmarks

The opinions or assertions contained herein are the private views of the authors and are not to be construed as official or as representing the views of the Department of the Army or Department of Defense.

* Corresponding author.
E-mail address: lee.cancio@us.army.mil (C.L.C. Cancio).

as reference points, the classification of burns based on depth of injury becomes more intelligible.

Thermal injury may be conceived as producing three concentric volumes of tissue damage (Fig. 1) [4]. The volume injured most severely, in the center of the wound, is the zone of coagulation. Outside the zone of coagulation is the zone of stasis. Beyond the zone of stasis lies the zone of hyperemia. In theory, the zone of coagulation is destroyed permanently; the zone of stasis is ischemic but potentially salvageable; and the zone of hyperemia features increased blood flow resulting from inflammation. In practice, attentive wound care and careful fluid resuscitation may salvage the zone of stasis and prevent a superficial injury from becoming full thickness.

Depth of burn and burn size

Depth of injury depends on the temperature and heat capacity of the causative agent, the duration of exposure, and the thickness of the skin. For example, hot grease, a substance with a high heat capacity, is likely to cause deep burns. Gasoline flame burns usually are full thickness, reflecting the high temperature. Patients who have underdeveloped skin, such as children, and patients who have atrophic skin, such as the elderly, are more likely to sustain full-thickness injuries than are young adults.

Determining the depth of burns on initial presentation may prove difficult even for experienced burn specialists (Fig. 2, Table 1). A burn that remains confined to the epidermis is termed a first-degree burn. An example of this is a nonblistering sunburn. Such burns rarely are of immediate medical consequence, heal rapidly, and are not included in burn size estimations for the

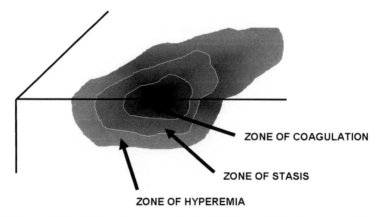

ZONE OF COAGULATION

ZONE OF STASIS

ZONE OF HYPEREMIA

Fig. 1. Zones of injury. Thermal energy can be visualized as producing three concentric spheres of injury. The innermost is the zone of coagulation, the middle sphere is the zone of stasis, and the outermost is the zone of hyperemia.

Table 1
Classification of burn depth

	First-degree	Second-degree	Third-degree
Cause	Sun, hot liquids, brief flash burns	Hot liquids, flash or flame	Flame, prolonged contact with hot liquid or hot object, electricity, chemical
Color	Pink or red	Pink or mottled red	Dark brown, charred, translucent with visible thrombosed veins, pearly white
Surface	Dry	Moist, weeping, blisters	Dry and inelastic
Sensation	Painful	Very painful	Anesthetic
Depth	Epidermis	Epidermis and portions of the dermis	Epidermis, dermis, and possibly deep structures
Time to healing[a]	A few days	One or more weeks	(Heals by contraction)

  [a] In the absence of excision and grafting.
  Data from Sabiston DC Jr, editor. Textbook of surgery. 15th edition. Philadelphia: WB Saunders; 1997.

purpose of determining fluid resuscitation requirements. They may, however, be of legal significance. A burn that extends into the dermis is termed a second-degree or partial-thickness burn. Blistering scald burns are a common example. If only the superficial layer of the dermis is involved, it is termed a superficial partial-thickness burn. These burns heal in less than approximately 21 days and generally do not require skin grafting. Deeper involvement in dermis classifies the burn as a deep partial-thickness burn. These burns heal by re-epithelialization after more than 21 days and generally benefit from skin grafting. A burn involving the entire depth of the dermis and the epidermal appendages is termed a third-degree or full-thickness burn. These burns heal only by contraction from the edges, if at all, over a prolonged period of time. Thus, skin grafting is required. Because the nerve endings are found at the dermal level, the depth of an anesthetic burn is deeper than the depth of a sensate burn. Likewise, lack of blanching in a burn implies injury to the dermal blood vessels. Technologies to estimate burn depth have been developed [5], but these methods have not found widespread use in the clinical arena.

  Estimation of the total body surface area burned (TBSA) as a percentage of the body surface area can be done using the rule of nines (Fig. 3) and refined with a Lund-Browder or Berkow chart [6] correlating the percentage of TBSA of different regions of the body as a function of developmental age (Table 2). Most emergency departments and burn units have one of these body surface charts available for use. Another useful rule is the rule of hands, whereby the patient's hand (palm and fingers) comprises approximately 1 percent of his body surface area. This facilitates estimation of the size of irregularly shaped burns. Careful estimation of TBSA is essential

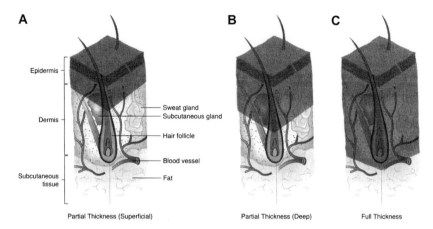

A   **B**   **C**

Epidermis

Sweat gland
Subcutaneous gland

Dermis

Hair follicle

Blood vessel

Subcutaneous
tissue

Fat

Partial Thickness (Superficial)   Partial Thickness (Deep)   Full Thickness

Fig. 2. Classification of burn wounds based on depth of injury. First-degree burns, limited to the epidermis, are not shown. Second-degree or partial-thickness burns commonly are divided into superficial and deep partial-thickness burns, based on healing time. Third-degree burns also are referred to as full-thickness burns. (*From* Edlich RF, Martin ML, Long WB. Thermal burns. In: Marx J, Hockberger R, Walls R, editors. Rosen's emergency medicine: concepts and clinical practice. 6th edition. St. Louis: Mosby; 2006; with permission.)

in the early management of burn patients, because burn size determines fluid requirements and triage and transfer criteria. Overestimation of the burn size by referring hospitals is common and may result from overzealous application of the rule of nines.

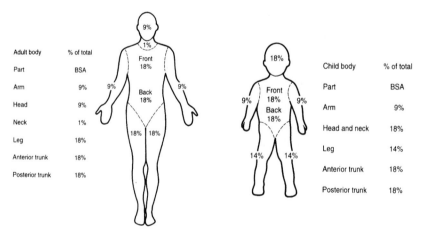

Adult body	% of total
Part	BSA
Arm	9%
Head	9%
Neck	1%
Leg	18%
Anterior trunk	18%
Posterior trunk	18%

Child body	% of total
Part	BSA
Arm	9%
Head and neck	18%
Leg	14%
Anterior trunk	18%
Posterior trunk	18%

Estimation of burn size using the Rule of Nines.

Fig. 3. The rule of nines. Areas of the body are partitioned into areas, each of which constitutes 9% of the TBSA or a multiple thereof. The exception is the genital/perineal area, which is allotted 1%. (*Reprinted from* Herndon DN, editor. Total burn care. 2nd edition. London: Saunders; 2002; with permission.)

Table 2
An example of a Berkow chart

Body part	0–1 year	1–4 years	5–9 years	10–14 years	15–18 years	Adult
Head	19	17	13	11	9	7
Neck	2	2	2	2	2	2
Anterior trunk	13	13	13	13	13	13
Posterior trunk	13	13	13	13	13	13
Right buttock	2.5	2.5	2.5	2.5	2.5	2.5
Left buttock	2.5	2.5	2.5	2.5	2.5	2.5
Genitalia	1	1	1	1	1	1
Right upper arm	4	4	4	4	4	4
Left upper arm	4	4	4	4	4	4
Right lower arm	3	3	3	3	3	3
Left lower arm	3	3	3	3	3	3
Right hand	2.5	2.5	2.5	2.5	2.5	2.5
Left hand	2.5	2.5	2.5	2.5	2.5	2.5
Right thigh	5.5	6.5	8	8.5	9	9.5
Left thigh	5.5	6.5	8	8.5	9	9.5
Right leg	5	5	5.5	6	6.5	7
Left leg	5	5	5.5	6	6.5	7
Right foot	3.5	3.5	3.5	3.5	3.5	3.5
Left foot	3.5	3.5	3.5	3.5	3.5	3.5

Estimates for each body part made and then summed to provide an accurate estimate of the TBSA.

Data from Townsend CM, Beauchamp DR, Evers BM, et al. Sabiston textbook of surgery: the biological basis of modern surgical practice. Philadelphia: Elsevier Saunders; 2004. Available at: http://home.medconsult.com/. Accessed September 2006.

Triage and treatment

What constitutes a major burn? The American Burn Association has written criteria for burn center referral (Box 1) [7]. Burn center referral does not necessarily imply burn center admission. Often, the referral should be made because the anatomic location of the burn requires evaluation by an experienced burn doctor. Some patients who require burn center referral, however, have burns severe enough to require immediate attention in an emergency department and probable admission to a burn ICU. Patients in this category include those patients who have inhalation injury, burns of more than 10% to 20% TBSA, high-voltage electrical injury, or extensive chemical injury.

Some burn patients also have associated nonthermal injuries. These patients should be approached diagnostically and therapeutically as nonthermal trauma victims with an initial evaluation, as in the American College of Surgeons Advanced Trauma Life Support algorithm [8]. Depending on severity of injury, the nonthermal injuries may take precedence over thermal injuries. If patients do not have serious nonthermal injuries, the decision should be made for burn center referral.

Patients who have burns of more than 20% TBSA commonly require intravenous fluid resuscitation [9]. The commonly used formulas predict

---

Box 1. Burn unit referral criteria

A burn unit may treat adults or children or both.
Burn injuries that should be referred to a burn unit include the following:

1. Partial-thickness burns greater than 10% TBSA
2. Burns that involve the face, hands, feet, genitalia, perineum, or major joints
3. Third-degree burns in any age group
4. Electrical burns, including lightning injury
5. Chemical burns
6. Inhalation injury
7. Burn injury in patients who have pre-existing medical disorders that could complicate management, prolong recovery, or affect mortality
8. Burns and concomitant trauma (such as fractures) in which the burn injury poses the greatest risk of morbidity or mortality. In such cases, if the trauma poses the greater immediate risk, patients may be stabilized initially in a trauma center before being transferred to a burn unit. Physician judgment is necessary in such situations and should be in concert with the regional medical control plan and triage protocols.
9. Burns in children who are in hospitals without qualified personnel or equipment for the care of children
10. Burn injury in patients who require special social, emotional, or long-term rehabilitative intervention

---

Excerpted from American College of Surgeons Committee on Trauma. Guidelines for the operations of burn units. Resources for optimal care of the injured patient. Chicago (IL): American College of Surgeons; 1999. p. 55–62.

---

a total fluid intake of 2 to 4 mL/kg/TBSA for the first 24 hours post burn (3–4 mL/kg/TBSA for children), with half of this total volume programmed for delivery over the first 8 hours post burn and half over the second 16 hours post burn. Lactated Ringer's solution is used commonly. The most important point is to then adjust the fluid rate based on physiologic response, mainly the urine output. Enough fluid should be given to maintain a urine output of 30 to 50 mL/hour in adults and approximately 1 mL/kg/hour in children weighing less than 30 kg—but no more. (The target urine output for children varies by age: 0.5–1 mL/kg/h for patients older than 2 years of age and 1–2 mL/kg/h for children under 2 years of age.) Children also require additional 5% dextrose in one-half normal saline at a maintenance rate.

Fluids actually infused often are in excess of formula predictions, in many cases because of failure to decrease fluid intake when the urine output increases. This exposes patients to the potentially disastrous risks of over-resuscitation, such as extremity and abdominal compartment syndromes [10]. The intravenous fluid rate should be changed, using urine output as the endpoint, by 20% to 30% every 1 or 2 hours. The patient also should have a clear sensorium, warm and well-perfused skin, and a heart rate of not more than approximately 120 per minute in adults. Blood pressure is not an established fluid resuscitation endpoint, but low blood pressure (mean arterial pressure < 60 mm Hg) may indicate hypovolemia. Careful documentation of fluid input and output, beginning in the emergency department, is vitally important in the management of burn resuscitation. A burn flow sheet, such as that provided in Fig. 4, assists in this process.

Deep partial-thickness to full-thickness burns cause damage to the dermal layer of the skin, which contains elastin and collagen fibrils and provides elasticity to the skin. If such a burn encompasses a limb, the inelastic burned skin (eschar) and the burn edema fluid that builds up beneath it act like a tourniquet, compressing the vascular supply and compromising nerve function. These types of burns require frequent and vigilant assessment of peripheral pulses, skin perfusion, and neurologic function. Edema should be reduced by elevating the extremity above the level of the heart. Many such patients require escharotomies, however, to relieve the tourniquet-like circumferential burn. If the burn occurs on the thorax or upper abdomen, the eschar likewise can compromise respiratory excursions; this situation also requires an escharotomy. An escharotomy usually is performed by a burn specialist or surgical consultant.

Other important caveats in the treatment of major burn patients in the immediate hours after injury include the following: keep the patient warm, do not apply wet linens, do not apply ice, and do not cool the patient. There is no need to apply topical antimicrobials before transfer to a burn center, provided transfer can be accomplished within 24 hours. Remove all jewelry and rings to protect limbs, hands, and digits. Prophylactic antibiotics are not indicated in burn injuries [11]. Do not use oral, intravenous, or topical steroids [12]. Use frequent, small doses of intravenous narcotics for pain management.

Special burns

Burn center referral is advised for patients who have electrical injuries. Patients who have high-voltage electrical injuries (contact with > 1000 V) are at elevated risk of spinal injury and require complete immobilization until this is ruled out. Direct muscle damage may cause gross myoglobinuria, requiring more aggressive fluid resuscitation [13]. In the presence of gross myoglobinuria, fluids should be administered at a rate sufficient to produce a urine output of 75 to 100 mL/hour in adults. If this does not produce

JTTS Burn Resuscitation Flow Sheet   Page 1

Date: [   ]   Initial Treatment Facility: [   ]

Name	SSN	Pre-burn Est. Wt (kg)	%TBSA	Estimated fluid vol. pat. should receive		
				1st 8 hrs	2nd 16th hr	Est. Total 24 hrs

Date & Time of Inury   BAMC/ISR Burn Team DSN 312-429-2876

Tx Site/ Team	HR from burn	Local Time	Crystalloid / Colloid	TOTAL	UOP	Basez	BP	MAP (>55) / CVP	Pressors (Vasopressin) 0.04 u/min)
1st									
2nd									
3rd									
4th									
5th									
6th									
7th									
8th									
Total Fluids:									
9th									
10th									
11th									
12th									
13th									
14th									
15th									
16th									
17th									
18th									
19th									
20th									
21st									
22nd									
23rd									
24th									
Total Fluids:									

Fig. 4. Burn fluid resuscitation flow sheet. This flow sheet was developed for use during the current conflict in Iraq and Afghanistan but is equally useful in civilian practice. MAP, mean arterial pressure; UOP, urine output.

gradual clearing of the urine over, for example, 3 hours, mannitol (25 g) should be given every 6 hours (and central monitoring should be considered). In addition, an infusion of sodium bicarbonate (150 m EQ/L) may be used to alkalinize the urine and reduce tubular pigment deposition. Gross myoglobinuria is an indication of severe muscle damage; these patients often require urgent fasciotomy in the operating room [14]. A severely injured electrical injury patient usually requires ICU care for resuscitation and monitoring. In severe electrical injuries, cardiac dysrhythmias are not uncommon; almost any type of dysrhythmia may be seen [15].

Chemical burns are another indication for burn center referral. One of the most important points in treating patients who have a chemical injury is protection of the treating team from the chemical that caused the injury to the patients [16]. The other important point is to irrigate the patients copiously with water, beginning at the scene and en route. If the chemical is in a powder form, it should be brushed off before irrigation is begun. For ocular irrigations, Morgan lenses and 0.9 normal saline solution should be used for irrigation.

Patients who have inhalation injury also should be referred to a burn center. Such patients constitute 10% to 20% of burn center admissions. Patients who have isolated inhalation injury (without cutaneous burns) may have an obscure or perplexing presentation [17]. On examination, singed nasal, facial, or scalp hairs, intraoral mucosal edema or blisters, or changes in the character of the voice may suggest but are not specific for inhalation injury. Inhalation injury is more common in patients who have large burns, are at the extremes of ages, who have facial burns, and who were injured in enclosed spaces [18]. The severity of inhalation injury cannot be judged on outward physical findings [19]. Fiberoptic bronchoscopy enables assessment of airway patency, permits the diagnosis of subglottic injury, and may facilitate endotracheal intubation. It is important to obtain carboxyhemoglobin levels in patients who have inhalation injury and to give the patients 100% oxygen for support until the level is less than 10% [20]. Early, prophylactic endotracheal intubation is essential for patients who have suspected inhalation injury, because laryngeal edema may progress rapidly. Even patients who have large burns and do not have inhalation injury may require intubation to guard against progressive airway edema.

Outpatient burn care

Patients who have minor burns (less than 10% TBSA) make up the majority of patients who have burns seen in emergency departments. By definition, patients who have a minor burn should not need fluid resuscitation for shock. If such a patient is in shock, there should be serious concern for a missed nonthermal injury or another problem.

Not all patients who have minor burns are candidates for outpatient management of their wounds. A family support structure is required to engage in dressing changes, to participate in range-of-motion exercises, and to transport patients for outpatient appointments and occupational and physical therapy visits.

Steps in the outpatient management of burns include the following:

- Even for minor burns, tetanus immunization status should be evaluated and brought up to date as needed [21].

- Provide adequate analgesia. For initial débridement, a narcotic, such as fentanyl or morphine, commonly is used. Some patients may require conscious sedation (eg, with ketamine). For home care, consider nonsteroidal anti-inflammatory drugs for background pain and an oral narcotic for dressing changes.
- Clean the burn with a mild surgical detergent, such as chlorhexidene gluconate [22].
- Débride dead skin with moist gauze or by sharp dissection with scissors and forceps. In general, blisters in excess of 2 cm diameter should be unroofed [23].
- Apply a dressing (discussed later).
- Ensure that patients are re-evaluated within 24 hours in a burn center, clinic, or other venue where the wound can be re-evaluated for progression and where patient compliance with instructions can be assessed.
- A mechanism should be in place allowing patients access to care for untoward events, such as wound infections.

Topical antimicrobials with efficacy against gram-negative organisms, such as mafenide acetate and silver sulfadiazine, are shown to exert a significant impact on postburn survival, particularly in patients who have large burns [24]. For small burns, the choice of topical agent is less important. Moist dressings are superior to dry dressings, however, in that moisture fosters re-epitheliazation of a wound [25]. For outpatient purposes, commonly used topical antimicrobials include silver sulfadiazine cream, bacitracin, and neomycin. For these, a coat of the substance is applied to the débrided burn wound; a nonadherent material, such as Adaptic (Johnson & Johnson, New Brunswick, New Jersey) is placed over the cream, and a gauze dressing is placed over this. The dressing can be held in place with an elastic dressing, such as an ACE bandage (BD, Franklin Lakes, New Jersey). For areas that have irregular contours, burns can be treated in open fashion. This means that the cream is applied to a burn, but no gauze is applied. Patients then must be instructed to reapply the cream as frequently as needed.

Silver ion is the active component in silver sulfadiazine and recently has been impregnated into dressings [26]. Available formulations include Silverlon (Argentum Medical, Libertyville, Illinois) and Acticoat (Smith & Nephew, Fort Saskatchewan, Alberta, Canada). These dressings may be left in place for several days, facilitating outpatient care.

Biobrane (Berkek Pharmaceuticals, Morgantown, West Virginia) is a dressing without active antimicrobial properties but that works well for superficial partial-thickness burns. This is a bilaminar material with an outer layer of silicone and an inner layer of collagen-impregenanted nylon mesh that lies against the burn wound. The inner layer acts as a scaffolding for reepitheliazation of the burn wound bed. The dressing reduces pain and promotes healing. Typically, this dressing is applied in an emergency department; the patient is instructed to leave the dressing in place and to return for a follow-up office visit in approximately 2 days for inspection. The Biobrane separates as the burn heals. If the burn wound is deeper than superficial partial thickness, purulent material may accumulate under the dressing. If this occurs, the Biobrane should be removed where it overlies the purulent collection, and the wound should be treated as deep partial or full thickness in depth.

Average laypersons require some training in products, such as Biobrane, Silverlon, and Acticoat. In addition, these dressings should not be used on patients who are not likely to return for follow-up visits.

Summary

- Evaluate patients for nonthermal injuries.
- Triage patients by severity of injury, based primarily on burn size and the presence of inhalation injury.
- Accurate estimation of the burn size is crucial in early management decisions.
- The selection of the fluid resuscitation protocol is less important than the execution of the protocol and the assessment of patients during the process, in order to avoid over-resuscitation.
- Patients who have electrical, chemical, or inhalation injuries also merit burn center referral.
- High-voltage electrical injuries often produce more damage than is apparent by inspection; gross myoglobinuria mandates more aggressive resuscitation and, possibly, urgent fasciotomy.
- Protection of health care personnel and early decontamination is paramount in treating patients who have chemical injuries.
- Early prophylactic endotracheal intubation of patients who have inhalation injury or large burns prevents airway obstruction during resuscitation.
- Selection of patients who may be treated as outpatient burn patients hinges as much on social issues as on medical concerns.

References

[1] American Burn Association. Burn incidence and treatment in the US: 2000 fact sheet. Available at: http://www.ameriburn.org/resources_factsheet.php. Accessed September 15, 2006.
[2] Reith EJ, Ross MH. Integument. In: Reith EJ, Ross MH, editors. Atlas of descriptive histology. 3rd edition. New York: Harper and Row; 1977. p. 136–41.
[3] Chung KC, Wilkins EG, Rees RS, et al. Skin and subcutaneous tissue. In: O'Leary JP, editor. The physiologic basis of surgery. 3rd edition. Philadelphia: Lippincott Williams & Wilkins; 2002. p. 637–55.
[4] Jackson DM. The diagnosis of the depth of burning. Br J Surg 1953;40:588–96.
[5] Atiles L, Muleski W, Sparrn K, et al. Early assessment of pediatric burn wounds by laser Doppler flowmetry. J Burn Care Rehabil 1995;16:596–601.
[6] Lund CC, Browder NC. The estimation of areas of burn. Surg Gynecol Obstet 1944;79: 352–8.

[7] American College of Surgeons Committee on Trauma. Resources for optimal care of the injured patient. Chicago: American College of Surgeons; 1999.

[8] American College of Surgeons Committee on Trauma. Advanced trauma life support for doctors. 7th edition. Chicago: American College of Surgeons; 2004.

[9] Pruitt BA Jr, Mason AD Jr, Moncrief JA. Hemodynamic changes in the early postburn patient: the influence of fluid administration and of a vasodilator (hydralazine). J Trauma 1971;11:36–46.

[10] Cancio LC, Chavez S, Alvarado-Ortega M, et al. Predicting increased fluid requirements during the resuscitation of thermally injured patients. J Trauma 2004;56:404–14.

[11] Dacso CC, Luterman A, Curreri PW. Systemic antibiotic treatment in burned patients. Surg Clin North Am 1987;67:57–68.

[12] Robinson NB, Hudson LD, Riem M, et al. Steroid therapy following isolated smoke inhalation injury. J Trauma 1982;22:876–9.

[13] DiVincenti FC, Moncrief JA, Pruitt BA Jr. Electrical injuries: a review of 65 cases. J Trauma 1969;9:497–507.

[14] Cancio LC, Jimenez-Reyna JF, Barillo DJ, et al. One hundred ninety-five cases of high-voltage electric injury. J Burn Care Rehabil 2005;26:331–40.

[15] Solem L, Fischer RP, Strate RG. The natural history of electrical injury. J Trauma 1977;17:487–92.

[16] Barillo DJ, Cancio LC, Goodwin CW. Treatment of white phosphorus and other chemical burn injuries at one burn center over a 51-year period. Burns 2004;30:448–52.

[17] Heimbach DM, Waeckerle JF. Inhalation injury. Ann Emerg Med 1988;17:1316–20.

[18] Cancio LC. Current concepts in the pathophysiology and treatment of inhalation injury. Trauma 2005;7:19–35.

[19] Park MS, Cancio LC, Batchinsky AI, et al. Assessment of the severity of ovine smoke inhalation injury by analysis of CT scans. J Trauma 2003;55:417–27.

[20] Weaver LK, Howe S, Hopkins R, et al. Carboxyhemoglobin half-life in carbon monoxide poisoned patients treated with 100% oxygen at atmospheric pressure. Chest 2000;117:801–8.

[21] Karyoute SM, Badran IZ. Tetanus following a burn injury. Burns Incl Therm Inj 1988;14:241–3.

[22] Mertens DM, Jenkins ME, Warden GD. Outpatient burn management. Nurs Clin North Am 1997;32:343–64.

[23] Rockwell WB, Ehrlich HP. Should burn blister fluid be evacuated? J Burn Care Rehabil 1990;11:93–5.

[24] Brown TP, Cancio LC, McManus AT, et al. Survival benefit conferred by topical antimicrobial preparations in burn patients: a historical perspective. J Trauma 2004;56:863–6.

[25] Winter GD. Formation of the scab and rate of epithelialization of superficial wounds in the skin of the young domestic pig. Nature 1962;193:293–4.

[26] Russell AD, Hugo WB. Antimicrobial activity and action of silver. Prog Med Chem 1994;31:351–70.

ELSEVIER
SAUNDERS

Emerg Med Clin N Am
25 (2007) 147–158

EMERGENCY
MEDICINE
CLINICS OF
NORTH AMERICA

Postcare Recommendations for Emergency Department Wounds

Paresh R. Patel, MD, FAAEM[a],
Michael A. Miller, MD, FAAEM[a,b,*]

[a]*Department of Emergency Medicine, Darnall Army Medical Center,*
36000 Darnall Loop, Fort Hood, Temple, TX 76544, USA
[b]*Central Texas Poison Center, Temple, TX 76508, USA*

Historical perspective

An often underappreciated but essential step in emergency department wound care is the posttreatment discharge instructions. Improper care throughout the healing phases can adversely affect outcome, despite the best initial emergency room management. Still, such an important aspect of practice often is based on anecdotal teachings. History shows this practice does not necessarily lend itself to the best possible outcome. Gone are the days of butter on burns. This article provides a concise review of evidence-based posttreatment wound care.

Methods of wound care are well documented throughout history. Wound dressings and salves were chiseled into a Sumerian clay tablet as two of "three healing gestures" in 2100 BC. Ancient salves were bactericidal. In fact, a combination of honey and grease would decrease bacterial counts threefold. The "healing effects" and antiseptic properties of wine have been well documented. Homer notes bandaging in both *The Odyssey* and *The Iliad* around 800 BC [1,2].

Wound pathophysiology

The human response to wounds is centered on healing. There are four phases of wound healing: hemostasis, inflammation, granulation, and tissue remodeling. Hemostasis generally occurs within minutes, allowing

Paresh Patel owns 129 shares of Pfizer.
* Corresponding author. Department of Emergency Medicine, Darnall Army Medical Center, 36000 Darnall Loop, Fort Hood, TX 76544.
E-mail address: Michael.adam.miller@us.army.mil (M.A. Miller).

vasospasm and clot formation. The inflammatory phase begins soon there-after, often peaking in the first 24 hours, although it can last for several days. In this phase, granulocytic activity promotes the destruction of bacteria and the removal of debris [3]. Re-epithelialization also begins within the first 24 hours, and by 48 hours the wound is considered watertight [4]. Macrophages arrive between 72 and 96 hours for wound reorganization and clean up of inflammatory debris, prompting the granulation phase, in which new tissue growth is achieved. This process involves further re-epithelialization, which begins within hours of injury, neovascularization, and matrix deposition. Finally tissue remodeling begins with collagen formation, approximately 5 to 7 days from initial injury. This phase lasts an average of 6 to 18 months, confers tensile strength, and affects scar size and appearance [3,4].

Utility of the dressing

The ancient Greeks made such elaborate dressings to cover wounds that they were considered an art form [1]. In modern medicine, the necessity of dressings for posttreatment wound care is more controversial. Since the 1940s, literature has been published demonstrating the utility of dressings in the clinical setting [5]. In the 1960s, Winter's [6] porcine model studies and subsequently Hinman and Maibach's [7] human studies supported a moist environment created by an occlusive dressing to promote more rapid re-epithelialization and wound healing. This method prompted a revolution in the development of occlusive dressings, although today's occlusive dressings are in fact semiocclusive [8].

An American College of Emergency Physicians survey of physicians on outpatient wound care showed that the most common dressing is gauze and a topical antimicrobial product. A wide variety of dressings are used: simple dry gauze, bio-occlusive dressings, petrolatum-impregnated dressings, and others [9]. Despite the increase in types of dressings available to emergency physicians, there is no consensus that a particular dressing is superior to another [5,10–12]. Ideally, the dressing should be semiocclusive, nonadherent, and semiabsorbable to maintain a moist, clean environment for 48 hours while epithelialization occurs [8,11,12]. Because nonadherent dressings do not stick to healings wounds, they cause less pain than gauze dressings [10]. Although some studies suggest a hypoxic wound environment created by an impermeable dressing is favorable for wound healing, others favor semipermeability, particularly in an ischemic wound, to maintain an appropriate level of oxygenation in the wound to expedite healing [13,14]. Studies have found no difference in healing between permeable and impermeable dressings [15,16]. Other special dressings, such as negative-pressure dressing, currently have no role in acute wound care but may offer enhanced healing in chronic or poorly healing wounds [17]. The classic wet-to-dry dressings also have not shown benefit over other forms of dressings [18].

Many studies have challenged the practice of dressing wounds in any manner. In 1966 Howells and Young [4] demonstrated that the omission of a dressing on surgical wounds did not increase the rate of infection. More recently, an Australian-based study revealed similar findings. It assessed 857 patients whose minor, uncomplicated skin lesion excisions were sutured. Those who kept their wounds dry and covered for 48 hours had an 8.9% infection rate; those who removed their dressings and were allowed to wash the wounds within 12 hours had a similar rate of 8.4%. This study also demonstrated that it is safe to wet wounds before 24 to 48 hours, a practice that is rarely taught [19]. Patients who had facial wounds were excluded from this Australian study, but Goldberg and colleagues [20] have shown that wounds to the head and neck do well without wound dressings; this area typically has a relatively low infection rate. Furthermore, they did not find evidence that cleansing with soap and water interferes with wound healing.

These studies mainly involved wounds closed to heal by primary intention with sutures and partial-thickness wounds healing by secondary intention. Few studies have addressed the need for dressings in larger wounds and puncture wounds. A Cochrane review reports that insufficient evidence exists to recommend one dressing over another for surgical wounds healing by secondary intention [10]. Another circumstance to consider is wounds closed with surgical tapes. Surgical tapes typically serve as dressings in and of themselves; therefore, studies evaluating their efficacy generally do not involve or recommend additional dressings [21–23]. It is recommended that wounds closed with tissue adhesives remain uncovered for maximal effectiveness, although after polymerization occurs, a dry protective dressing may be applied judiciously [24–26].

Most simple wounds closed in the emergency room do not require dressings. Simple antibiotic ointment or petroleum jelly (discussed in the next section) is sufficient for simple sutured wounds or abrasions. Keeping wounds open is less expensive, allows patients to monitor their wounds continuously, and removes fear about what lies beneath the dressing. A simple nonadherent occlusive dressing may provide the optimal environment and keep contaminants out of larger and complex wounds left open to heal by secondary intention. Wounds left open to close by delayed primary closure should be kept covered with a nonadherent dressing and should be re-evaluated for closure on day four or five, when bacterial counts have dropped significantly [27].

Special situations

Certain wounds do require specific posttreatment wound care. Auricular hematomas, for example, should have a pressure dressing to prevent formation of a cauliflower ear deformity, although a Cochrane review could not definitively recommend its use based on current evidence [28]. For oral lacerations, chlorhexidine and other oral antiseptics have been shown to reduce oral bacterial and viral counts [29,30]. Further studies on infection rates in oral lacerations treated with antimicrobial antiseptics such as Listerine (Pfizer, Morris Plains, New Jersey) are needed. Until such studies are available, warm-water rinses after meals are sufficient to prevent further wound contamination by food or other foreign material.

Packing incised and drained wounds is controversial also. Packing has been advocated to prevent dead space formation and premature wound closure, but it may delay healing and increase rates of infection [31–33]. Despite the controversy, there is not enough evidence to dismiss the practice of packing completely. Prolonged packing is unnecessary and often is detrimental. The best approach is light packing for a limited time of 48 hours or until granulation tissue has formed. Patients should be educated about methods of daily packing as needed. If patients are unable to perform changes, timely follow-up should be arranged for repacking.

The role of topical antibiotics/ointments

It is well known that oral antibiotic prophylaxis is not needed for simple, clean lacerations seen in the emergency department [34]. Topical antibiotic ointment, however, is routinely used for aftercare of wounds, serving as an antibacterial barrier to facilitate wound repair. In addition, ointments maintain a moist environment for wound healing and prevent tissue adherence to dressings. Multiple studies show topical antibiotics significantly decrease bacterial counts in wounds [35–37]. Whether this decrease translates into clinical benefit is widely debated in the literature. Berger and colleagues [38] showed that topical antibiotics might minimize the appearance of scarring more effectively than a simple gauze dressing alone. In 1995, Dire and colleagues [39] published a study demonstrating a statistically significantly lower infection rate in when antibiotic ointment rather than petroleum jelly was applied to sutured traumatic wounds. In a randomized trial examining procedural wounds in a dermatology clinic, however, petroleum jelly was as effective as antibiotic ointment in preventing infections. Additional benefits cited were cost savings and decreased allergenic potential [40]. Of note, this study compared procedurally inflicted wounds, not traumatic wounds.

Although the use of topical antibiotics may be controversial, they are widely used in aftercare wound management [9]. There are many antibiotics ointments from which to choose. Dire and colleague's [39] study further compared infection rates among several different antibiotic ointments, including bacitracin (5.5%), triple antibiotic ointment (neomycin sulfate, bacitracin zinc, and polymyxin B sulfate) (4.5%), and sulfadiazine cream (12.1%). Although the use of the first two did demonstrate a lower infection rate than sulfadiazine, the findings were not statistically significant. In addition, the potential for local and systemic toxicity, the potential for emergence of resistant organisms, and the allergenic potential must be considered. For example, neomycin is highly allergenic; bacitracin is better tolerated [15]. In general, safety profiles for all the topical antibiotics ointments are good, so choosing an ointment for the desired antimicrobial effect becomes important. Gram-negative bacteria make up the majority of pathogens found in wounds, although *Staphylococcus aureus* is most commonly isolated [41]. In healing wounds methicillin-resistant *S aureus* has become a potential complication of particular concern but currently is susceptible to mupirocin [42,43]. Overall the use of topical antibiotics is good practice for wounds seen in the emergency department, which usually are traumatic in nature. The use of ointment keeps patients involved in the daily care of their wounds and also may decrease the rate of infection. Ointments serve as a moist dressing, reduce dressing attachment to the wound, and are inexpensive. Based on cost, its low rate of allergenicity, and antimicrobial coverage, bacitracin is a good choice for most lacerations. A special exception involves adhesive closure. According to one manufacturer of Dermabond (Ethicon, Somerville, New Jersey) (2-octyl-cyanoacrylate adhesive), ointments and liquids must not be applied, because they weaken the polymerized film and increase the risk of wound dehiscence [24].

There is limited evidence for the routine use of other commonly used ointments without antibiotic properties in traumatic wound care. Aloe vera, a commonly used over-the-counter agent, has received mixed reviews in small studies [44,45]. Topical steroids have been shown to impede wound healing [46]. Vitamin E, zinc oxide, heparinoid ointments, and imiquimod are among other topical therapies with insufficient evidence to support their use [47–53]. Topical epidermal growth factors are promising but do not have a current role in acute wound care [54]. Proteolytic enzymes may have some utility in nonhealing and chronic wounds [55]. In addition, antiseptics are not recommended. In particular, the use of hydrogen peroxide for continued care of the healing wound has fallen out of favor. Its application causes tissue disruption and has been shown to impede wound healing in several studies [56,57].

The sun poses an interesting threat to the healing wound as well and requires special consideration. In a small, commonly cited study of patients undergoing dermabrasion, patients exposed to the sun had unfavorable pigmentation compared with those who abstained from sun exposure [58]. Sunscreens may be a helpful alternative when sun avoidance is not possible; they are safe, effective, and have limited toxicity [59].

Treatment adjuncts

Elevation, compression, and splinting often have been touted for aftercare wound management. Although preliminary reviews suggest a possible role for these treatment modalities, the studies in emergency medicine literature are sparse. No current clinical trials are available to document the efficacy of elevation, but in considering its overall risk-to-potential benefit ratio, its recommendation is reasonable based on current knowledge about wound healing. Elevation in the initial phases of wound healing may be beneficial by decreasing the edema associated with trauma and inflammation, but no well-designed studies particularly address this treatment for emergency wounds [60]. A Cochran review suggests compression may be of limited benefit to the healing of chronic ulcer wounds [61]. The orthopedic literature shows compression dressing may result in decreased postoperative pain and blood loss [62,63]. Data are needed, however, for the role of compression dressing in traumatic wound healing. Splinting throughout the healing process is particularly important with wounds overlying joints, in which repeated movement may impede a timely healing process. Other extremity wounds may benefit from splinting by immobilizing the extremity and promoting healing and patient comfort [60].

Splinting, elevation, and compression are simple techniques and may affect healing. For simple lacerations over nonjoints these methods seem to have limited utility. For suture wounds over joints splinting may prevent delayed healing and a larger scar formation from excessive movement. Compression and elevation may be more useful for complex wounds on extremities with significant edema from contused skin than for simple lacerations.

Plan for pain

An integral part of the wound aftercare plan is ongoing pain control, but often pain control is overlooked in emergency department discharge planning. Although the degree and nature of the pain depends on individual patient and wound factors, some basic principles can be applied. For most minor wounds, oral acetaminophen or nonsteroidal anti-inflammatory drugs (NSAIDs) provide adequate pain control. Although some animal research suggests that ibuprofen delays wound healing, the clinical data in humans remain poor, and NSAIDs remain accepted in the treatment of pain for minor wounds [64]. A short course of oral narcotics may be necessary for larger, more complex wounds, those with soft tissue contusions, or those following a significant incision and drainage.

The topical use of cold compresses, or even ice, has been reported to serve as an analgesic [62,63,65]. On the other hand, preliminary studies in the surgical literature have shown benefits of warming on healing wounds [66,67]. In a small, randomized study of postoperative hernia surgical wounds, Melling and Leaper demonstrated a decrease in pain and improvement in wound healing using special heating devices. No increased risk of infection was noted [66]. Although the routine use of temperature-based adjuncts for simple lacerations and puncture wounds is not necessary, particularly given the variable factors of compliance and practicality, their simplicity and minimal cost do make them useful adjuncts for pain control of more complex wounds involving significantly contused tissue and edema.

Discharge instructions

No all wounds are treated the same in the emergency department. Wound care may be achieved with no closure, sutures, staples, adhesive glue, or surgical tape. The initial method of treatment should affect the discharge management and follow-up plan. Postcare wound instructions must be reinforced during repair and when the patient is discharged home. Clear instructions outlining reasons to return must be given. In general, the use of structured, preformatted instructions for all emergency department patients with exact days for suture removal and follow-up is recommended [68].

Austin and colleagues [69] conducted a small, randomized, blinded, prospective study of patients discharged with lacerations and found that the addition of illustrations improves patients' comprehension, especially among nonwhite patients, women, and patients with no more than a high school education. Wounds remodeling usually takes 6 to 12 months, and it is important to educate the patient that the short-term appearance does not predict the long-term cosmetic outcome of the wound [70]. Physical examination and basic radiographic imaging cannot rule out the presence of all foreign bodies, and patients should always be told of this possibility [66].

There is little literature addressing when and if wound checks are needed. Seaman and Lammers [71] found patients were unable to recognize wound infections. In their study of 433 patients who had a sutured wound repair, 21 cases of infection were found, with only 11 cases diagnosed by patients and a 48% false-negative rate. The false-positive rate was only 8%. They concluded that, unless the wounds involved very low risk, all patients who had traumatic wounds should have follow-up examinations performed by medical examiners before suture removal. Patients who had simple, cleaned wounds, however, need only return at the time of suture or staple removal. All high-risk wounds or wounds infected on initial presentation should be considered for close follow up within 24 to 72 hours. The exact time should be determined by the concern over the type of wound, social situation, and logistics of follow-up.

Before a patient is discharged from the emergency department, a plan to return for suture or staple removal must be outlined clearly. Estimating the date of return can be difficult, because wounds heal at varying rates depending on individual host factors. If sutures or staples are removed too early, the risk of wound dehiscence and poor cosmetic outcome increases. Sutures left in too long also may result in poor cosmetic outcome, including an unsightly sinus tract or permanent suture imprints [72]. Thus, it is important to base recommendations on the general principles of wound healing.

Patients who have sutured or stapled head or facial wounds should return for removal in 3 to 5 days. For wounds on the rest of the body, removal can take place after 7 to 10 days. Scalp sutures and sutures or staples over joints can remain in place for as long as 14 days [73,74].

Wounds closed with adhesive or surgical tape do not need follow-up unless a concern arises. Adhesives have an increased risk of dehiscence, and signs heralding this complication must be addressed with the patient before discharge [75–77]. Steri-strips (3M, Minneapolis, Minnesota) generally peel off in a few weeks and can be left untouched. Edges that peel can be trimmed with scissors. If they are still present after 2 weeks, they can be removed gently with nail polish remover, soap and water, or adhesive remover.

Summary

The plan for posttreatment wound care is as important as the emergency department interventions. To date, there are limited, and often conflicting, recommendations in the literature to guide management plans. Further studies are needed to direct care more effectively. Nevertheless specific instructions must be given to patients to complete wound care. Table 1 provides basic guidance for wound care.

These instructions should include whether a dressing is indicated, which dressing should be used, and the duration of use. Patients also should understand the method of application. Generally, if a dressing is required, 48 hours of dressing is sufficient. Patients who have sutured primary closures may bathe or swim in uncontaminated water 24 hours after discharge. Some studies suggest that wetting as early as 8 to 12 hours will not have detrimental effects. Soap and water may be used to clean the area. Topical antibiotic ointments are useful in traumatic wounds and can eliminate the need for a dressing entirely in many instances. The type of ointment selected must depend on the wound and individual factors.

Table 1
Recommendations for wound care

Wound Type	Dressing	Follow-up
Simple lacerations/abrasions	Vaseline or topical antibiotic ointment and sunscreen or clothing if exposed to sunlight	None required
Complex lacerations and wounds healing by secondary intention and delayed primary closure	Topical antibiotic ointment and simple nonadherent dressing with elastic wrap to secure in place	3–5 days
Complex hematoma/contusions	Elastic wrap for gentle compression	1 week
Puncture and bite wounds	Topical antibiotic ointment and nonadherent dressing	3–5 days
Abscesses	Loose packing/nonadherent dressing	24–48 hours

One may consider recommending adjunctive therapies, such as elevation, compression, or splinting as indicated. A plan for pain control must be in place. NSAIDs and acetaminophen are prescribed most often, although attention must be paid to the type and location of the wound. Warm and cold compresses may have a role in treating particular types of complex wounds.

Perhaps most importantly, the plan must explain clearly the reasons for returning for further medical attention, for follow-up, for routine removal of sutures/staples, and an earlier return for possible concerns of infection or dehiscence. Preprinted discharge instruction sheets are useful, and illustrations can be helpful also. Diligent posttreatment wound care management undoubtedly will improve wound outcome and patient satisfaction.

References

[1] Broughton G 2nd, Janis JE, Attinger CE. A brief history of wound care. Plast Reconstr Surg 2006;117(7 Suppl):6S–11S.
[2] Majno G. The healing hand: man and wound in the ancient world. Cambridge (MA): Harvard University Press; 1975. p. 570.
[3] Cho CY, Lo JS. Dressing the part. Dermatol Clin 1998;16(1):25–47.
[4] Howells CHL, Young HB. A study of completely undressed surgical wounds. Br J Surg 1966;53:436–8.
[5] Jones J. Winter's concept of moist wound healing: a review of the evidence and impact on clinical practice. J Wound Care 2005;14(6):273–6.
[6] Winter GD. Formation of the scab and the rate of epithelisation in the skin of the young domestic pig. Nature 1962;193:293–4.
[7] Hinman CD, Maibach H. Effect of air exposure and occlusion on experimental human skin wounds. Nature 1963;200:377–8.
[8] Eaglstein WH. Moist wound healing with occlusive dressings: a clinical focus. Dermatol Surg 2001;27(2):175–81.
[9] Howell JM, Chisholm CD. Outpatient wound preparation and care: a national survey. Ann Emerg Med 1992;21:976–81.
[10] Vermeulen H, Ubbink D, Goossens A, et al. Dressings and topical agents for surgical wounds healing by secondary intention. Cochrane Database Syst Rev 2004;2:CD003554.
[11] James H. Wound dressings in accident and emergency departments. Accid Emerg Nurs 1994; 2(2):87–93.
[12] Jones AM, San Miguel L. Are modern wound dressings a clinical and cost-effective alternative to the use of gauze? J Wound Care 2006;15(2):65–9.
[13] Ueno C, Hunt TK, Hopf HW. Using physiology to improve surgical wound outcomes. Plast Reconstr Surg 2006;117(7 Suppl):59S–71S.
[14] Hopf HW, Gibson JJ, Angeles AP, et al. Hyperoxia and angiogenesis. Wound Repair Regen 2005;13(6):558–64.
[15] Brown CD, Zitelli JA. Choice of wound dressings and ointments. Otolaryngol Clin North Am 1995;28(5):1081–91.
[16] Eaglestein WH. Occlusive dressings. J Dermatol Surg Oncol 1993;19:716–20.
[17] Evans D, Land L. Topical negative pressure for treating chronic wounds. Cochrane Database Syst Rev 2001;1:CD001898.
[18] Ovington LG. Hanging wet-to-dry dressings out to dry. Home Healthc Nurse 2001;19(8): 477–83.
[19] Heal C, Buettner P, Raasch B, et al. Can sutures get wet? Prospective randomized controlled trail of wound management in general practice. BMJ 2006;332:1053–4.

[20] Goldberg HM, Rosenthal SAE, Nemetz JC. Effect of washing closed head and neck wound on wound healing and infection. Am J Surg 1981;141:358–9.

[21] Rodeheaver GT, Matthew Halverson J, Edlich RF. Mechanical performance of wound closure tapes. Ann Emerg Med 1983;12(4):203–7.

[22] Moy RL, Quan MB. An evaluation of wound closure tapes. J Dermatol Surg Oncol 1990; 16(8):721–3.

[23] 3M Company. Available at: http://multimedia.mmm.com/mws/mediawebserver. dyn?6666660Zjcf6lVs6EVs666_sMCOrrrrQ-. Accessed October 14, 2006.

[24] Dermabond information. Available at: http://www.ethicon.com. Accessed October 14, 2006.

[25] Available at: http://www.dermabond.com, dermabond information. Accessed October 14, 2006.

[26] Available at: http://www.mypreceptor.com. dermabond information. Accessed October 14, 2006.

[27] Edlich RF, Rogers W, Kasper G, et al. Studies in the management of the contaminated wound: I. Optimal time for closure of contaminated open wounds: II. Comparison of resistance to infection of open and closed wounds during healing. Am J Surg 1969;117: 323–9.

[28] Jones SEM, Mahendran S. Interventions for acute auricular haematoma. Cochrane Database Syst Rev 2004;2:CD004166.

[29] Sreenivasan PK, Gittins E. Effects of low dose chlorhexidine mouthrinses on oral bacteria and salivary microflora including those producing hydrogen sulfide. Oral Microbiol Immunol 2004;19(5):309–13.

[30] Meiller TF, Silva A, Ferreira SM, et al. Efficacy of Listerine antiseptic in reducing viral contamination of saliva. J Clin Periodontol 2005;32(4):341–6.

[31] Barnes SM, Milsom PL. Abscesses: an open and shut case. Arch Emerg Med 1988;5(4): 200–5.

[32] Sorensen C, Hjortrup A, Moesgaard F, et al. Linear incision and curettage vs. deroofing and drainage in subcutaneous abscess. A randomized clinical trial. Acta Chir Scand 1987; 153(11–12):659–60.

[33] Stewart MP, Laing MR, Krukowski ZH. Treatment of acute abscesses by incision, curettage and primary suture without antibiotics: a controlled clinical trial. Br J Surg 1985; 72(1):66–7.

[34] Cummings P, Del Beccaro MA. Antibiotics to prevent infection of simple wounds: a meta analysis of randomized studies. Am J Emerg Med 1995;13:396–400.

[35] Mack RM, Cantrell JR. Quantitative studies of bacterial flora on open skin wounds. The effects of topical antibiotics. Ann Surg 1967;166:886–95.

[36] Hirschmann JV. Topical antibiotics in dermatology. Arch Dermatol 1988;124:1691–700.

[37] Saik RP, Walz CA, Rhoads JE. Evaluation of a bacitracin-neomycin surgical skin preparation. Am J Surg 1971;121:557–60.

[38] Berger RS, Pappert AS, Van Zile PS, et al. A newly formulated topical triple-antibiotic ointment minimizes scarring. Cutis 2000;65(6):401–4.

[39] Dire DJ, Coppola M, Dwyer DA, et al. A prospective evaluation of topical antibiotics for preventing infections in uncomplicated soft-tissue wounds repaired in the ED. Acad Emerg Med 1995;2:4–10.

[40] Smack DP, Harrington AC, Dunn C, et al. Infection and allergy incidence in ambulatory surgery patients using white petrolatum vs. bacitracin ointment. JAMA 1996;276:972–7.

[41] Sebben JE. Surgical antiseptics. J Am Acad Dermatol 1983;9:759–65.

[42] Strock LL, Lee MM, Rutan RL, et al. Topical Bactroban (mupirocin): efficacy in treating burn wounds infected with methicillin-resistant staphylococci. J Burn Care Rehabil 1990; 11(5):454–9.

[43] Lykova EA, Eremina LV, Sterkhova GV, et al. The results and characteristics of the mupirocin (Bactroban) sanative treatment of intranasal Staphylococcus carriers in a large hospital. Antibiot Khimioter 2000;45(6):25–8.

[44] Gallagher J, Gray M. Evidence-based report card from the Center for Clinical Investigation. Is aloe vera effective for healing chronic wounds? J Wound Ostomy Continence Nurs 2003; 30(2):68–71.

[45] Davis RH, Leitner MG, Russo JM, et al. Wound healing. Oral and topical activity of aloe vera. J Am Podiatr Med Assoc 1989;79:559.

[46] Hengge UR, Ruzicka T. Schwartz RA, et al. Adverse effects of topical glucocorticosteroids. J Am Acad Dermatol 2006;54(1), 1–15; [quiz: 16–8].

[47] Kloth LC, McCulloch JM, Feeder JA. Would and healing: alternatives in management. Philadelphia: F.A. Davis Co.; 1990.

[48] Mukherjee PK, Mukherjee K, Rajesh Kumar M, et al. Evaluation of wound healing activity of some herbal formulations. Phytother Res 2003;17(3):265–8.

[49] Baumann LS, Spencer J. The effects of topical vitamin E on the cosmetic appearance of scars. Dermatol Surg 1999;25(4):311–5.

[50] Agren MS. Studies on zinc in wound healing. Acta Derm Venereol Suppl (Stockh). 1990;154: 1–36.

[51] Williams KJ, Meltzer R, Brown RA, et al. The effect of topically applied zinc on the healing of open wounds. J Surg Res 1979;27(1):62–7.

[52] Skipworth JF, Mouzas GL. The value of heparinoid ointments in the accident department. Br J Clin Pract 1971;25(11):505–6.

[53] Berman B, Frankel S, Villa AM, et al. Double-blind, randomized, placebo-controlled, prospective study evaluating the tolerability and effectiveness of imiquimod applied to postsurgical excisions on scar cosmesis. Randomized controlled trial. Dermatol Surg 2005; 31(11 Pt 1):1399–403.

[54] Grazul-Bilska AT, Johnson ML, Bilski JJ, et al. Wound healing: the role of growth factors. Drugs Today 2003;39(10):787–800.

[55] Yager DR, Nwomeh BC. The proteolytic environment of chronic wounds. Wound Repair Regen 1999;7(6):433–41.

[56] Tur E, Bolton L, Constantine BE. Topical hydrogen peroxide treatment of ischemic ulcers in the guinea pig: blood recruitment in multiple skin sites. J Am Acad Dermatol 1995;33:217–21.

[57] Lineaweaver W, Howard R, Soucy D, et al. Topical antimicrobial toxicity. Arch Surg. 1985; 120:267–70.

[58] Moloney FJ, Collins S, Murphy GM. Sunscreens: safety, efficacy and appropriate use. Am J Clin Dermatol 2002;3(3):185–91.

[59] Ship AG, Weiss PR. Pigmentation after dermabrasion: an avoidable complication. Plast Reconstr Surg 1985;75:528–32.

[60] Edlich RF, Thacker JG, Buchanan L, et al. Modern concepts of treatment of traumatic wounds. Adv Surg 1979;13:169–97.

[61] Cullum N, Nelson EA, Fletcher AW, et al. Compression for venous leg ulcers. Cochrane Database Syst Rev 2001;2:CD000265.

[62] Levy AS, Marmar E. The role of cold compression dressings in the postoperative treatment of total knee arthroplasty. Clin Orthop Relat Res 1993;(297):174–8.

[63] Webb JM, Williams D, Ivory JP, et al. The use of cold compression dressings after total knee replacement: a randomized controlled trial. Orthopedics 1998;21(1):59–61.

[64] Clarke S, Lecky F. Best evidence topic report. Do non-steroidal anti-inflammatory drugs cause a delay in fracture healing? Emerg Med J 2005;22(9):652–3.

[65] Akan M, Misirlioglu A, Yildirim S, et al. Ice application to minimize pain in the split-thickness skin graft donor site. Aesthetic Plast Surg 2003;27(4):305–7.

[66] Melling AC, Leaper DJ. The impact of warming on pain and wound healing after hernia surgery: a preliminary study. J Wound Care 2006;15(3):104–8.

[67] MacFie CC, Melling AC, Leaper DJ. Effects of warming on healing. J Wound Care 2005; 14(3):133–6.

[68] Taylor DM, Cameron PA. Discharge instructions for emergency department patients: what should we provide? J Accid Emerg Med 2000;17:86–90.

[69] Austin PE, Matlack R II, Dun KA, et al. Discharge instructions: do illustrations help our patients understand them? Ann Emerg Med 1995;25:317–20.
[70] Hollander JE, Blasko B, Singer AJ, et al. Poor correlation of short and long term appearance of repaired lacerations. Acad Emerg Med 1995;2(11):983–7.
[71] Seaman M, Lammers R. Inability of patients to self diagnose wound infections. J Emerg Med 1991;9:215–9.
[72] Crikelair GF. Skin suture marks. Am J Surg 1958;96:631–9.
[73] Singer AJ, Hollander JE, Quinn JV. Evaluation and management of traumatic lacerations. New Engl J Med 1997;337:1142–8.
[74] Hollander JE, Singer AJ. Laceration management. Ann Emerg Med 1999;34:356–67.
[75] Singer AJ, Thode HC Jr. A review of the literature on octylcyanoacrylate tissue adhesive. Am J Surg 2004;187(2):238–48.
[76] Farion KJ, Osmond MH, Hartling L, et al. Tissue adhesives for traumatic lacerations: a systematic review of randomized controlled trials. Acad Emerg Med 2003;10(2):110–8.
[77] Ginsburg MJ, Ellis GL, Flom LL. Detection of soft-tissue foreign bodies by plain radiography, xerography, computed tomography, and ultrasonography. Ann Emerg Med 1990; 19(6):701–3.

ELSEVIER
SAUNDERS

Emerg Med Clin N Am
25 (2007) 159–176

EMERGENCY
MEDICINE
CLINICS OF
NORTH AMERICA

Use of Appropriate Antimicrobials in Wound Management

Yoko Nakamura, MD[a], Mohamud Daya, MD, MS[b],*

[a]*Department of Emergency Medicine, Oregon Health & Science University,
2730 NW Pettygrove Street, Portland, OR 97210-2449, USA*
[b]*Department of Emergency Medicine, Oregon Health & Science University, Mail Code:
CDW-EM, 3181 SW Sam Jackson Park Road, Portland, OR 97239-3098, USA*

The primary goal of wound management in the emergency department (ED) is to achieve a functional closure with minimal scarring. Prevention of infection is important to facilitate the healing process. Although antibiotics can help reduce infection risk and promote healing, they are not a substitute for good local wound care, in particular irrigation and surgical débridement. Furthermore, judicious use of antibiotics prevents adverse effects and reduces the development of resistance. This article reviews the role of antibiotics in ED wound management.

Wound irrigation

In animal models, wound infections have been shown to correlate with tissue bacterial counts of more than $10^5/g$ of tissue [1]. In these models, the use of irrigation has been found to be an effective means of decreasing the incidence of infection by removing bacterial and other contaminants. Such studies have driven much of the initial approach to reducing infection rates, although their extrapolation has been questioned because the bacterial counts of many wounds seen in the ED are less than 10^2 colonies [2,3].

The optimal irrigation solution also has been the subject of considerable study. Important factors to consider include availability, tissue toxicity, and cost of the solution. In recent years, several comparative trials have found no difference when tap water was used instead of normal saline for wound cleansing in the ED [4,5]. Unfortunately, these studies have been small and

* Corresponding author.
E-mail address: dayam@ohsu.edu (M. Daya).

0733-8627/07/$ - see front matter © 2007 Elsevier Inc. All rights reserved.
doi:10.1016/j.emc.2007.01.007
emed.theclinics.com

have excluded high-risk wounds. Wilson and colleagues [6] recently studied the toxicity of commercially available skin, wound, and skin/wound cleansers on cultured fibroblasts and keratinocytes. With regards to fibroblasts, Shur-Clens, SAF-Clens, and saline were the least toxic (toxicity index 0), and Dial Antibacterial Soap and Ivory Liqui-Gel were the most toxic (toxicity index 100,000). For keratinocytes, Biolex, Shur-Clens, and Techni-Care were the least toxic (toxicity index 0), and hydrogen peroxide, modified Dakin's solution, and povidone (10%) were the most toxic (toxicity index 100,000). Although povidone-iodine 10% solutions have not been shown to reduce the infection rate [7,8], a prospective ED study of sutured traumatic lacerations did report reduced infection rates when wounds were routinely irrigated for 60 seconds with a dilute (1%) povidone-iodine solution [9]. Finally, antibiotic-containing solutions also have been studied in animals and humans with limited evidence for efficacy [10].

Pending further randomized, controlled trials, the ideal irrigation solution at this time is sterile normal saline or, in selected low-risk wounds, running tap water [4]. An alternative option is to use normal saline irrigation for clean uncomplicated wounds and dilute povidone-iodine (1%) for dirty or bite wounds [11]. In addition to irrigation, the sharp surgical removal of devitalized tissue is essential to reduce the risk of infection.

Established risk factors for infection

When considering the role of antibiotics in wound management, it is useful to appreciate the host, wound, and treatment factors that have been found to be associated with increased infection risk. Established host risk factors include the extremes of age, diabetes mellitus, chronic renal failure, obesity, malnutrition, and immunocompromising illnesses or therapies such as corticosteroids and chemotherapeutic agents [12,13]. Most of these risk factors have been established through the study of postoperative wound infection rates in surgical patients. Animal studies have established high bacterial counts, soil contamination, crush injury, and stellate lacerations as wound risk factors for infection [2]. It also is generally accepted that wounds involving normally sterile sites such as tendons, joints, or bones are at increased wound risk for infection. Finally, puncture wounds, intraoral lacerations, and most mammalian bites are considered to be infection-prone wounds. Treatment factors associated with increased risk of infection include the use of epinephrine-containing solutions, the number of sutures placed, and the experience of the treating physician [14].

Only a limited number of studies have examined risk factors for wound infection in the ED. Hollander and colleagues [2] studied risk factors for infection in 5121 consecutive patients who had traumatic lacerations repaired over a 4-year period. Complicating medical conditions were infrequent, and 763 patients (14%) received prophylactic antibiotics on the index visit.

Infections developed in 194 patients (3.5%). Infected lacerations tended to be longer, wider, deeper, and jagged. Infected lacerations also were more likely to have visible contamination and to be associated with the finding of a foreign body. Additional risk factors for infection included older age and a history of diabetes mellitus. Of note, lacerations involving the hand or neck or a blunt mechanism of injury were associated with reduced rates of infection. Adjustment for treatment technique and prescription of oral antibiotics did not change the findings of this study. More recently, Lammers and colleagues [14] studied risk factors in uncomplicated wounds that required suturing in the ED as part of an effort to develop and validate a neural network–derived decision model that could predict infection. They analyzed 1142 wounds with a 7.2% infection rate. The most predictive factors for infection were wound location, wound age, depth (down to muscle), configuration, and contamination. Of these, wound location was the strongest predictor, with infection rates being the highest in the extremities, especially the lower limb. An important limitation of this study is that bites, puncture wounds, and intraoral lacerations were excluded.

In summary, many of the established host and wound risk factors for infection can be identified before treatment in the ED and used to guide wound-treatment decisions including the use of antibiotics.

Role of systemic antibiotics in emergency department wound management

In wound care, antibiotics can be used for either prophylaxis or therapy. Prophylactic use implies an absence of established infection and gross contamination of the tissues [15,16]. Several randomized, controlled trials have examined the ability of antibiotics to prevent infection of simple nonbite wounds managed in the ED. In 1995, Cummings and Del Beccaro [17] reported a meta-analysis of nine studies, seven of which were included in the final assessment. The wound infection rates in the control populations ranged from 1.1% to 12% with a mean of 6%. Patients treated with antibiotics had a slightly greater risk of infection than untreated controls (odds ratio [OR], 1.16; 95% confidence interval [CI], 0.77 –1.78). More detailed analysis of several subgroups based on whether the wounds were sutured, located on the hands, route of antibiotic administration (oral versus intramuscular), and antibiotic type also failed to show any benefit. The authors concluded that there was little justification for the routine administration of antibiotics to patients who had simple nonbite wounds managed in the ED. Unfortunately, these authors were unable to examine the potential benefits of antibiotics in high-risk groups because most of these individuals were excluded from these clinical trials. Selection bias remains a problematic issue with most of the published studies of the role of antibiotics in ED wound management [18].

Established indications for antibiotic prophylaxis and therapy in the ED include wounds associated with open joints or fractures, human or animal bites, and intraoral lacerations (Table 1). Despite limited evidence, antibiotics also are used for high-risk groups or heavily contaminated wounds (eg, soil, feces, or other contaminants) [18]. They also are advocated occasionally for patients who have prosthetic devices or who are at risk for developing endocarditis [18]. The following sections review the evidence for the established indications and antibiotic recommendations in greater detail.

Open fractures and joint wounds

Microbial contamination of open fracture and joint wounds is a recognized risk factor for infection. In addition to irrigation and surgical débridement, antibiotic therapy is important to decrease tissue bacterial load. Open fractures are classified into three categories according to the mechanism of injury, severity of soft tissue damage, configuration of the fracture, and degree of contamination [19,20]. Type I includes open fractures with a skin wound that is clean and less than 1 cm long. Type II includes open fractures with a laceration that is more than 1 cm long but without evidence of extensive soft tissue damage, flaps, or avulsions. Type III fractures are either open segmental fractures or open fractures with extensive soft tissue damage or a traumatic amputation. The importance of antibiotics in the treatment of open fractures was established first by Patzakis and colleagues [21] in a prospective, randomized, controlled trial. In this study, infection rates were 13.9%, 10%, and 2.3% in the placebo, penicillin, and cephalosporin groups, respectively. Other investigators have confirmed these results, and the evidence has been summarized by the Eastern Association for Surgery on Trauma [19]. In a follow-up study, Patzakis and Wilkins [22] reported that the single most important factor in reducing the infection rate was early (<3 hours) administration of antibiotics that provide antibacterial activity against both gram-positive and gram-negative organisms. Although the efficacy of antibiotics in the management of open fracture and joint wounds is clear, the duration of therapy and the optimal antibiotic choices remain unresolved issues [15]. Current recommendations with regards to duration are for 24 hours after wound closure in Type I and II injuries and for 72 hours or for 24 hours after wound closure in Type III [19,23]. For Type I and II open fractures, *Staphylococcus aureus*, Streptococci species, and aerobic gram-negative bacilli are the most common infecting organisms, and the antibiotic of choice is a first- or second-generation cephalosporin (see Table 1) [19,24]. An extended-spectrum quinolone (eg, gatifloxacin or moxifloxacin) is a reasonable alternative and currently is the preferred choice in the military [25,26]. Type III open fractures must have better coverage for gram-negative organisms, and the addition of an aminoglycoside to a cephalosporin is recommended (see Table 1) [19]. For severe injuries with soil or fecal contamination and tissue damage with areas of ischemia, penicillin should be added to provide coverage against anaerobes, particularly Clostridia species [15]. Antibiotic coverage for other bacteria also may be needed for special environmental exposures including farm accidents (*Clostridium*), combat casualty wounds (*Acinetobacter, Pseudomonas, Clostridium*), freshwater exposure (*Aeromonas, Pseudomonas*), and saltwater exposure (*Aeromonas, Vibrio*) [24,27].

Extremity gunshot wounds are also classified as a type of open fracture. Recommendations for antibiotic therapy depend in part on whether the injury was caused by a low- or high-velocity missile [15]. The role of antibiotics in low-velocity gunshot wounds remains controversial. In 1989, Dickey and colleagues [28] compared infection rate in 67 patients who had fractures associated with low-velocity wounds that were treated with a closed technique. Patients were randomly assigned prospectively to either an antibiotic or a nonantibiotic group. There was no significant difference in infection rate (3% in both groups). Wounds caused by high-velocity gunshot injuries are associated with increased risk of infection, and antibiotic therapy is recommended for 48 to 72 hours [29]. Although a first-generation cephalosporin with or without an aminoglycoside is recommended for most patients, a penicillin should be added to provide additional anaerobic coverage of Clostridia species in grossly contaminated wounds [30].

Intraoral wounds

Intraoral and tongue lacerations are commonly encountered in the ED. Intraoral wounds can involve the mucosa only or the mucosa and adjacent skin, so-called "through-and-through" lacerations. They usually are the result of puncture and penetration of the lips by the patient's teeth following minor trauma or seizures. All intraoral wounds are dirty and at high risk for infection. Infection has been reported in up to 12% of wounds involving the mucosa only and in up to 33% of through-an-through lacerations [31]. Alteri and Brasch [32] studied the benefits of 3 days of penicillin prophylaxis in a randomized, controlled trial of 100 intraoral lacerations managed in a pediatric ED. The overall infection rate was 6.4% with no statistically significant differences between the control (8%) and the penicillin (4%) groups. This underpowered study concluded that routine antibiotic prophylaxis is unwarranted for simple intraoral lacerations in children although it may be beneficial in sutured wounds. In 1989, Steele and colleagues [31] conducted a prospective, randomized, double-blind, controlled study of 5 days of penicillin in adults who had full-thickness injuries of the oral mucosa or through-and-through lacerations, most of which were repaired. They found a statistically significant difference ($P = .03$) in the infection rates between compliant patients in the two groups (6.7% for penicillin versus 20% for control). The value of antibiotic prophylaxis for lacerations of the tongue is less well studied, although one underpowered study reported no infections in 28 children managed without antibiotics [33].

Table 1
Antibiotic prophylaxis and therapy

Type of wound	Antibiotic prophylaxis and therapy
Open fracture wounds Indications: all patients Antibiotics should be started within 3 h of injury	**Adults** Type I and II: A first-generation cephalosporin (eg, cefazolin, 1–2 g IV, q 8 h) for 24 h after wound closure. Type III: A first-generation cephalosporin (eg, cefazolin 1–2 g IV, q 8 h) plus an aminoglycoside (eg gentamicin, 7 mg/kg/d or 1.75–3 mg/kg IV q 8–12 h) for 72 h or for 24 hours after wound closure Farmyard injuries (fecal or clostridial contamination): Add high dose penicillin **Children** Type I and II: > 4 y/o: a first-generation cephalosporin (eg cefazolin 100 mg/kg/d IV divided q 8 h) for 24 h after wound closure. Type III: > 4 y/o: a first-generation cephalosporin (eg, cefazolin 100 mg/kg/d IV divided q 8 h) plus tobramycin (7.5 mg/kg/d IV divided q 8 h) for 72 h or for 24 h after wound closure Farmyard injuries (fecal or clostridial contamination): Add high-dose penicillin
Intraoral wounds Indications: Full-thickness wounds, through-and-through wounds	**Adults** Penicillin VK (500 mg PO q 6 h) for 5 d or Clindamycin (150–450 mg PO q 6 h) for 5 d

Human bites
Indications: Hand bites, high-risk bites

Adults

First parental dose, ampicillin-sulbactam (3 g) or cefoxitin (1 g) or ertapenam (1 g); then amoxicillin-clavulanate (875/125 mg PO q 12 h) for 3–5 d

or

First parental dose, clindamycin (600 mg); then clindamycin (300 mg PO q 8 h) plus a fluoroquinolone (ciprofloxacin, 500 mg PO q 12 h, or levofloxacin, 750 mg/d PO, or moxifloxacin, 400 mg/d PO) for 3–5 d

or

If parental therapy cannot be given, appropriate oral antibiotics (eg, amoxicillin-clavulanate, 875/125 mg PO q 12h) for 3–5 d

Children

First parental dose: ampicillin-sulbactam (50 mg/kg as ampicillin to a maximum of 3 g); then amoxicillin-clavulanate (> 40 kg: 875/125 mg PO q 12 h; ≥ 3 mo and < 40 kg: 45 mg/kg/d PO divided q 12 h or 40 mg/kg/d PO divided q 8 h) for 3–5 d

or

First parental dose: clindamycin (5–10 mg/kg IV to a maximum of 600 mg) followed by clindamycin (10–30 mg/kg/d PO divided q 6–8 h to a maximum of 300 mg/dose) plus trimethoprim-sulfamethoxazole (8–10 mg/kg of trimethoprim/d PO divided q 12 h) for 3–5 d

Human bites, infected

Adults

Ampicillin-sulbactam (3 g IV q 4–6 h) or cefoxitin (1 g IV q 6–8 h) or ertapenam (1 g/d IV)

Subsequent oral therapy or initial therapy for minor infection: amoxicillin-clavulanate (875/125 mg PO q 12 h)

Children

Ampicillin-sulbactam (100–200 mg/kg/d IV divided q 6 h to a maximum of 3 g/dose)

or

Cefoxitin or ticarcillin-clavulanate can be alternative

Subsequent oral therapy or initial therapy for minor infection: amoxicillin-clavulanate (> 40 kg: 875/125 mg PO q 12 h; ≥ 3 mo and < 40 kg: 45 mg/kg/d divided q12 h or 40 mg/kg/d divided q 8 h)

(continued on next page)

Table 1 (*continued*)

Type of wound	Antibiotic prophylaxis and therapy
Dog and cat bites Indications: High-risk dog bites, all cat bites	**Adults** First parental dose: ampicillin-sulbactam (3 g) or a carbapenem (imipenem, 500 mg, or meropenem, 1 g, or ertapenam, 1 g); then amoxicillin-clavulanate (875/125 mg PO q 12 h) can be given for 3–5 d or First parental dose: clindamycin, 600 mg IV; then clindamycin (300 mg PO q 8 h) plus a fluoroquinolone (ciprofloxacin, 500 mg PO q 12 h, or levofloxacin, 750 mg/d PO, or moxifloxacin, 400 mg/d PO) for 3–5 d or If parental therapy cannot be given, appropriate oral antibiotics (eg, amoxicillin-clavulanate 875/125 mg PO q 12 h) should be given for 3–5 d **Children** First parental dose: ampicillin-sulbactam (50 mg/kg as ampicillin to a maximum of 3 g); then amoxicillin-clavulanate (> 40 kg: 875/125 mg PO q 12 h; ≥ 3 months and < 40 kg: 45 mg/kg/d divided q 12 h or 40 mg/kg/d divided q 8 h) for 3–5 d or First parental dose: clindamycin (5–10 mg/kg IV to a maximum of 600 mg) followed by clindamycin (10–30 mg/kg/d PO divided q 6–8 h to a maximum of 300 mg/dose) plus trimethoprim-sulfamethoxazole (8–10 mg/kg/d trimethoprim divided q 12 h) for 3–5 d
Dog and cat bites, infected	**Adults** Ampicillin-sulbactam (3 g IV q 6 h) or ticarcillin-clavulanate (3.1 g IV q 4 h) or piperacillin-tazobactam (3.375 g IV q 6 h) or cefoxitin (1 g IV q 6–8 h) Subsequent oral therapy or initial therapy for minor infection: amoxicillin-clavulanate (875/125 mg PO q 12 h) **Children** Ampicillin-sulbactam (100–200 mg/kg/d divvied q 6 h to maximum of 3 g/dose) or Piperacillin-tazobactam can be alternative Subsequent oral therapy or initial therapy for minor infection: amoxicillin-clavulanate (> 40 kg: 875/125 mg PO q 12 h; ≥ 3 mo and < 40 kg: 45 mg/kg/d divided q 12 h or 40 mg/kg/d divided q 8 h)

Data from Refs. [18,19,23,31,34,40,45,76].

In summary, a 5-day course of prophylactic penicillin is indicated for intraoral full-thickness mucosal and through-and-through lacerations in adults (see Table 1). Penicillin-allergic patients should receive clindamycin. In addition, patients should be encouraged to use saltwater rinses. There is insufficient evidence to make any definitive recommendations with regards to antibiotic prophylaxis for tongue or intraoral lacerations in children [18].

Mammalian bites

Human and animal bites are believed to account for 1% of ED visits annually in the United States [34]. These wounds can result in serious infections, and prophylactic antibiotics frequently are prescribed in the ED although the evidence to support this approach is limited. The most common organisms associated with these infections originate from the oral cavity of the biting mammal or the skin flora of the victim and occasionally the environment. The choice of antibiotics should be based on the susceptibility patterns of the pathogens most likely to be encountered.

Human bites

Most human bites occur as a result of a clenched-fist injury or an occlusive bite. In addition, exposure to mouth flora can also occur through toothpick injuries and finger- or thumb-sucking [35]. Commonly encountered organisms include anaerobes and aerobes. In a multicenter prospective study of 50 infected human bites [36], the affected individuals were primarily male (70%) with a median age of 27 years. The hands were involved in 86% of cases; most of which were caused by clenched-fist (56%) and occlusive bite (44%) injuries. The most frequent pathogens isolated in this study were *Streptococcus anginosus, Staphylococcccus aureus, Eikenella corrodens, Fusobacterium nucleatum,* and *Prevotella melaninogenica.* Many strains of *Prevotella* and *Staphylococcccus. aureus* were found to be β-lactamase producers.

In patients with human bite wounds who present early, before there is any evidence of infection, the role of antibiotics remains unclear. A prospective, double-blind, placebo-controlled trial found that infection rates were low, with or without antibiotics (combination of cephalexin and penicillin) in 127 immunocompetent adults who had low-risk wounds and who presented within 24 hours of sustaining a human bite [37]. This study characterized low-risk wounds as involving the epidermis only. Bites involving the hands, feet, or skin overlying joints or cartilaginous structures were excluded. In comparison, antibiotic prophylaxis was found to be beneficial in a small, randomized trial of human bites involving the hand [38]. This finding is consistent with a meta-analysis reported in the Cochrane library [39]. Using data from the aforementioned trial of human bites and three trials of dog bites involving the hand, antibiotic prophylaxis markedly reduced the rate of infection (2% in patients receiving antibiotics versus 28% in patients receiving placebo; OR, 0.1; 95% CI, 0.01–0.86). Unfortunately, most of the studies were small or methodologically deficient. In addition to hand bites, antibiotic prophylaxis also is recommended for patients at high risk for infection.

If patients are to receive antimicrobial prophylaxis, the first dose ideally should be given parenterally to obtain effective tissue levels as quickly as possible. Appropriate oral antibiotics should be given and continued for 3 to 5 days [40]. Current recommendations are summarized in Table 1. Ampicillin-sulbactam, cefoxitin, and ertapenem are the drugs of choice for the initial parental dose; amoxicillin-clavulanate is the recommended oral drug. For patients who have penicillin sensitivity, alternative options include clindamycin plus a fluoroquinolones in adults or clindamycin plus trimethoprim-sulfamethoxazole in children.

Dog bites

The majority of dog bites occur in children [41]. Dog bites usually affect the upper extremities, and males are bitten more often than females [42]. The routine use of antibiotics prophylaxis for dog-bite wounds is controversial because infection rates are 2% to 5% [43]. A meta-analysis of eight randomized trials found an absolute benefit of one infection prevented for every 14 patients treated [44]. Antibiotic prophylaxis currently is recommended in the following circumstances following dog bites [45]:

Hand wounds
Deep puncture wounds
Wounds requiring surgical débridement
Wounds in older patients
Wounds in immunocompromised patients
Bite wound near or in a prosthetic joint
Bite wound in an extremity with underlying venous and/or lymphatic compromise

As with human bites, the isolates recovered from clinical cultures of dog-bite wounds include both aerobes and anaerobes. Common aerobes include *Staphylococcus aureus* and Pasteurella species including *Pasteurella multocida* and *Pasteurella canis*. Common anaerobes include Prevotella, Bacteroides, and Fusobacterium species. An important organism occasionally associated with dog bites is *Capnocytophaga canimorsus* [46]. Prophylactic antibiotic recommendations are the same as for human bites and are summarized in Table 1.

Cat bites

Wound infection rates as high as 50% have been reported following cat bites [35]. In a prospective study of 216 cat bite/scratch wounds, Dire [47] reported a wound infection rate of 14.4%. Fifty-five percent of the time, the cat was a pet, and women are bitten more often than men. It is thought that cat's slender, sharp teeth produce deep puncture wounds that are more likely to be complicated by infection. Of particular concern with cat bites is contamination of bone and joint resulting in osteomyelitis or septic arthritis, respectively. *Pasteurella multocida* subspecies *multocida* and *septica* were the predominant aerobic organisms recovered in one study [45]. Anaerobes isolated included Fusobacterium, Bacteroides, Porphyromonas, Prevotella, and Proprionibacterium species. Prophylactic antibiotics are recommended for all cat bites (see Table 1) but not for cat-scratch wounds.

Infected mammalian bites

Clinical evidence of wound infection that develops within a few hours of a bite injury is strongly suggestive of *Pasteurella multocida* infection [46,47]. Pending culture data, polymicrobial coverage directed against aerobic and anaerobic organisms should be administrated empirically (see Table 1) [48].

Topical antibiotics

The routine use of topical antibiotics after wound treatment is a common practice in the ED, although research in this area is limited. In 1992, a national survey of wound-care practices found that 71% of the respondents used gauze and a topical antibiotic as part of their after-care for simple lacerations [49]. Many of these topical preparations contain several antibacterial agents. In 1995, Dire and colleagues [50] prospectively studied the differences in infection rates among uncomplicated repaired wounds managed prophylactically with topical bacitracin zinc (BAC); neomycin sulfate, bacitracin zinc, and polymyxin B sulfate combination (triple antibiotic ointment or TAO); silver sulfadiazine; or petrolatum. This trial was double-blinded, randomized, and controlled, and subjects were asked to apply the provided preparation three times a day until the sutures were removed or the patient developed an infection. The follow-up wound infection rates were 5.5% for BAC, 4.5% for TAO, 12.2% for silver sulfadiazine, and 17.6% for petrolatum ($P = .0034$). More recently, Hood and colleagues [51] compared the safety, efficacy, and cost effectiveness of TAO and mupirocin in a similarly designed but smaller pilot trial. They reported similar rates of infections between these two groups and concluded that the less expensive TAO is preferable for wound prophylaxis following the repair of uncomplicated wounds in the ED. High-risk wounds were excluded from both these studies.

BAC is an inexpensive, readily available bactericidal topical antibiotic that blocks cell wall synthesis by inhibiting peptidoglycan synthesis. BAC is effective against gram-positive organisms, anaerobic cocci, and Clostridia, Neisseria, and Haemophilus species, but most gram-negative bacteria are resistant. Allergic reactions to BAC are rare, but cross-sensitization with neomycin has been reported. TAO is compounded from three antibacterial agents to provide more adequate antibacterial coverage. It is bactericidal and covers most gram-positive and gram-negative organisms, including anaerobes, *P aeruginosa*, and Staphylococcus species. Polymyxins are decapeptides that disrupt the phospholipids of cell membranes through a surfactant-like action. They are active primarily against gram-negative bacteria. Neomycin is an aminoglycoside that interferes with protein synthesis. Allergic sensitization to the neomycin is a concern and has a reported incidence of 1% to 6%. Frequent use of TAO can lead to neutropenia, leucopenia, and hyperpigmentation [52]. Another popular compound formulation in the ED is double antibiotic ointment containing bacitracin and polymyxin. This preparation may be less likely to cause allergic sensitization, but the coverage it provides is inferior to that of TAO, and it was less effective in an in vitro study [53].

Additional benefits of topical antibiotic agents include decreased formation of the crust that covers and separates the edges of a wound [54]. This action helps maintain a moist environment that permits optimal re-epithelialization and wound healing [55] and may facilitate suture removal. Finally, topical agents may help prevent dressings from adhering to the wound, decreasing pain at the time of dressing change [50].

In summary, the prophylactic use of topical antibiotic agents such as TAO, BAC, or double antibiotic ointment is reasonable for uncomplicated soft tissue wounds repaired in the ED. Bandages impregnated with antimicrobial agents are available as over-the-counter products [56].

High-risk bacteria

Capnocytophaga canimorsus

Capnocytophaga canimorsus (Latin for "dog bite"), originally called "dysgonic fermenter 2," is a gram-negative, non–spore-forming, facultative aerobic bacillus that was first isolated from the blood and cerebrospinal fluid of a septic patient who had a dog bite in 1976. Host risk factors for infection with this organism include splenectomy and alcoholism [57]. Janda and colleagues [58] recently reviewed the clinical and epidemiologic features of 56 human *C canimorsus* isolates submitted over a 32-year period and submitted to the California Microbial Disease Laboratory for identification. Most of the patients were males older than 50 years of age with a history of a recent dog bite or prolonged exposure to dogs. More than 60% of patients presented with sepsis, sepsis and meningitis, or fever of unknown origin. Disseminated intravascular coagulation or septic shock developed in seven patients (13%) and was associated with a poor prognosis. In six patients (11%) the admitting diagnosis was cellulitis, but in each case *C canimorsus* was isolated subsequently from blood but not from wounds. The median time from a dog bite to onset of symptoms was 3 days (range,

1–10 days), and the case-fatality rate was 33%. Only one third (32%) of the isolates were identified correctly by the initial laboratory. Many strains were reported out as unidentified gram-negative rod or "identification unknown" (55%). Identification of *C canimorsus* requires an extended incubation period because the organism is slow growing and requires carbon dioxide. *C canimorsus* is susceptible to most antibiotics with the exception of aztreonam and should be suspected in any patient who has fulminant sepsis following a dog bite [58]. High-risk individuals should receive antibiotic prophylaxis to reduce the morbidity and mortality associated with this organism [58,59].

Eikenella corrodens

Eikenella corrodens is a slow-growing gram-negative obligate or facultative anaerobic organism that is part of the endogenous flora in humans. It can found in the mucous membranes of the oral cavity, respiratory tract, gastrointestinal tract, and genitourinary tract and has been recovered from 15% to 30% of human bite infections [36,60–62]. Infection develops within 24 to 36 hours after a human bite; presenting features include localized pain, cellulitis, and purulent or malodorous discharge. Systemic signs such as fever and adenopathy usually are absent [63]. *E corrodens* also has been associated with abscesses of the abdominal cavity, head, and neck and with meningitis, endocarditis, osteomyelitis, and fatal gram-negative sepsis. *E corrodens* is an opportunistic pathogen that reduces nitrates and requires a low-oxygen environment for growth. The contaminant presence of oxygen-consuming organisms such as alpha hemolytic Streptococci, Staphylococcus, Bactericides, and other gram-negative species within a wound facilitates its growth [61,64]. It usually is susceptible to penicillin, amoxicillin/clavulanic acid, cefoxitin, trimethoprim-sulfamethoxazole, ceftriaxone, tetracycline, and ciprofloxacin but is resistant to dicloxacillin, nafcillin, first-generation cephalosporins, clindamycin, aminoglycosides, and erythromycin [61]. A recent study found that 100% and 92% of isolates were susceptible to amoxicillin and tetracycline, respectively [65].

Pasteurella multocida

Pasteurella are aerobic, non–spore-forming, gram-negative coccobacilli that are primarily animal pathogens [66]. The frequency of asymptomatic carriage varies among species: 50% to 90% in cats, 50% to 66% in dogs, 51% in swine, and 14% in rats [67]. Human *Pasteurella multocida* infections are associated most often with bites, scratches, or licks from cats and dogs [68]. Although dog bites account for 70% to 90% of animal bites, 65% of bite-associated *P multocida* infections are caused by cats [35,46]. The greater risk of infection associated with cat bites may be related to the higher incidence of *P multocida* colonization of cats and to the fact that cat teeth are extremely sharp and more likely to penetrate into tendons, joints, and bone. The higher incidence of infection following cat bites also might be attributable to a higher virulence of the cat-associated strains of *P multocida*, in particular subspecies *septica* and *multocida*. *P multocida* infections also have been reported following the bites of lions, panthers, rabbits, opossums, and rats [66]. Infections with *P multocida* are characterized by the acute onset of erythema, pain, and swelling, usually within hours of the bite [46,47]. Serosanguinous drainage from the lesion often is present within 24 to 48 hours after onset of symptoms. Bite wounds usually are located on the hands and arms, legs, or head and neck area. A low-grade fever, lymphangitis, and regional lymphadenitis may be present in 10% to 20% of cases [68]. Local complications of infected bites, including osteomyelitis, tenosynovitis, and septic arthritis, occur in about 40% of cases and often are responsible for prolonged residual disability [67,69,70]. Children who have sustained cat bites to the hand have, on occasion, developed *P multocida* brain abscesses [66]. Penicillin is the drug of choice. Other oral agents that have good in vitro activity include ampicillin, amoxicillin-clavulanic acid, cefuroxime, trimethoprim-sulfamethoxazole, tetracycline, and ciprofloxacin. Amoxicillin-clavulanic acid has been shown to be clinically effective in the treatment of cat-bite wound infections [71]. Dicloxacillin, cephalexin, cefadroxil, cefaclor, erythromycin, and clindamycin have poor activity against *P multocida* in vitro [67,71,72].

Staphylococcus aureus *and methicillin-resistant* Staphylococcus aureus

Staphylococcus aureus is very hardy aerobic gram-positive cocci that colonizes and infects hospitalized patients with decreased host defenses as well as healthy immunocompetent people in the community. Children and adults are intermittently colonized and can harbor the organism in their nasopharynx and skin [73]. It also is a common isolate from the oral flora of many mammals globally. Most Staphylococci infections are characterized by abscess formation and are usually responsive to β–lactam antibiotics. Methicillin-resistant *Staphylococcus aureus* (MRSA) emerged in the 1960s as an infection among patients exposed to the bacteria in health care settings (hospital acquired or HA-MRSA). More recently, MRSA infections have been reported among persons without such exposure (community-acquired or CA-MRSA). All MRSA harbor the *mec*A gene that encodes a modified cell protein that does not bind β–lactam antibiotics [74]. In a recent study, Moran and colleagues [75] reported on the prevalence of CA-MRSA as a cause of skin infections among adult patients presenting to the ED in 11 United States cities. *Staphylococcus aureus* was isolated from skin and soft tissue infections in 320 patients, and 249 isolates (78%) were methicillin resistant. As compared with patients who had other bacterial infections of the skin, patients who had CA-MRSA infection were more likely to report a spider bite as the reason for their skin lesion. All MRSA isolates were susceptible to trimethoprim-sulfamethoxazole, and 95% were susceptible to clindamycin. Because inducible resistance to clindamycin is a concern with CA-MRSA, the prevailing antibiotic susceptibility patterns in the community should be followed whenever possible. If a patient provides a history of CA-MRSA infection or exposure, antibiotic selection should be adjusted accordingly [74].

Summary

Antibiotic prophylaxis and therapy are indicated for open fracture and joint injuries, intraoral lacerations, and mammalian bites. Antibiotics also are generally recommended for patients who have increased risk factors for infection. Antibiotic selection should be based on the most likely pathogens and prevailing susceptibility patterns. Most simple, uncomplicated wounds treated in the ED do not need systemic antibiotics but do benefit from the use of topical antibiotics. Judicious use of antibiotics will reduce unnecessary adverse events and help reduce the development of resistance.

References

[1] Hamer ML, Robson MC, Krizek TJ, et al. Quantitative bacterial analysis of comparative wound irrigations. Ann Surg 1975;181:819–22.
[2] Hollander JE, Singer AJ, Valentine SM, et al. Risk factors for infection in patients with traumatic lacerations. Acad Emerg Med 2001;8:716–20.
[3] Hollander JE, Richman PB, Werblud M, et al. Irrigation in facial and scalp lacerations: does it alter outcome? Ann Emerg Med 1998;31:73–7.
[4] Beam JW. Wound cleaning: water of saline? J Athl Train 2006;41:196–7.
[5] Valente JH, Forti RJ, Freundlich LF, et al. Wound irrigation in children: saline solution or tap water? Ann Emerg Med 2003;41:609–16.
[6] Wilson JR, Mills JG, Prather ID, et al. A toxicity index of skin and wound cleansers used on in vitro fibroblasts and keratinocytes. Adv Skin Wound Care 2005;18:373–8.
[7] Rogers DM, Blouin GS, O'Leary JP. Povidone-iodine wound irrigation and sepsis. Surg Gynecol Obstet 1983;157:426–30.
[8] Galle PC, Homesley HD. Ineffectiveness of povidone-iodine irrigation of abdominal incisions. Obstet Gynecol 1980;55:744–7.
[9] Gravett A, Sterner S, Clinton JE, et al. A trial of povidone-iodine in the prevention of infection in sutured laceration. Ann Emerg Med 1987;16:167–71.
[10] Anglen JO. Comparison of soap and antibiotic solutions for irrigation of lower-limb open fracture wounds: a prospective, randomized study. J Bone Joint Surg Am 2005;87:1415–22.
[11] Brancato JC. Minor wound preparation and irrigation. UpToDate 2006; version 14.2. Available at: www.uptodate.com. Accessed October 19, 2006.
[12] Singer AJ, Hollander JE, Quinn JV. Evaluation and management of traumatic lacerations. N Engl J Med 1997;337:1142–8.
[13] Cruse PJE, Foord R. A five-year prospective study of 23,469 surgical wounds. Arch Surg 1973;107:206–9.
[14] Lammers RL, Hudson DL, Seaman ME. Prediction of traumatic wound infection with a neural network-derived decision model. Am J Emerg Med 2003;21:1–7.
[15] Holtom PD. Antibiotic prophylaxis: current recommendations. J Am Acad Orthop Surg 2006;14:S98–100.

[16] Mangram AJ, Horan TC, Pearson ML, et al. Guideline for prevention of surgical site infection. 1999: Hospital infection control practices advisory committee. Infect Control Hosp Epidemiol 1999;20:250–78.

[17] Cummings P, Del Beccaro MA. Antibiotics to prevent infection of simple wounds: a meta-analysis of randomized studies. Am J Emerg Med 1995;13:396–400.

[18] Wedmore IS. Wound care: modern evidence in the treatment of man's age-old injuries. Emerg Med Practice 2005;7:1–24.

[19] Luchette FA, Bone LB, Born CT, et al. East practice management guidelines work group: practice management guidelines for prophylactic antibiotic use in open fractures. Available at: http://www.east.org/. Accessed November18, 2006.

[20] Gustilo RB, Mendoza RM, Williams DN. Problems in the management of type III (severe) open fractures. A new classification of type III open fractures. J Trauma 1984;24:742–6.

[21] Patzakis MJ, Harvey JP Jr, Ivler D. The role of antibiotics in the management of open fractures. J Bone Joint Surg Am 1974;56:532–41.

[22] Patzakis MJ, Wilkins J. Factors influencing infection rate in open fracture wounds. Clin Orthop Relat Res 1989;243:36–40.

[23] Calhoun J, Sexton DJ, et al. Adult posttraumatic osteomyelitis. UpToDate 2006; ver 14.3. Avalilable at: www.uptodate.com. Accessed November 16, 2006.

[24] Templeman DC, Gulli B, Tsukayama DT, et al. Update on the management of open fractures of the tibial shaft. Clin Orthop Relat Res 1998;350:18–25.

[25] Patzakis MJ, Banis RS, Lee J, et al. Prospective randomized, double-blind study comparing single-agent antibiotic therapy, ciprofloxacin, to combination antibiotic therapy in open fracture wounds. J Orthop Trauma 2000;14:529–33.

[26] Butler F. Antibiotics in tactical combat casualty care 2002. Mil Med. 2003;168:911–4.

[27] Davis KA, Moran KA, McAllister K, et al. Multidrug-resistant Acinetobacter extremity infection in soldiers. Emerg Infect Dis 2005;11:1218–24.

[28] Dickey RL, Barnes BC, Kearns RJ, et al. Efficacy of antibiotics in low-velocity gunshot fractures. J Orthop Trauma 1989;3:6–10.

[29] Heenessy MJ, Banks HH, Leach RB. Extremity gunshot wound and gunshot fracture in civilian practice. Clin Orthop Relat Res 1976;114:296–303.

[30] Simpson BM, Wilson RH, Grant RE. Antibiotic therapy in gunshot wound injuries. Clin Orthop Relat Res 2003;408:82–5.

[31] Steele MT, Sainsbury CR, Robinson WA, et al. Prophylactic penicillin for intraoral wounds. Ann Emerg Med 1989;18:847–52.

[32] Altieri M, Brasch L. Antibiotic prophylaxis in intraoral wounds. Am J Emerg Med. 1986;6: 507–10.

[33] Lamell CW, Fraone G, Casamassimo MS, et al. Presenting characteristics and treatment outcomes for tongue lacerations in children. Pediatr Dent 1999;21:34–8.

[34] Endom EE. Animal and human bites in children. UpToDate. 2006; ver 14.3. Available at: www.uptodate.com. Accessed October 19, 2006.

[35] Goldstein EJ. Bite wounds and infection. Clin Infect Dis 1992;14:633–8.

[36] Talan DA, Abrahamian FM, Moral GJ, et al. Clinical presentation and bacteriologic analysis of infected human bites in patients presenting to emergency departments. Clin Infect Dis 2003;37:1481–9.

[37] Broder J, Jerrard D, Olshaker J, et al. Low risk of infection in selected human bites treated without antibiotics. Am J Emerg Med 2004;22:10–3.

[38] Zubowicz VN, Gravier M. Management of early human bites of the hand: a prospective randomized study. Plast Reconstr Surg 1991;88:111–4.

[39] Medeirous I, Saconato IF. Antibiotic prophylaxis for mammalian bites. Cochrane Database Syst Rev 2001;2 CD001738.

[40] Larry MB. Soft tissue infections due to human bite. UpToDate. 2006; ver 14.2. Available at: www.uptodate.com. Accessed October 19, 2006.

[41] Weiss HB, Friedman DI, Coben JH. Incidence of dog bites injuries treated in emergency department. JAMA 1998;279:51–3.

[42] Dire DJ, Hogan DE, Riggs MW. A prospective evaluation of risk factors for infections from dog-bite wounds. Acad Emerg Med 1994;1:258–66.

[43] Brook I. Management of human and animal bite wounds: an overview. Adv Skin Wound Care 2005;18:197–203.

[44] Cummings P. Antibiotics to prevent infection in patients with dog bite wounds: a meta-analysis of randomized trials. Ann Emerg Med 1994;23:535–40.

[45] Larry MB. Soft tissue infections due to dog and cat bites in adults. UpToDate. 2006; ver 14.2. Available at: www.uptodate.com. Accessed October 19, 2006.

[46] Talan DA, Citron DM, Abrahamian FM, et al. Bacteriological analysis of infected dog and cat bites. N Engl J Med 1999;340:85–92.

[47] Dire DJ. Cat bite wounds: risk factors for infection. Ann Emerg Med 1991;20:973–9.

[48] Duke Orthopedics. Wheeless' textbook of orthopedics. Available at: http://www.wheelessonline.com/ortho/open_fractures. Accessed November 18, 2006.

[49] Howell JM, Chisholm CD. Outpatient wound preparation and care: a national survey. Ann Emerg Med 1992;24:976–81.

[50] Dire DJ, Coppola M, Dwyer DA, et al. Prospective evaluation of topical antibiotics for preventing infection in uncomplicated soft-tissue wounds repaired in the ED. Acad Emerg Med 1995;2:4–10.

[51] Hood R, Shermock KM, Emerman C. A prospective, randomized pilot evaluation of topical triple antibiotic versus mupirocin for the prevention of uncomplicated soft tissue wound infection. Am J Emerg Med 2004;22:1–3.

[52] Spann CT, Tutrone WD, Weinberg JM, et al. Topical antibacterial agents for wound care: a primer. Dermatol Surg 2003;29:620–6.

[53] Hendley JO, Ashe KM. Eradication of resident bacteria of normal human skin by antimicrobial ointment. Antimicrob Agents Chemother 2003;47:1988–90.

[54] Lammers RL. Principals of wound management. In: Roberts JR, Hedges JR, editors. Clinical procedures in emergency medicine. 2nd edition. Philadelphia: W.B. Saunders; 1991. p. 515–65.

[55] Markovchick V. Suture material and mechanical aftercare. Emerg Med Clin North Am 1992;10:673–89.

[56] Davis SC, Cazzaniga AL, Eaglstein WH, et al. Over-the-counter topical antimicrobials: effective treatments? Arch Dermatol Res 2005;297:190–5.

[57] Brenner DJ, Hollis DG, Fanning GR, et al. *Capnocytophaga canimorsus* sp, nov. (formerly CDC Group DF-2), a cause of septicemia following dog bite, and *C. cynodengmi* sp. nov., a cause of localized wound infection following dog bite. J Clin Microbial 1989;27: 231–5.

[58] Janda JM, Graves MH, Lindquist D, et al. Diagnosing *Capnocytophaga canimorsus* infection. Emerg Infect Dis 2006;12:340–2.

[59] Verghese A, Hamati F, Berk S, et al. Susceptibility of dysgonic fermenter 2 to antimicrobial agents in vitro. Antimicrob Agents Chemother 1988;32:78–80.

[60] Rosen T, Conrad N. Genital ulcer caused by human bite to the penis. Sex Transm Dis 1999; 26:527–30.

[61] Griego R, Rosen T, Orengo IF, et al. Dog, cat, and human bites: a review. J Am Acad Dermatol 1995;33:1019–29.

[62] Brook I. Microbiology of human and animal bite wounds in children. Pediatr Infect Dis J 1987;6:29–32.

[63] Smith RF, Meadowcroft AM, May DB. Treating mammalian bite wounds. J Clin Pharm Ther 2000;25:85–99.

[64] Schmidt D, Heckman J. *Eikenella corrodens* in human bites infection of the hand. J Trauma 1983;23:478–82.

[65] Luong N, Tsai J, Chen C. Susceptibilities of Eikenella corrodens, Prevotella inteermedia, and *Prevotella nigrtescens* clinical isolates to amoxicillin and tetracycline. Antimicrob Agents Chemother 2001;45:3253–5.

[66] John MB. Pasteurella species. In: Mandell GL, Bennett JE, Dolin R, editors. Principles and practice of infectious disease. 4th edition. New York: Churchill Livingstone; 1995. p. 2068–70.

[67] Weber DJ, Wolfson JS, Swartz MN, et al. *Pasteurella multocida* infections. Report of 34 cases and review of the literature. Medicine 1984;63:133–54.

[68] Weber DJ, Hansen AR. Infections resulting from animal bites. Infect Dis Clin North Am 1991;5:663–80.

[69] Ewing R, Fainstein V, Musher DM, et al. Articular and skeletal infections caused by *Pasteurella multocida*. South Med J 1980;73:1349–52.

[70] Lucas GL, Bartlett DH. *Pasteurella multocida* infection in the hand. Plast Reconstr Surg 1981;67:49–53.

[71] Goldstein EJC, Citron DM. Comparative activities of cefuroxime, amoxicillin-clavulanic acid, ciprofloxacin, enoxacin, and ofloxacin against aerobic and anaerobic bacteria isolated from bite wounds. Antimicrob Agents Chemother 1988;32:1143–8.

[72] Goldstein EJC, Citron DM, Richwald GA. Lack of in vitro efficacy of oral forms of certain cephalosporins, erythromycin and oxacillin against Pasteurella multocida. Antimicrob Agents Chemother 1988;32:213–5.

[73] Waldvogel FA. *Staphylococcus aureus*. In: Mandell GL, Bennett JE, Dolin R, editors. Pinciples and practice of infectious disease. 4th edition. New York: Churchill Livingstone; 1995. p. 1754–77.

[74] Johnson PDR, Howden BP, Bennett CM. *Staphylococcus aureus*: a guide for the perplexed. The differences between community-acquired and health care-associated MRSA explained. Med J Aust 2006;184:374–5.

[75] Moran GJ, Krishnadasan A, Gorwitz RJ, et al. Methicillin-resistant *S. aureus* Infections among patients in the emergency department. N Engl J Med 2006;355:666–74.

ELSEVIER
SAUNDERS

Emerg Med Clin N Am
25 (2007) 177–188

EMERGENCY
MEDICINE
CLINICS OF
NORTH AMERICA

Hyperbaric Oxygen Therapy in the Treatment of Open Fractures and Crush Injuries

Mark F. Buettner, DO, ABEM*,
Derek Wolkenhauer, RRT, CHT

*Great River Wound and Hyperbaric Clinic, Center for Rehabilitation,
1401 West Agency Road, West Burlington, IA 52655, USA*

Traumatic injuries to the extremities that involve tissue ischemia are known to share a common dynamic pathophysiology. In the practice of hyperbaric medicine such injuries fall within a group known as the acute traumatic peripheral ischemias (ATPIs). These injuries include open fractures and crush injuries, skeletal muscle compartment syndromes, thermal burns, frost bite and threatened flaps, and grafts and replantations. In their various forms, these injuries share a common pathophysiology involving (1) a triad of tissue ischemia, hypoxia, and edema, (2) a gradient of tissue injury, and (3) a capacity for the injury to become self perpetuating. Early administration of hyperbaric oxygen therapy (HBOt) is reported to be beneficial when provided as an adjunct to appropriate surgical interventions for the ATPIs. Emergency department management of these injuries is part of the core curriculum of emergency medicine residency training. Emergency physicians should familiarize themselves with this treatment modality because of their role in the early management of these injuries. The focus of this article is on the use of HBOt in the treatment of open fractures and crush injuries.

Background

Hyperbaric oxygen is a therapy in which a patient breathes 100% oxygen while inside a treatment chamber at a pressure greater than that of sea level. The earliest cited application of treating patients under pressure dates back to 1662 when the British clergyman Henshaw [1] constructed a sealed

---

* Corresponding author.
E-mail address: mbuettner@pol.net (M.F. Buettner).

0733-8627/07/$ - see front matter © 2007 Elsevier Inc. All rights reserved.
doi:10.1016/j.emc.2007.01.008   *emed.theclinics.com*

chamber he called a "domicilium." By connecting his vessel to valved organ bellows, he was able to increase or decrease the air pressure within. Without any scientific basis he treated a variety of acute and chronic illnesses. In the nineteenth century discoveries were made allowing safer and more effective delivery of anesthesia within a compressed air environment. Decompression sickness was first identified among bridge caisson workers in the 1850s. Compression therapy for this disorder was first provided in 1889. Modern-day use of hyperbaric oxygen therapy emerged in 1955 with the work of Churchill-Davidson [2]. The high-oxygen environment was used to potentiate the effects of radiation therapy in cancer patients. That same year, the Dutch surgeon Ite Boerema [3] proposed using HBOt to enhance tolerance to circulatory arrest during cardiac surgery. The promising results of his animal studies led to the construction of a large hyperbaric operating chamber at the University of Amsterdam. Boerema [3] performed a variety of surgeries within this chamber for conditions such as transposition of the great vessels, tetralogy of Fallot, and pulmonic stenosis. His first publication appeared in 1956. In the early 1960s the first reports on the positive effects of HBOt for anaerobic infections and carbon monoxide poisonings were published [4,5]. The 1970s witnessed both degradation and decline in the field. On the heels of the discoveries found in the 1960s researchers eagerly sought other applications for HBOt. Experiments were performed using it in a variety of debilitating conditions. Positive reports were largely anecdotal, touting the "good results" without regard for scientific methodology [6]. Indiscriminate use of HBOt led to the need for regulation. There were no formal guidelines for insurers to reference regarding payment for the valid use of HBOt. In 1976, the Undersea Medical Society formed an ad hoc committee to work with Medicare and Blue Cross. As a result, the first edition of the Hyperbaric Oxygen Therapy Committee Report was published. Formal indications for the valid use of HBOt were established based on scientific merit. With periodic revisions, the committee report remains the authority on approved indications for HBOt within the United States (Fig. 1).

Physiology

The primary means for oxygen transport is in the form of oxyhemoglobin bound within the erythrocyte. At sea level the barometric pressure is 1 atmosphere absolute (ata). At 1 ata the partial pressure of alveolar oxygen (P_{AO_2}) is about 100 mm Hg. Also at 1 ata hemoglobin is about 97% oxygen saturated ($SaO_2 = 97$) and yields an oxygen content (HbO_2 + plasma dissolved O_2) of about 19.8 mL oxygen per dL blood. Under pressure, as the P_{AO_2} reaches 200 mm Hg, hemoglobin becomes fully saturated with oxygen ($SaO_2 = 100\%$). Further increases in pressure beyond a P_{AO_2} of 200 mm Hg will not result in an increase in oxyhemoglobin. Therefore, the superoxygenated state achieved in a hyperbaric oxygen environment is attributed to the amount of oxygen physically dissolved in the plasma. When air is breathed

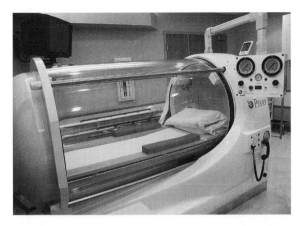

Fig. 1. Monoplace hyperbaric oxygen chamber at Great River Wound and Hyperbaric Clinic West Burlington, Iowa. (Courtesy of Perry Baromedical, Riviera Beach, FL; with permission.)

at sea level (1 ata), only 1.5% of the oxygen content is related to oxygen dissolved in plasma. Comparatively, when 100% oxygen is breathed at a pressure of 3 ata, a P_{AO_2} of 2200 mm Hg is generated, dissolving another 6.8 mL of oxygen into each dL of blood, resulting in an arterial oxygen tension (PaO_2) of about 2000 mm Hg (Fig. 2). A healthy adult at rest uses about 6 mL of oxygen per dL of circulating blood. Therefore, as demonstrated in Boerema's 1960 study "Life Without Blood" [7], life can be sustained without the need for erythrocytes while in a hyperbaric oxygen environment at a pressure of 3 ata.

Crush injury pathophysiology

If the amount of energy transfer during a crush injury is sufficient, a gradient of tissue injury expands from the impact site (Fig. 3). The most immediate injury is the primary zone of tissue destruction. This region of

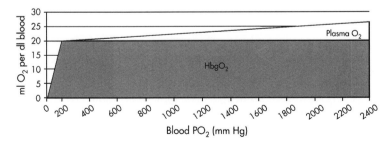

Fig. 2. Combined blood oxygen content bound to hemoglobin and dissolved in plasma at high levels of blood PO_2. (*From* Sheffield PJ, Smith PS. Physiologic and pharmacological basis of hyperbaric oxygen therapy. In: Bakker DJ, Cramer FS, editors. Hyperbaric surgery perioperative care. Flagstaff (AZ): Best Publishing Company; 2002. p. 68; with permission.)

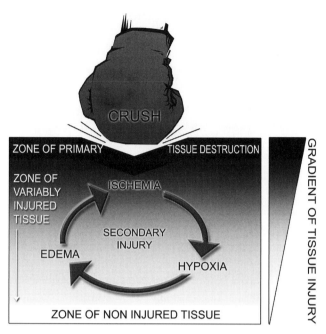

Fig. 3. Zones of injured tissues relative to the crush impact and the secondary perpetuation of injury.

injured tissue may be rendered nonviable regardless of intervention. The next zone along the gradient of injury is composed of variably injured or variably ischemic tissues. Most therapeutic interventions are targeted within this penumbra of tissues. The outermost zone along the gradient of injury is composed of minimally injured to noninjured tissues. A self-perpetuating secondary injury may occur to tissues at any point along the injury gradient.

Secondary injury

Ischemia

A decrease in blood perfusion to the variably injured tissues is the initial event leading to secondary injury. Ischemia may result from direct traumatic injury to blood vessels. Ischemia also may arise indirectly. The indirect mechanism for ischemia often is multifactorial and may include one or more of the following: fluid leakage (edema, hemorrhage) with or without vascular collapse from the external pressure of the tissue fluid (compartment syndrome); vasoconstriction; stasis; occlusion. The indirect mechanisms for ischemia within the microcirculation are the largest contributor to the secondary injury.

Hypoxia

Cellular processes involved in wound repair are heavily oxygen dependant. The zone of variably injured tissues has an increased oxygen demand at a time of diminished perfusion. Oxygen demands may increase by a factor of greater than 20 [8]. Wound-repair mechanisms such as fibroblast activity and collagen formation are compromised under hypoxic conditions [9]. An increased risk of infection develops with the failure of oxygen-dependant host immune functions. Hypoxic cells cannot retain intracellular water, leading to cytogenic edema.

Edema

Edema is a profound contributor to tissue hypoxia. When fluid accumulates within the extracellular space, the distance from the capillary wall to the injured cell is greater. Therefore, less oxygen reaches the injured cell to exert repair. Vasodilatation of the proximal arterial vasculature increases blood flow to the site of injury. This reflex results in vasogenic edema. When combined with increased bleeding from the injured vessels, fluid accumulates in the interstitial space. Collapse of the capillary bed occurs as the pressure within the interstitial space exceeds capillary filling pressures (12–32 mm Hg). Cellular hypoxia is propagated.

Reperfusion injury

Reperfusion contributes to the perpetuation of the secondary injury. Neutrophils adhere to postcapillary venules after a period of ischemia and during reperfusion. This process results in a release of toxic oxygen free radicals. Oxygen free radicals are destructive to tissues in several ways: the induction of a no-reflow phenomenon by the vasoconstriction of precapillary arterioles, lipid peroxidation of cell membranes, and the formation of peroxynitrite when the oxygen free radicals react with endothelial-generated nitric oxide.

The net result is a self-perpetuating secondary injury. If left unchecked, this secondary injury may result in a volume of tissue necrosis much larger than and remote from the primary zone of tissue destruction. When the drug oxygen is delivered within a hyperbaric environment, its pharmacodynamics mitigates the pathophysiology of ischemia.

Pharmacodynamics of hyperbaric oxygen therapy

Diffusion radius

To exert its effects, oxygen must travel out of the arterial end of the capillary wall through the interstitial space to the injured cell. This diffusion radius of oxygen from the arterial end of the capillary into the interstitial space has been calculated to traverse a distance of 64 μm. With HBOt at 3 ata, this diffusion radius has been calculated to traverse a distance of 247 μm (Fig. 4) [10]. During the immediate postinjury period of a crush injury the maintenance of tissue oxygenation is critical [11].

Vascular response

Oxygen breathing results in smooth muscle contraction of the arterial vasculature resulting in up to a 20% reduction of blood flow to the limb [12]. This response is physiologic, and it is observed in healthy tissues. With an increase in upstream arterial resistance comes a drop in downstream capillary hydrostatic pressure. The drop in local capillary hydrostatic pressure creates an environment that favors absorption. The increase in oxygen dissolved in plasma compensates for the reduction in blood flow. Conversely, Hammerlund and colleagues [13,14] have shown that with oxygen breathing blood flow increases within the local microvasculature of both acute and chronic wounds. The net response to HBOt within the variably injured tissues is a redistribution of perfusion and physiologic resorption of edema.

Cellular function

Cellular function is restored when HBOt corrects the Po_2 to normal or slightly elevated values. This restoration is manifested by enhanced

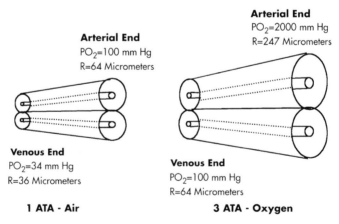

Arterial End
PO_2=2000 mm Hg
R=247 Micrometers

Arterial End
PO_2=100 mm Hg
R=64 Micrometers

Venous End
PO_2=34 mm Hg
R=36 Micrometers

1 ATA - Air

Venous End
PO_2=100 mm Hg
R=64 Micrometers

3 ATA - Oxygen

Fig. 4. Krogh-Erlang oxygen diffusion model used to estimate oxygen diffusion from the capillaries to surrounding tissue and the potential increase in oxygen diffusion distances with hyperbaric oxygenation. ATA, atmosphere absolute; R, radius. (*From* Sheffield PJ, Smith PS. Physiologic and pharmacological basis of hyperbaric oxygen therapy. In: Bakker DJ, Cramer FS, editors. Hyperbaric surgery perioperative care. Flagstaff (AZ): Best Publishing Company; 2002. p. 68; with permission.)

epithelialization, fibroplasia, collagen synthesis, angiogenesis, and leukocyte bactericidal-killing mechanisms [15,16]. The enhanced fibroblast activity can last up to 72 hours following a hyperbaric oxygen exposure. HBOt reduces the secondary injury by blunting the release of oxygen free radicals. More specifically, the Beta2 integrin system is disrupted, preventing neutrophil adherence to the postcapillary venules [17]. Hyperbaric oxygen also antagonizes lipid peroxidation of the cell membrane [18]. Erythrocyte sludging is reduced because of enhanced erythrocyte deformability in response to HBOt (Fig. 5) [19].

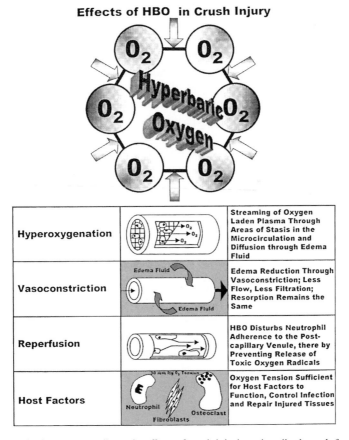

Fig. 5. Hyperbaric oxygen mediates the effects of crush injuries primarily through four mechanisms. These mechanisms also are useful adjuncts in managing the injuries in the other acute traumatic peripheral ischemias. HBO, hyperbaric oxygen. (*From* Strauss B. Crush injury, compartment syndrome and other acute traumatic peripheral ischemias. In: Kindwall E, Whalen H, editors. Hyperbaric medicine practice. 2nd (revised) edition. Flagstaff (AZ): Best Publishing Company; 2002. p. 760; with permission.

Clinical application

Despite all that is understood about the physiologic and pharmacody-namic properties of hyperbaric oxygen, guidelines for its clinical application in the treatment of the ATPIs as a group are limited. The lack of guidelines is related to a noticeable paucity of randomized clinical trials in the litera-ture. The vast majority of the clinical literature is in the form of case reports. A well-designed clinical trial allows comparison between treatment groups so that it is possible to identify which patients actually need the therapy to heal and which ones do not. Clinical guidelines are derived more accu-rately from such studies. Unfortunately, the complex and variable nature of these injuries as a group makes it difficult to develop well-designed clinical trials.

The clinical recommendations for the use of HBOt in open fractures and crush injuries are perhaps the best founded. In 1979 Strauss [20] had sum-marized more than 700 positive case reports in the use of HBOt for crush injuries. Perhaps the highest level of evidence for its use was reported in the results of Bouachour's [21] 1996 randomized, clinical trial of hyperbaric oxygen therapy in the management of crush injuries [21]. The severity of in-jury was graded objectively using the widely accepted Gustilo classification scheme (Table 1). The more severe injuries (Gustilo grade III-B and III-C) have been associated with a 50% complication rate (infection, non-union, nonhealing, amputation) [22–24]. Thirty-six patients who had Gustilo grade II or III injuries were assigned in a blinded, randomized fashion to the HBOt treatment group or the placebo group. All the patients received the same standard therapies (antibiotics, anticoagulants, and wound dressings). The two groups were similar in terms of subject age, risk factors, number,

Table 1
Gustilo classification of open fractures and crush injuries

Grade	Findings	Complications (infections, nonhealing, amputation)
I	Puncture type wound, usually from inside to out	Almost nil
II	Laceration associated with the open fracture	10%
III	Crush component to the injury	Vary with the subtype
A	Sufficient soft tissue to cover the bone	~ 10%
B	Exposed bone remains after débridement	~ 50%
C	Concomitant major vascular injury to the extremity	> 50%

Data from Gustilo R. Management of open fractures and their complications. Philadelphia: WB Saunders; 1962. p. 202–8; Gustilo R, Williams DN. The use of antibiotics in the manage-ment of open fractures. Orthopedics 1984;7:1617–9; and Gustilo RB, Mendoza RM, Williams DN. Problems in the management of type III (severe) open fractures: a new classification of type III open fractures. J Trauma 1984;24:742.

type and location of vascular injuries, neurologic injuries, or fractures. They were similar as well in type, location, and timing of surgical procedures. The results revealed complete healing in 94% of the HBOt group versus 59% of the controls ($P < .01$). Subsequent surgeries were required in 6% of the HBOt group versus 33% of the controls ($P < .05$). The healing of fractures in patients over the age of 40 years was significantly improved within the HBOt group ($P < .05$). Finally, transcutaneous oxygen measurements were significantly improved in the HBOt group as compared with the control group. The patients who healed had higher transcutaneous oxygen levels than those who did not heal.

The results of Bouachour's clinical trial revealed which crush-injured patients benefit from HBOt. Such information provides the basis for formulating objective guidelines for patient selection. Factors to consider are severity of injury, age, and host comorbidities. Strauss [11] has published the most comprehensive guidelines. The Strauss guidelines incorporate the Gustilo grade of injury with a five-criteria 10-point host assessment (Table 2). Because of the 50% complication rate, HBOt is recommended for all Gustilo grade III-B and III-C injuries regardless of host status (Table 3). With this high grade of injury, however, a primary amputation should be considered in severely compromised hosts (host score, 0–3). For the moderately compromised host (host score, 4–7) HBOt is indicated for both Gustilo grades II and III–A. HBOt should be considered for a Gustilo grade I fracture if the host is severely compromised. Finally, the decisions regarding surgical management should be made independently of whether HBOt is provided. Although HBOt should not delay any necessary surgical intervention, it should be provided as soon after the injury as possible [11]. Clinical

Table 2
Strauss evaluation system: five criteria, 10-point host assessment

Criteria	Findings			Interpretation
	2 Points[a]	1 Point[a]	0 Points[a]	
Age in years	< 40	40–60	>60	Healthy 8-10 Points
Ambulation[b]	Community	Household	None	
Cardiovascular/renal function[c]	Normal	Imparted	Decompensate	Impaired 8-10 Points
Smoking/steroid use[c]	None	Past	Current	
Neuropathy/deformity[c]	None	Mild-to-Moderate	Severe	Marginal 3-10 Points

[a] Use half-points if observations fall between two findings.
[b] Subtract one-half point if walking aids required.
[c] Whichever gives the lower score.
From Strauss MB. Hyperbaric oxygen for crush injuries and compartment syndromes. In: Bakker DJ, Cramer FS, editors. Hyperbaric surgery perioperative care. Flagstaff (AZ): Best Publishing Company; 2002. p. 344; with permission.

Table 3
Objective indications for using hyperbaric oxygen in open fracture–crush injuries

Gustilo Grade	Host status		
	Normal	Impaired	Marginal (severely compromised)
I	—	—	Yes
II	—	Yes	Yes
III -A	—	Yes	Yes
III-B	Yes	Yes	Yes/No[a]
III-C	Yes	Yes/No[a]	Yes/No[a]

[a] Consider primary amputation.

From Strauss MB. Hyperbaric oxygen for crush injuries and compartment syndromes. In: Bakker DJ, Cramer FS, editors. Hyperbaric surgery perioperative care. Flagstaff (AZ): Best Publishing Company; 2002. p. 344; with permission.

guidelines for patient selection are now well defined, but there is no single standard treatment protocol for HBOt in crush-injured patients. The Bouachour study called for two hyperbaric oxygen treatments per day for 6 days to be initiated within 24 hours of injury. Each treatment provided a pressure of 2.5 ata for 90 minutes. Strauss [11] has published his recommended treatment protocol with consideration for maintenance of tissue oxygenation during the immediate injury period, edema reduction, host responses to injury, and metabolic state stabilization. This protocol calls for three treatments per day for the first 2 days, two treatments per day for the next 2 days, and once-daily treatments for the last 2 days. Each of the 12 treatments is to be delivered at a pressure of 2 to 2.4 ata.

Cost impact

The cost impact of treating crush-injured patients with HBOt is favorable. In 1977 Brighton [25] reported that in the United States the average cost was $140,000.00 to resolve each case of crush-type fracture that failed to heal primarily. When projected to today's costs, that amount would be significantly higher. The Gustilo grade III-B and III-C injuries are associated with a 50% complication rate. The grade II injuries are associated with a 10% complication rate. For these fractures, Bouachour's [21] study demonstrated an overall 35% improvement in primary healing and a 27% decrease in the need for additional surgeries within the group treated with hyperbaric oxygen. At the authors' institution the total Medicare reimbursement cost for a patient to receive one hyperbaric oxygen treatment is $466.00.

Summary

In crush injuries, HBOt has objective indications based on the highest level of clinical evidence supporting its use. It meets the American Heart

Association's criteria for a category 1 indication. Both Medicare and Undersea and Hyperbaric Medical Society guidelines list crush injuries as an approved indication for HBOt [26,27]. Based on the clinical evidence and cost analysis, medical institutions that treat these types of injuries are justified in incorporating HBOt as a standard of care. As more hyperbaric programs go online, emergency physicians increasingly will be involved in coordinating the early administration of HBOt with the plans for surgical intervention. In such cases the phrase "time is muscle" also applies to skeletal muscle. The United States has recently witnessed a resurgence in the use of HBOt coinciding, in large part, with the technological advances in the treatment of chronic wounds. The practice of hyperbaric medicine as a whole remains challenged to develop evidence-based guidelines like those derived for the treatment of crush injuries.

Acknowledgments

The authors acknowledge the efforts of Craig Borchard and Shawn Mears, Great River Medical Center Public Relations, Lynette Collier and the talented GRMC wound clinic staff, and Derek and Jen, for the quality delivery of HBOt.

References

[1] Henshaw IN, Simpson A. Compressed air as a therapeutic agent in the treatment of consumption, asthma, chronic bronchitis and other diseases. Edinburgh (UK): Sutherland and Knox; 1857.

[2] Churchill-Davidson I, Sanger C, Thomlinson RH. High-pressure oxygen and radiotherapy. Lancet 1955;1:1091–5.

[3] Boerema I, Kroll JA, Meijne NG, et al. High atmospheric pressure as an aid to cardiac surgery. Arch Chir Neerl 1956;8:193–211.

[4] Brummelkamp WH, Hogendijk J, Boerema I. Treatment of anaerobic infections (clostridial myositis) by drenching the tissues with oxygen under high atmospheric pressure. Surgery 1961;49:299–302.

[5] Smith G, Sharp GR. Treatment of coal gas poisoning with oxygen at two atmospheres pressure. Lancet 1962;1:816–9.

[6] Kindwall Eric. A history of hyperbaric medicine. In: Kindwall E, Whalen H, editors. Hyperbaric medicine practice. 2nd (revised) edition. Flagstaff (AZ): Best Publishing Company; 2002. p. 1–20.

[7] Boerema I, Meyne NG, Brummelkamp WH, et al. Life without blood: a study of the influence of high atmospheric pressure and hypothermia on dilution of blood. J Cardiovasc Surg 1960;1:133–46.

[8] Strauss MB. Introduction to nonhealing wounds. Current concepts in wound care. 1986;Fall:5–6.

[9] Hunt TK, Niinikoski J, Zederfeldt BH, et al. Oxygen in wound healing enhancement: cellular effects of oxygen. In: Davis JC, Hunt TK, editors. Hyperbaric oxygen therapy. Bethesda (MD): The Undersea Medical Society; 1977. p. 111–2.

[10] Krogh A. The number and distribution of capillaries in muscle with calculations of the oxygen pressure head necessary for supplying the tissue. J Physiol 1919;52:409–15.

[11] Strauss MB. Hyperbaric oxygen for crush injuries and compartment syndromes; surgical considerations. In: Bakker DJ, Cramer FS, editors. Hyperbaric surgery perioperative care. Flagstaff (AZ): Best Publishing Company; 2002. p. 341–57.

[12] Bird AD, Telfer ABM. Effect of hyperbaric oxygen on limb circulation. Lancet 1965;(1): 355–6.

[13] Hammerlund C, Kutlu N. Effects of oxygen breathing on blister wound microcirculation in man. In: Hyperbaric oxygenation and wound repair. Effects on the dermal microcirculation [dissertation]. Lund University, Sweden; 1995.

[14] Hammerlund C, Castenfors J, Svedman P. Dermal vascular response to hyperoxia in healthy volunteers. In: Bakker DJ, Schmutz J, editors. Proceedings of the second Swiss symposium on hyperbaric medicine. Basel (Switzerland): Foundation for Hyperbaric Medicine; 1988. p. 55–9.

[15] Sheffield PJ, Smith PS. Physiologic and parmacological basis of hyperbaric oxygen therapy. In: Bakker DJ, Cramer FS, editors. Hyperbaric surgery perioperative care. Flagstaff (AZ): Best Publishing Company; 2002. p. 63–109.

[16] Hunt TK, Pai MP. The effect of varying ambient oxygen tensions on wound metabolism and collagen synthesis. Surg Gynecol Obstet 1972;135:561–7.

[17] Thom SR. Functional inhibition of neutrophil B2 integrins by hyperbaric oxygen in carbon monoxide mediated brain injury. Toxicol Appl Pharmacol 1993:123:248–56.

[18] Thom SR. Antagonism of co-mediated brain lipid peroxidation by hyperbaric oxygen. Toxicol Appl Pharmacol 1990;105:340–4.

[19] Mathieu D, Coget J, Vinkier L, et al. Red blood cell deformability and hyperbaric oxygen therapy [abstract]. HBO Review 1985;6(4):280.

[20] Strauss MB. Role of hyperbaric oxygen therapy in acute ischemias and crush injuries—an orthopedic perspective. HBO Review 1981;2:87–108.

[21] Bouachour G, Cronier P, Gouello JP, et al. Hyperbaric oxygen therapy in the management of crush injuries: a randomized double-blinded placebo-controlled clinical trial. J Trauma 1996;41:333–9.

[22] Gustilo R. Management of open fractures and their complications. Philadelphia: WB Saunders; 1982. p. 202–8.

[23] Gustilo R, Williams DN. The use of antibiotics in the management of open fractures. Orthopedics 1984;7:1617–9.

[24] Gustilo RB, Mendoza RM, Williams DN. Problems in the management of type III (severe) open fractures: a new classification of type III open fractures. J Trauma 1984;24:742–6.

[25] Brighton CT. Hospital Tribune. May 9, 1977:4.

[26] Medicare bulletin 424. Hyperbaric oxygen (HBO) therapy. May 11, 1999.

[27] Hampson NB, editor. Hyperbaric oxygen therapy: 1999 committee report. Kensington (MD): Undersea and Hyperbaric Medical Society, Inc; 1999. p. 17–21.

ELSEVIER
SAUNDERS

Emerg Med Clin N Am
25 (2007) 189–201

EMERGENCY
MEDICINE
CLINICS OF
NORTH AMERICA

Reducing Risk in Emergency Department Wound Management

James A. Pfaff, MD, FACEP, FAAEM[a,b,*], Gregory P. Moore, MD, JD[c,d]

[a]San Antonio Uniformed Health Services Health Education Consortium Emergency
Medicine Residency, San Antonio, TX, USA
[b]Uniformed Services University of the Health Sciences, San Antonio, TX, USA
[c]Emergency Department, Kaiser Permanente Sacramento/Roseville, CA, USA
[d]Emergency Medicine Residency, University of California at Davis School of Medicine,
Sacramento, CA, USA

Overview of malpractice issues in wounds

There are more than 12 million visits a year to emergency departments (EDs) throughout the United States for traumatic wounds, making them one of the most common reasons for ED visits [1]. Most of the wounds are located on the head and neck or upper extremities, usually involving the fingers [2]. More than 50% of wounds are caused by blunt force, and most others are caused by sharp objects such as metal, glass, and wood [1]. Animal and human bites are responsible for less than 10% of wounds for which emergency care is sought [3].

Wound care is one of the most common areas of emergency medicine malpractice suits. Wound care accounts for 5% to 20% of all ED malpractice claims and 3% to 11% of all dollars paid out [4]. The individual case awards are not relatively high [5–7]. The most common reason for litigation involves failure to diagnose foreign bodies, wound infections, and failure to detect underlying injury to nerves, tendons, or violation of a joint capsule [4].

Although the economic impact may be small, when a wound malpractice case is lost by the defendant, mandatory reporting to regulatory agencies can be source of significant loss of professional standing. The time spent

The opinions expressed in this article are those of the authors and should not be construed as official or as reflecting the views of the Department of Defense.

* Corresponding author. 3400 Rawley E. Chambers Avenue, Suite B, US Army ISR/BAMC, Fort Sam Houston, Texas 78234.

E-mail address: james.pfaff@amedd.army.mil (J.A. Pfaff).

both in responding to the case and in explaining it in future credentialing processes is another real personal cost.

To be successful in a malpractice action, the plaintiff's lawyer must prove four elements. All of the elements must be shown, or the suit fails. These elements are

1. The defendant had a duty to the patient.
2. The defendant breached the duty to the patient (the standard of care was not met).
3. Harm occurred to the patient.
4. The harm was directly a result of the breach in the duty (proximate cause).

A review of the four legal elements with regards to wound care generally leaves room for optimism by the provider. Of course, when there is a bad outcome, it will be maintained that the physician owed the duty to the patient (element 1). With wounds, however, ancillary hospital staff often are responsible for significant parts of the overall care. For example in a wound infection, the staff may be responsible for the cleaning process. The hospital, through vicarious liability, then will be named in the suit. To avoid excessive legal expenses in a relatively low-cost settlement, the hospital may take responsibility, settle, and absolve the individual physician.

The second element requires the physician to practice according to the standard of care. Wound care has many controversial areas, and the lack of scientific evidence to guide some of the management leaves room for a variety of professional expert opinions. Many different experts can testify in a wound case. To be an expert, one usually must show only that he or she has special knowledge in the area. A surgeon, plastic surgeon, orthopedist, hand surgeon, radiologist, or infectious disease specialist could testify against an emergency medicine physician in given situations. A plastic surgeon is very knowledgeable in suturing, as is a surgeon. An orthopedist or hand surgeon may have great experience in handling emergent cases of dirty wounds or foreign bodies. An infectious disease specialist may have vast experience with managing animal bites and other infection-prone wounds. The court often has allowed expert testimony by specialists in fields other than that of the defendant when the deponents have special knowledge (proven education, skill, and experience) in the area. For example, an orthopedist has been allowed to provide expert testimony in testifying against a radiologist [8], and a cardiovascular surgeon was allowed to testify against an orthopedic surgeon [9]. These examples are only a couple of a multitude of similar court decisions in this area. Wound care crosses a variety of potential areas of specialty care. It behooves the emergency medicine provider to be aware of the practice of the specialists in the area. One should realize, for example, that although the emergency medicine literature may not support the use of prophylactic antibiotics in certain wound care situations, the local plastic or hand surgeon may practice differently. It also may be critical to enlist opinions from appropriate local specialists as consultants in the more high-risk and controversial areas of wound management.

A likely reason for the low amounts recovered in litigation centers around the third element of malpractice, harm. It is difficult to prove harm in many cases. For example, if a tendon injury, nerve injury, or foreign body is missed, there may be no harm. The patient may require a surgery, but surgery would have been necessary anyway. Although there may be permanent damage, that damage also might have occurred anyway. When the plaintiff is successful in winning the case, the recovery often is focused only on the delay in definitive care with the associated patient pain and inconvenience.

The fourth element is proximate cause. In a recent case, *Brown v Brennan* [10], a 25-year-old woman came to the ED with a wound to the back of her leg. The wound was cleaned and dressed, and follow-up instructions were given. The wound became infected and required surgery with skin grafting. The plaintiff claimed that a failure to prescribe antibiotics caused the infection. The defendant claimed that infection is a known risk with all wounds. A defense verdict was returned. It is widely known that a certain percentage of wounds will become infected despite fastidious care, so it often is difficult to prove the defendant was the direct cause of the infection. Thus the fourth element of proximate cause may be difficult to prove in wound care malpractice suits.

Discharge instructions are critical in treating patients who have wounds. In recognizing that wounds are at risk for infection or missed injury, the physician must warn clearly about signs of infection, expected course of recovery, hallmarks of tendon or nerve damage, and the potential for a residual foreign body despite exploration or radiographic imaging. In high-risk wounds, specific follow-up is optimal. It is much better to have a patient later state, "They told me that could happen," rather than, "I had no idea what was going on."

Wound preparation

The goals of laceration management are to avoid infection and to achieve a functional and aesthetically pleasing scar [1]. These goals can be achieved by reducing tissue contamination, débriding devitalized tissue, restoring perfusion in poorly perfused tissues, and establishing a well-approximated skin closer [2].

Wound repair requires anesthesia and may require procedural sedation. It is incumbent upon the emergency physician to be familiar with all the local anesthetics used and pay particular attention to the dosage recommendation. Local anesthetics have a multitude of side effects including central nervous effects such as paresthesias and seizures, cardiovascular effects including bradycardia and dysrhymias, and methemoglobinemia. Patients may become toxic with doses smaller than the recommended doses [11].

Procedural sedation may be necessary in children who have certain wounds. The equipment and protocols in place to ensure the safety of the procedure should include oxygen, suction, and airway equipment, resuscitation medications, monitoring equipment, reversal agents, and dedicated nursing personnel to monitor the patient. There are many medications available, and their use depends upon the practitioner's experience and comfort level. Ketamine or a combination of narcotics and benzodiazepines is commonly used.

Visually inspecting the wound to its complete depth is required to search for foreign bodies and any anatomic injuries. Probing the wound with forceps will prevent potential injuries to the examiner. After exploration of the wound, irrigation can be performed. High-pressure irrigation is an effective method for removing bacteria and other potentially infective material; most authorities recommend irrigation with 5 to 8 psi. A 19-gauge needle with a 35- to 65-cm^3 syringe has been shown to generate this amount of pressure and more [12].

Normal saline is the most commonly used irrigant, although tap water has been shown to be just as effective and is readily available and cheaper [13,14]. Chlorhexidine, hydrogen peroxide, benzalkonium chloride, and detergent-containing products such as povidone-iodine should not be used for wound cleansing because they can result in local tissue injury and, in some instances, are less effective antimicrobials [12]. Most authorities recommend using 50 to 100 mL of irrigant per centimeter of wound length [15]. High-pressure irrigation is not necessary in all wounds, particularly in highly vascular wounds such as the scalp and face where there is no difference in the rate or infection or cosmetic appearance [16]. Soaking wounds is not effective and may be detrimental to repair and healing.

Hair removal may make closing the wound edges easier but is not required. Shaving should be avoided because of the potential for increased infection [17]. Hair removal should be avoided in the eyebrows because they are important as cosmetic landmarks in closure. In conjunction with irrigation and before skin closure, débridement may be necessary. The goal of débridement is removal of devitalized tissue that could increase the risk of infection. Additionally, removing any nonviable tissue around the wound edges may improve cosmetic appearance.

The timing of wound closure depends on a number factors including the location of the wound, the degree of contamination, and the amount of time that has elapsed from the injury to closure. It has been a generally accepted standard that wounds on the extremities can be open for 6 hours before closure, whereas wounds on the head and neck can remain open up to 24 hours. Wounds that are at high risk for infection even after copious irrigation and cleansing techniques may be candidates for delayed primary closure. Physician judgment is key in this decision making. When in doubt, "one is never wrong not closing a wound." Patients also should be informed that all wound repair leaves scars, that scars sometimes can be revised, and that it will be months before the ultimate result is known. It should be emphasized that "closing a wound loosely" or using surgical tape instead of suture is considered primary closure of a wound with all the associated risks of infection and their sequelae.

Standard of care

Much of wound preparation and closure decisions are anecdotal with few good evidence-based studies in existence. It therefore is difficult to define a true standard of care. Practice among emergency physicians varies both in the methods of closure and the use of cleaning techniques. One study of board-certified emergency medicine physicians demonstrated that 38% soak wounds, 21% use full-strength (10%) povidone-iodine or hydrogen peroxide, 67% scrub wounds using cotton gauze or coarse sponges, 27% irrigate wounds with other than recommended irrigation, and 76% never or infrequently practice delayed primary closure [18].

Tendon and nerve injuries

Alexander Herrerra v New York City Health and Hospitals Corporation

A 22-year-old male slipped on a staircase at work and lacerated his left forearm in November 2001 [19]. Sutures were used to close the laceration. Soon afterwards he lost mobility of his left (dominant) hand. He developed a permanent claw-hand and cannot perform fine motor movement. He was forced to learn to write with his right hand. He claimed the laceration involved the ulnar nerve, and the involvement was undetected. The case settled for $1.5 million.

Joseph and Tonya Luby v. H Arthur Heafer MD and Susan Galbele

The plaintiff sustained a laceration to the distal joint of his left index finger when he accidentally closed the finger in a bank night-deposit drawer [20]. He presented to Presbyterian Hospital-Kaufman ED for treatment. The wound was cleaned and sutured by a physician's assistant under the supervision of Dr. Heafer. When the plaintiff failed to regain movement of the distal finger joint after 30 days, he was sent to a hand surgeon who discovered a previously undiagnosed rupture to the flexor profundus tendon at the site of the previous injury. A complex tendon transplant procedure followed but left the plaintiff with a deformed and disabled finger. The plaintiff claimed the tendon injury should have been discovered on the original visit when a simple repair could have been done easily and successfully. He also claimed the delay led to a more complicated surgery that was unsuccessful. The case was settled for a confidential amount.

Before exploration and before anesthesia, a functional examination should be performed to determine the extent of injury. The mechanism of injury should be elicited before the examination, and, in the case of hand injuries, the patient's dominant hand should be documented. Careful attention should be paid to the effects of fight bites, pain on movement, numbness, or weakness.

The exploration should be performed in a relatively bloodless field after anesthesia with optimal lighting. Methods used include increasing the blood pressure cuff to 20 to 30 mm above the patient's systolic blood pressure for upper- or lower-extremity injuries. In the case of hand injuries, putting a plastic glove on the involved hand, cutting the finger tips, and rolling the glove down past the wound creates a tourniquet. Commercially available finger tourniquets can be used instead. Tourniquets should not be in place for longer than 30 to 60 minutes in the ED [21].

Examine the wound with good range of motion because the location or mechanism of injury may prevent easy visual inspection of the tendons. As much as possible, recreate the mechanism of injury. Inspect the wounds for any degree of tendon sheath or tendon involvement. Tendon repair may be done either primarily or in a secondary fashion depending on the type of wound involvement, the presence of foreign matter, involvement of the flexor or extensor tendon, and any other injury the patient may have. Flexor tendon injuries to the hand need to be repaired by a hand specialist or orthopedic surgeon. Primary repair is recommended, with most injuries being repaired in 12 to 24 hours [22,23]. In the event of excessive contamination, skin loss, unstable bony injuries, or missing tissue, delayed closure up to 2 to 3 weeks is possible with little difference in outcomes [22,23].

Extensor tendon injuries can be repaired by emergency physicians depending on the location and the physician's comfort level. If the laceration is between the distal wrist and metacarpal joint and is less than 8 hours old, and the skin and tendon wounds are sharp, easily visualized, and not heavily contaminated, the emergency physician can perform the repair if he or she feels qualified to do so and can arrange appropriate follow-up [23]. Not all tendon injuries need repair. Most tendon lacerations that are less than 50% can be treated without surgery [22].

Nerve repair, like tendon repair, can be done either primarily or in a secondary fashion. By definition, primary repair is done within 5 to 7 days of the injury and is most effective when the nerve ends can be reapproximated without tension in a well-vascularized area [24]. Secondary repair generally is performed about 2 to 3 weeks after injury and can involve either reapproximating the nerve ends or grafting. Most repairs are done in the upper extremities, although repairs can be performed in the lower extremities with mixed results [24]. For all nerve injuries, there is better likelihood of success in younger patients and those who have a cleaner mechanism of injury.

Patients should be involved in the decision-making process as much as possible. Explaining the potential for infections, the type of repair, and the expectation of function after repair are important elements. Practices may vary among consultants, and the emergency physician should discuss these differences of opinion with the patient. Although many of these injuries may be repaired acutely, it is possible that the orthopedic surgeon will want the skin closed primarily and the injured extremity splinted with follow-up arranged as an outpatient. Most patients requiring surgical intervention can be discharged after appropriate follow-up is arranged [25].

Foreign bodies

Nelson v Richter- Mich 2003

A 17-year-old male cut his foot when a glass fell from a counter. In eth ED wth wound was examined, cleaned, and dressed [26]. The wound was too small to be explored visually. Ten days later the patient returned with continued pain and stiffness. He ultimately went to surgery to remove a piece of glass from between his third and fourth metatarsals. The plaintiff's contention was that a radiograph should have been obtained. The defense stated that the patient returned for suture removal and not for problems, and that surgery might have been required anyway. There was a jury verdict for the defense.

Ashley v Gustafson and colleagues Jackson County (Missouri) Circuit Court

The 44-year-old plaintiff broke a glass and put the pieces in a trash bag but failed to notice that a piece of broken glass was jutting out from the bag [27]. While walking past the bag, she cut her ankle on the protruding glass. A doctor saw her and sutured the wound. No radiograph was performed. A second doctor saw her 9 months later for persistent pain and removed a 2.5-cm piece of glass from the wound. He did not obtain radiographs either. Seven months later she returned to the ED with more pain, and a radiograph was performed. It revealed three more pieces of glass. The plaintiff claimed a radiograph was required for this type of wound. The defendants claimed no radiograph was needed. A verdict for $179,000 was returned but was reduced to $119,930 after fault was allocated. Fault was designated as 42% to one ED physician, 25% to other ED physician, and 33% to the plaintiff.

In every patient presenting with a traumatic wound, there should be a concern for foreign bodies, with a high index of suspicion in certain animal bites or grossly contaminated wounds. The mechanism of injury may be a clue to the presence of foreign bodies. For example, a wound caused by sliding on gravel should heighten suspicion for retained fragments, whereas a puncture with a knife will be less suggestive. Additional clues would be wounds that have persistent pain, drainage, or that otherwise fail to heal. Patients who have glass injury may be able to feel the presence of the foreign body, and it may be useful to ask them [28].

A number of imaging techniques are used for foreign bodies. Their effectiveness is variable and depends on the material of the foreign body. Radiography is readily available and may locate a number of materials, including metal, bone, teeth, pencil graphite, certain plastics, glass, gravel, sand, some fish bones, some wood, and some aluminum [29]. Glass does not need to contain lead to be visible on a radiograph, and glass fragments 2 mm or larger are visible radiographically [30]. There should be a low threshold for obtaining radiographs in glass wounds because they are one of the most common causes of foreign-body litigation. In one study, up to 7% of wounds caused by glass injury had retained glass, with puncture wounds being the most common cause [31]. Wounds at greatest risk included puncture wounds, head or foot wounds, wounds caused by stepping on glass, and those resulting from a motor vehicle accident [31].

CT scanning can detect more types of foreign material than radiographs and is 100 times more sensitive in differentiating densities [25]. Some wood, thorns, and spines not visible on plain radiographs have been identified with CT. Expense and radiation exposure does limit the usefulness of CT. Although ultrasonography is an option, its success is variable. The overall sensitivity ranges from 50% to 90%, and specificity is 70% to 97% for gravel, metal, glass, cactus spines, wood, and plastic [30]. The usefulness of MRI is limited in wounds that involve gravel or metal. It probably should be reserved for suspicion of vegetative matter that is not seen on other imaging techniques [29].

The need for foreign body removal depends on its location and type of material: vegetative material is markedly more reactive than metal. The benefits of removal need to be weighed against the trauma and tissue destruction that may occur with attempts at removal and the likelihood of successful recovery.

If one foreign body is found, it is important to be vigilant in searching for additional pieces, remembering the adage "where there's smoke there's fire." Educate the patient and the patient's family about the potential for foreign bodies and the potential for wound infection. Document that a search was performed and give good wound care and follow-up instructions.

High-risk wounds

Bessenyei v Raiti. US District Court- Maryland

Mr. Bessenyei had paint thinner injected into his thumb under high pressure and presented to the ED [32]. Dr. Raiti, the ED physician, consulted a hand surgeon, who was not on call but who previously had demonstrated a willingness to help. The hand surgeon recommended antibiotics and pain medications, which the patient was given. The patient's tetanus immunization was updated, and he was discharged with instructions to return if his condition worsened. The patient's thumb worsened, and subsequently a partial amputation was necessary. Mr. Bessenyei sued both physicians claiming they negligently failed to realize the seriousness of a high-pressure injection and did not appropriately incise and débride the thumb. The hand surgeon asked the judge to dismiss him from the case because he had no relationship with the patient or contractual duty; he simply provided advice. The judge agreed and held the ED physician solely liable. "It was Dr. Raiti (ED physician) who had direct contact with the patient, rendered care, and initiated contact with the consultant. He could override the consultant by accepting or rejecting his recommendations and made the final decision."

Although all wounds are at risk for infection and adverse outcomes, several types of wounds are associated with a considerably greater risk. These wounds include high-pressure injection injuries and wounds caused by human teeth, or "fight bites."

High-pressure injuries often present with a small puncture wound, primarily to the hand. The wound may seem innocuous to both the patient and the initial provider, but lack of vigilance in caring for these patients can result in substantial morbidity. The high-pressure spray guns in use discharge a variety of products including water, paint, thinners, solvents, and hydraulic oil and fluid.

Factors that affect morbidity include the site of injection and the type, amount, and viscosity and pressure of the material injected [33]. Solvents and paint thinner are significantly more damaging than grease and oil-based compounds because their lower viscosity allows the injected material to spread more easily [34]. If the material is injected into relatively nondistensible tissue such as the fingers, the increased tissue pressure can result in tissue damage and compromise of the microcirculation, causing a compartment-like syndrome [35]. The injury often occurs in the nondominant hand while a worker is clearing equipment or trying to steady in during it during its operation.

Plain-film radiographs may reveal varying distribution of radiopaque densities associated with paint or subcutaneous air from air or water injection. Although imaging may be important, a hand surgeon should be consulted expeditiously, because the amputation rate is significantly greater if surgical débridement occurs more than 6 hours from the time of injury and varies from 16% to 55% of patients [34].

Human bites can be divided into occlusional bites and bites of the hand involving the metacarpal phalangeal joint (clenched-fist injuries). Occlusional bites occur when the teeth break the skin, often tearing the tissue and leaving bite marks. When they occur in places other than the hand, they are no more dangerous than any other laceration or bite [36]. Injuries to the metacarpal phalangeal joint, on the other hand, often occur in younger men as a result of an altercation, and these are at substantial risk for infection. The extensor tendon often retracts proximally after the injury, seals the puncture, and creates an anaerobic environment for inoculated bacteria within the joint [37]. There is a basic axiom in emergency medicine that any wound over the metacarpal phalangeal joint of the hand joint is a fight bite until proven otherwise. Care must be taken to explore these wounds, and many of them may need timely involvement by the ED hand surgeon. The organisms involved include Streptococcus spp and *Staphylococcus aureus*, but there also is a high percentage of anaerobes [38].

Consultation

Lockard v. Lacker- Kentucky 2002

A 7-year-old boy tripped at school and had a minor cut on his middle finger. Later in the day he went swimming [39]. The mother looked at the cut and thought it did not need any attention. Later that night he awoke crying with vomiting and fever. He went to the ED at 2:30 AM. The physician performed a radiograph of the finger, which was normal, and examined the laceration, which looked "benign." The boy was diagnosed as having "stomach flu" and was released. Two days later his finger appeared swollen and purple with blisters. He was admitted with a necrotizing Strepotcoccus A infection, and ultimately the finger was amputated. The suit against the emergency medicine physician claimed that a plastic surgeon or orthopedist should have been consulted on the initial visit. The verdict found for the defense, deciding that the initial diagnosis was reasonable based on the presentation.

In general, a consultation over the telephone does not establish a physician–patient relationship; thus, the consultant cannot be held liable for malpractice related to advice. Most courts require an actual examination by the physician to establish a relationship or a specific and affirmative action by the physician that establishes that the doctor agrees to be involved in the patient's care. The courts are hesitant to have mere conversations (even in on-call situations) or an agreement to provide follow-up care represent the establishment of a formal relationship, because doing so would chill the normal communication between professionals that usually facilitates optimal patient care.

Antibiotics

Antibiotic prophylaxis has no usefulness in uncomplicated wounds [40]. Some practitioners give antibiotics for all wounds with the intent of avoiding litigation should an infection develop. This practice is not without consequence, because unneeded medications can result in selection of resistant organisms, side effects, allergies, or hypersensitivity. Litigation still can result even with this conservative and rather arbitrary approach. As mentioned previously, it may be prudent to find out how local specialists practice, because, depending on the injury, the emergency medicine physician's practices may be compared with their practice.

Certain factors are associated an increased likelihood of wound infection. These factors include advanced age, history of diabetes, the presence of foreign body in the wound, stellate shape of the wound, a wide laceration, jagged wound edges, and wounds deeper than the subcutaneous tissue [41]. Antibiotics also are sometimes recommended in an immunosuppressed host; an open fracture; a wound involving exposed tendon, bone, or joint;

grossly contaminated high-risk bite wounds (eg, puncture, crush, or extremity wounds); oral wounds; and wounds that have significant delay before presentation [42]. The location of the wound is also a factor; the incidence of infection ranges from 1% to 2% in head and neck wounds to as high as 7% in the lower extremities [21].

Discharge and follow-up instructions

Older Americans, particularly older women, some immigrants, intravenous drug users, and the poor are at risk for being underimmunized. The patient's status should be well documented in the medical record.

Patients may not have the ability to identify and assess wound healing properly [43]. Follow-up instructions should be explicit, especially for wounds that have a high risk of complications. All patients should be given specific wound-care instructions. These instructions are given most effectively best with a written form that identifies all potential complications and the need to return for any signs of swelling redness or fever. All wounds considered high risk should have a mandatory 24- to 48-hour recheck. Patients also should know that, even with meticulous treatment, wounds do get infected. Patients should be cautioned about using anything other than water to clean their wounds, because solutions such as hydrogen peroxide and Betadine are toxic to the tissues.

Summary

Although substantial dollar amounts are not involved, wound-care litigation constitutes a significant number of lawsuits to emergency medicine physicians resulting in an increased drain on the physician's time and exposing the physician to all the psychosocial effects involved in the medicolegal process. The procedures outlined in this article—paying attention to wound-care principles, involving patients in the medical decision-making process, and ensuring appropriate medical follow-up—can, it is hoped, reduce the incidence of medical claims.

References

[1] Singer AJ, Hollandr JE, Quinn JV. Evaluation and management of traumatic laceration. N Engl J Med 1997;337:1142–8.
[2] Hollander JE, Singer JE. Laceration management. Ann Emerg Med 1999;34:356–67.
[3] Hollander JE, Singer AJ, Valentine S, et al. Wound registry: development and validation. Ann Emerg Med 1995;25:675–85.
[4] Henry GL. Specific high risk medical-legal issues. In: Henry GL, Sullivan DJ, editors. Emergency medicine risk management. Dallas (TX): American College of Emergency Physicians; 1997. p. 475–94.
[5] Karcz A, Auerbach B, et al. Preventability of malpractice claims in emergency medicine: a closed claims study. Ann Emerg Med 1990;19:865–73.

[6] Karcz A, Holbrook J, et al. Massachusetts emergency medicine closed malpractice claims: 1988–1990. Ann Emerg Med 1993;22:553–9.

[7] Karcz A, Korn R, et al. Malpractice claims against emergency physicians in Massachusetts 1975-1993. Am J Emerg Med 1996;14:341–5.

[8] Silvas v Ghiatas, 954 S.W.2d 50 (Tes. App. San Antonio).

[9] Dempsy v Phelps, 700 So.2d 1340 (Ala 1997).

[10] Brown v Brennan. (Texas)

[11] Mulroy MF. Systemic toxicity and cardiotoxicity form local anesthetics: incidence and preventive measures. Reg Anesth Pain Med 2002;27:556–61.

[12] Singer AF, Hollander JE. Pressure dynamics of various irrigation techniques commonly used in the emergency department. Ann Emerg Med 1994;24:36–40.

[13] Valente JH, Forti RJ, Freundlich LF, et al. Wound irrigation in children: saline solution or tap water? Ann Emerg Med 2003;41:609–16.

[14] Howell JM, Chisolm CD. Wound care. Emerg Med Clin North Am 1997;15:417–25.

[15] Singer AJ, Hollander JE. Wound preperation. In: Singer AJ, Hollander JE, editors. Lacerations and cute wounds: an evidence-based guide. Philadelphia: FA Davis; 2003. p. 13–22.

[16] Hollander JA, Richman PB, Werblud MP, et al. Irrigation in facial and scalp lacerations: does is alter outcome? Ann Emerg Med 1998;31:73–7.

[17] Seropian R, Reynolds BM. Wound infections after pre-operative depilation vs. razor preparation. Am J Surg 1975;129:251–4.

[18] Howell JM, Chisolm CD. Outpatient wound preparation and care: a national survey. Ann Emerg Med 1992;21:976–81.

[19] Alexander Herrerra v New York City Health and Hospitals Corporation. NY Supreme Court Index Number 103063/03.

[20] Joseph and Tonya Luby v H. Arthur Heafer, MD and Susan Gabele- Kaufman County (Texas) District Court Case No. 58532.

[21] Hollander JE. Patient and wound assessment: basic concepts of the patient history and physical examination. Foreign bodies in wounds. In: Singer AJ, Hollander JE, editors. Lacerations and acute wounds: an evidence-based guide. Philadelphia: FA Davis; 2003. p. 9–12.

[22] Harrison BP, Hilliard MW. Emergency department evaluation and treatment of hand injuries. Emerg Med Clin North Am 1999;17:793–822.

[23] Trott A. The hand. In wounds and lacerations: emergency care and closure. St. Louis (MO): Mosby; 1991. p. 177–214.

[24] Allan CH. Functional results of primary nerve repair. Hand Clinics; 2000;16:67–72.

[25] Capellan MD, Hollandr JE. Management of lacerations in the emergency department. Emerg Med Clin North Am 2003;21:205–31.

[26] Nelson v Richter, Oakland County (MI) Circuit Court Case No. 03-048262-NH.

[27] Ashley v Gustafson et al. Jackson County (Missouri) Circuit Court, Case No. CV97–19936.

[28] Steele MT, Tran LV, Watson WA, et al. Retained glass foreign bodies in wounds: predictive value of wound characteristics, patient perception, and wound exploration. Am J Emerg Med 1998;16:627–30.

[29] Lammers R. Foreign bodies in wounds. In: Singer AJ, Hollander JE, editors. Lacerations and acute wounds: an evidence-based guide. Philadelphia: FA Davis; 2003. p. 147–57.

[30] Couter BI. Radiographic screening of glass foreign bodies. What does a "negative" foreign body series really mean? Ann Emerg Med 1990;19:997–1000.

[31] Montano JB, Steele MT, Watson WA. Foreign body retention in glass caused wounds. Ann Emerg Med 1992;21:1360–3.

[32] Bessenyei v Raiti. US District Court- Maryland No JFM-01-1029, June 9, 2003.

[33] Flotre M. High-pressure injection injuries of the hand. Am Fam Physician 1992;45:2230–4.

[34] Vasilevski D, Noorbergen M, Depierreux M, et al. High pressure injection injuries to the hand. Am J Emerg Med 2000;18:820–4.

[35] Karlbauer A, Gasperschitz A. High pressure injection injury: a hand threatening emergency. J Emerg Med 1987;5:375–9.

[36] Goldstein EJ. Management of human and animal bite wounds. J Am Acad Dermatol 1989;
     21:1275–9.
[37] Talan DA, Citron DM, Abrahamian FM, et al. Bacteriologic analysis of infected dog and cat
     bites. N Engl J Med 1999;340:85–92.
[38] Griego RD, Rosen T, Orengo IF, et al. Dog, cat and human bites: a review. J Am Acad Der-
     matol 1995;33:1019–29.
[39] Lockard v Lacher, Jefferson Couty (KY) Circuit Court, Case No. 02–8116.
[40] Cummings P, Del Beccaro MA. Antibiotics to prevent infection of simple wounds: a meta-
     analysis of randomized studies. Am J Emerg Med 1995;13:396–400.
[41] Hollander JE, Singer AJ, Valentine S, et al. Risk factors for infection in patients with trau-
     matic lacerations. Acad Emerg Med 2001;8:716–20.
[42] Moran GJ, House HR. Antibiotics in wound management. In: Singer AJ, Hollander JE,
     editors. Lacerations and acute wounds: an evidence-based guide. Philadelphia: FA Davis;
     2003. p. 194–204.
[43] Seaman M, Lammers R. Inability of patients to self-diagnose wound infections. J Emerg
     Med 1991;9:215–9.

ELSEVIER
SAUNDERS

Emerg Med Clin N Am
25 (2007) 203–221

EMERGENCY
MEDICINE
CLINICS OF
NORTH AMERICA

Emergency Management of Chronic Wounds

Richard S. Hartoch, MD[a,b,*],
LTC John G. McManus, MD, MCR, FACEP[c,d],
Sheri Knapp, FNP[a],
Mark F. Buettner, DO, ABEM[e]

[a]Department of Emergency Medicine, Oregon Health & Science University,
3181 Southwest Sam Jackson Park Road, Portland, OR 97239-7500, USA
[b]Veterans Administration Medical Center, Portland, OR, USA
[c]Emergency Medicine, The University of Texas Health
Science Center at San Antonio, San Antonio, TX, USA
[d]US Army Institute of Surgical Research, 3400 Rawley Chambers Avenue, Suite B,
Fort Sam Houston, San Antonio, TX 78234-6315, USA
[e]Great River Wound and Hyperbaric Clinic, Center for Rehabilitation,
1401 West Agency Road, West Burlington, IA 52655, USA

As America's emergency departments witness an escalation in care provided to an aging population, the emergency physician increasingly evaluates and treats manifestations of chronic disease. In 2004 the population of Americans over the age of 65 was 34 million. By the year 2030 this population is projected to reach 69 million. Nonhealing wounds are often a presenting manifestation of chronic disease. They are a source of pain and disability for this population. Emergency physicians should possess a fundamental knowledge in the management of chronic wounds. This article familiarizes the emergency physician with the epidemiology of chronic wounds, the physiology of tissue repair, the pathophysiology involved in wound healing failure, the common types of chronic wounds, and specific management strategies.

Epidemiology of chronic wounds

Acute wounds are wounds that proceed through an orderly and timely reparative process and result in a sustained restoration of anatomic and

---

* Corresponding author. Department of Emergency Medicine, Oregon Health & Science University, 3181 Southwest Sam Jackson Park Road, Portland, OR 97239-7500.
   E-mail address: rickhartoch@yahoo.com (R.S. Hartoch).

functional integrity. In chronic wounds, however, this process has been disrupted. Chronic wounds fail to proceed through the usual stepwise fashion and experience prolonged or incomplete healing, with lack of restoration of integrity. A chronic wound is generally defined as a wound that fails to progress over a period of 30 days [1]. Some wounds never heal. The financial impact for their treatment along with the emotional and physical impact can be devastating for patients and create a burden on the health care system as a whole. These wounds predominantly affect patients over the age of 60 [1]. It is estimated that chronic wounds affect 0.78% of the population, with a prevalence ranging from 0.18% to 0.32% [2]. The most common forms of chronic wounds are related to diabetes, venous stasis disease, peripheral vascular diseases, and pressure ulcerations. In 1999 it was estimated that the average cost for 2 years of treatment of a diabetic ulcer was $27,987 per patient [3]. More recently the cost for a single ulcer has increased to $8000, with the cost of an infected ulcer increasing to approximately $17,000 per year and the cost of a major amputation spiraling upward to approximately $45,000. In the year 1996 more than 86,000 lower extremity amputations were performed in the United States. Roughly half of these patients develop an infection or ulceration on the contralateral limb within 18 months [4]. The incidence of diabetes is on the rise in the United States. America currently spends an estimated $1.5 billion annually in the treatment of diabetic foot ulcers.

Normal tissue repair

The process of normal tissue repair is a complex but organized sequence of events mediated by cellular and biochemical activities. This process can be broken down into four characteristic stages. Each stage of repair involves a propagating series of events that lead to the next stage.

Stage I. Hemostasis

The process of hemostasis is initiated with tissue injury. There are three major steps that characterize this process. The first step is the formation of the fibrin clot. On exposure to type I collagen, the inactive proteases of the intrinsic and extrinsic pathways become activated. These activated proteases induce the conversion of prothrombin to thrombin, which in turn induces the conversion of fibrinogen to fibrin. The fibrin strands assemble into a network that traps red blood cells and platelets, forming a clot in the wound that blocks flow from injured blood vessels. Vasoconstriction further reduces the flow of blood from injured vessels. Platelet degranulation occurs in the second step. As the platelets become entrapped in the fibrin lattice, degranulation allows for the release of growth factors. Chief among these are platelet derived growth factor (PDGF), transforming growth factors (TGF), basic fibroblast growth factor (bFGF), and vascular endothelial growth factor (VEGF). These growth factors are chemotactic to fibroblasts, neutrophils, and monocytes. The third step in hemostasis is the formation of the provisional wound matrix. Type III collagen is synthesized by fibroblasts that serve to reinforce the matrix. More than just a fibrin clot, the provisional wound matrix is a dynamic environment of biochemical signaling. The transition to the next stage occurs as the cells of immune function and tissue repair migrate to the provisional wound matrix.

Stage II. Inflammation

The inflammatory phase begins approximately 24 hours after injury and normally lasts up to 2 weeks [5]. With the provisional wound matrix in place, white blood cells migrate to the region in response to chemotaxis. The marginating pool of neutrophils is the first line of defense against infection. Through phagocytosis they ingest and kill bacteria. They also play a role in removing foreign materials and devitalized tissue. Mast cells release histamine, which causes the rubor and calor noted about the peri-wound tissues. Edema ensues. Various chemokines are released that mediate the recruitment and activation of more neutrophils, eosinophils, lymphocytes, basophils, and macrophages. The T and B lymphocytes exert humoral and cell-mediated immune responses. Following migration into the wound matrix, neutrophils perform several activities. Oxygen free radicals are released that kill phagocytized bacteria. Proinflammatory cytokines are released that perpetuate the overall inflammatory process. Neutrophils also release high levels of proteases known as the matrix metalloproteases (MMPs). These proteases come in the form of elastase and collagenase that remove components of the damaged extracellular matrix within the wound. Activated macrophages play a similar role as the neutrophils early in the inflammatory stage. They ingest bacteria through phagocytosis and secrete MMPs. Late in the inflammatory stage the macrophage plays a key role in mediating the transition to the next stage of repair. By releasing protease inhibitors, macrophages turn off the furnace of proteolytic destruction. Growth factors (PDGF and TGFβ) and anti-inflammatory cytokines are released. A second call is made to recruit and activate fibroblasts to the wound matrix.

Stage III. Proliferation

Within the fibrin-rich wound matrix, the fibroblasts proliferate and begin synthesizing collagen, fibronectin, and proteoglycans. With the release of TGFβ and VEGF angiogenesis is stimulated. This combination of activities leads to the development of granulation tissue. Granulation tissue is composed of a density of collagen and capillaries. It serves as a transitional replacement for normal dermis. The process of epithelialization follows in this timed sequence of events.

Stage IV. Maturation

The final phase of healing takes place over the next year. Type III collagen is replaced with the deposition of type I collagen. The organization and cross-linking of collagen fibers increases their tensile strength. The density of the capillaries is reduced as the tissues begin to take on the characteristics of normal dermis.

Pathophysiology of chronic wounds

Unlike the organized sequence of events that occurs during normal tissue repair, the chronic wound environment is suspended in a stage of prolonged inflammation. The studies of wound fluid analysis have led to the understanding of three key concepts with regard to the molecular and cellular activities of chronic wounds. First, chronic wounds have decreased mitogenic activity within fibroblasts, keratinocytes, and vascular endothelial cells [4]. This decrease in cellular activity is known as cellular senescence. Second, chronic wounds have elevated levels of proinflammatory cytokines that perpetuate the inflammatory stage. Finally, chronic wounds have elevated levels of destructive protease activity.

Common pathways in the development of chronic wounds

Normal wound healing, as outlined previously, may be negatively impacted by numerous factors creating a state of perpetual imbalance. The vast majority of chronic wounds are a consequence of three basic conditions: vascular disease (venous disease, arterial insufficiency), diabetes mellitus, or inappropriate pressures (pressure ulcers). Factors that negatively affect wound healing are listed in Box 1. Inappropriate recognition or

---

Box 1. Factors that delay wound healing

- Advanced age/immobilization.
- Infection, poor hygiene.
- Malnutrition/chronic illness
- Diabetes
- Peripheral vascular disease
- Medications (corticosteroids, immunosuppressants etc.)
- Cigarette smoking
- Stress (mechanical/emotional)
- Inadequate/inappropriate wound care
- Excessive dryness/moisture
- Edema

treatment of the chronic wound may allow the wound to advance to deeper tissue layers, including muscle and bone, and eventually threaten limb and life.

Examples of chronic wounds

Diabetic foot ulcers

Foot ulcers develop in 15% to 20% of the 16 million people in the United States who have diabetes [6–8] and 85% of lower extremity amputations are preceded by foot ulcers. At least 50% of amputations within the population of people who have diabetes can be prevented [9]. People who have diabetes are prone to arterial insufficiency and generally diminished immunity but neuropathy (which develops in 42% of people who have diabetes after 20 years) is the most critical element in the development of nonhealing ulcers [10–12].

Although not all foot deformities are a direct result of diabetes (eg, bunion propensity is likely genetic), diabetic neuropathy affects motor innervation to muscle spindles and may lead to intrinsic foot muscle weakness [10]. The resulting imbalance between normal extrinsic and weak intrinsic muscle groups may lead to the development of claw or hammer toes, which shift pressure and frictional forces to vulnerable areas, particularly the plantar metatarsal heads. The top (dorsal surface) of the deformity is also at risk from rubbing on the shoe. Sensory and autonomic neuropathic changes give rise to dry, insensate feet unable to protect themselves from low-grade repetitive trauma. Charcot arthropathy may present initially as a diffusely erythematous, hot foot that eventually degenerates into a chronic deformity termed the Charcot "rocker bottom" foot. These numb, highly deformed feet are at particularly high risk for ulceration. Acute Charcot is a difficult diagnosis to make but vital to suspect early.

The combination of diabetic neuropathy, foot deformity, and minor trauma has been implicated as a basic recipe for foot ulceration [13,14]. A callus can increase underlying tissue pressure by as much as 30% [15] and may be the first indication of imminent woe [16]. A callus is classified by some practitioners as a pre-ulcerative state [17]. When whitish, macerated tissue appears beneath the callus, ulceration is looming. Diabetic ulcers may be avoidable to some extent through regular foot examination, correction of foot deformities, detection of sensory neuropathy with a monofilament, and identification of sources of trauma, often related to ill-fitting footwear (Fig. 1).

Venous stasis ulcers

Some 85% of chronic lower extremity skin ulcers are related to chronic venous insufficiency (CVI) [18]. It is estimated that 2.5 million Americans

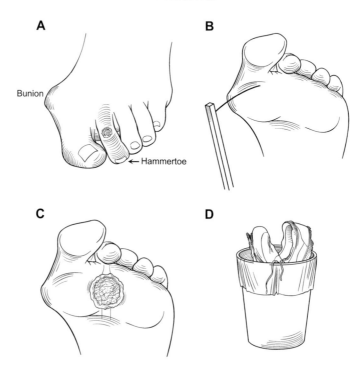

Fig. 1. Diabetic foot deformities allow shoes to rub on top of toe (*A*) and transfer pressure to plantar surface of metatarsal heads (*C*) resulting in callus development and ulceration. Semmes-Weinstein mono-filament (*B*) tests for neuropathy. Ill-fitting shoes (*D*) are a major factor in diabetic ulceration and should be discarded.

have CVI, of whom 20% develop venous ulcers. Therapy is required for 50% of these ulcers for more than 1 year with an estimated annual treatment expenditure of $3 billion [19,20]. To appreciate the serious sequelae of CVI it is worthwhile to examine normal venous physiology. The venous system of the lower extremities is divided into superficial and deep systems with an extensive series of perforator veins connecting the two (Fig. 2). All veins have delicate bicuspid valves that, when competent, allow venous blood to flow in one direction, returning deoxygenated blood to the central circulation.

CVI generally results from venous valve dysfunction causing pump failure, venous hypertension, and reflux [21–23]. Valve dysfunction usually originates in the deep system. Deep venous thrombosis (DVT) is a major cause of valve destruction. Initially the DVT causes obstruction to flow but in the process of recanalization valves are damaged, yielding essentially open tubes [24]. Five years after a significant DVT, 40% to 70% of patients have signs and/or symptoms of venous insufficiency as described in Box 2.

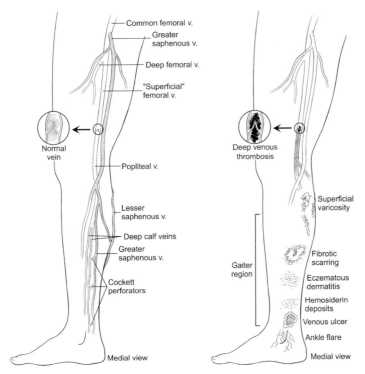

Fig. 2. The deep venous system is well supported within the muscle fascia. Disrupted deep valves allow pressure transmission through perforators to vulnerable superficial veins with resultant skin changes.

Pressure ulcers

A pressure ulcer, also termed decubitus (Latin for "lying down") ulcer, is a potentially avoidable lesion that is frequently seen and unfortunately occasionally develops in the emergency department setting. An estimated 2.5 million pressure ulcers are treated in acute care settings per year, costing billions of dollars [25]. An individual pressure ulcer may cost up to $60,000 to treat [26]. Some 60% of pressure ulcers develop during acute care hospitalizations [27], with patients more than 70 years of age and those who have spinal cord injuries accounting for the majority. The foundation of a pressure ulcer may develop following 2 hours of unmitigated soft tissue compression [28] but may not be clinically evident for 2 to 7 days. Risk factors for developing decubitus ulcer are listed in Box 3.

Pressure ulcers occur when pressure exerted on the tissues is greater than the pressure at the capillaries. This creates an area of ischemia. If the area of ischemia is prolonged an ulcer develops. Offloading the area after prolonged pressure can also result in damage from reperfusion and the release of toxic substances that arise from the initial inflammation response. The release of

---

Box 2. Chronic venous insufficiency

Symptoms
- Leg heaviness, aching pressure, throbbing burning pain
- Nocturnal leg cramps, restless legs
- Discomfort worse in dependent position

Signs
- Ankle edema
- Superficial varicosities
- Hyperpigmentation (hemosiderin deposition)
- Eczematous skin changes
- Lipodermatosclerosis (inflamed woody induration)
- Gaiter area ulcer (usually above medial malleolus)

---

these substances can expand the area of damage beyond the area of pressure. Muscle tissue needs more oxygen than skin and shows greater damage and tissue destruction from prolonged pressure. A small area of pressure on the skin is often concealing a deeper area of damage beneath.

The early pressure ulcer may be difficult to detect clinically. The underlying oxygen-hungry muscle and dermis are more susceptible to ischemic damage than the relatively resistant epidermis. A stage 1 pressure ulcer may present with nonblanchable erythema and intact skin similar to a bruise. This pre-ulcerative state is vital to recognize before further breakdown occurs. The stages of pressure ulceration are outlined in Box 4.

Emergency department evaluation

Although chronic wounds are by their very nature slowly progressive, complications can be emergently life and limb threatening. The most serious

---

Box 3. Pressure ulcer risk factors

- Immobility (inability to effectively shift weight)
- Paralysis (spinal cord, postintubation)
- Incontinence (excessive moisture)
- Altered mental status
- Exposure to hard surfaces, friction, shear forces
- Poor nutritional status/low protein diet
- Existing pressure ulcer
- Dry sacral skin
- Nonblanchable erythema of intact skin (Stage 1 ulcer)

Box 4. Pressure ulcer staging

Stage 1. Skin intact but reddened (nonblanchable erythema) for greater than 1 hour after pressure is relieved

Stage 2. Blister or abrasion up to dermal layer

Stage 3. Extension of ulcer into muscle layer

Stage 4. Extension into bone or joint

---

threats that the emergency physician must evaluate for include overwhelming sepsis, deep venous thrombosis, pulmonary embolus, advancing local tissue destruction, and stress-induced exacerbation of existing medical conditions.

Once the ABCs of the primary survey are complete a more thorough history and physical examination may proceed. The history should focus initially on the chief complaint, which may or may not explicitly be the chronic wound itself. The practitioner must sort out what role the ulcer is playing in the patient's presenting concern. Occasionally a patient may be unaware of the ulcer's existence.

History

The history is then focused on the ulcer and its consequences. A detailed review may suggest ulcer cause as outlined in Table 1. Is there a past history of ulcers? How were they managed? What is the time course of the current ulcer? What therapy has already been tried and has it been effective? Is the

Table 1
History pearls in chronic wound epidemiology

	Location	Appearance	Pain?	Findings	Therapy
Venous	Medial leg above malleolus	Large but shallow, irregular border	Some, relieved with elevation and walking	Characteristic skin changes, edema	Graduated compression, elevation
Diabetic	Plantar surface foot, metatarsals	Punched out	None	Absent ankle reflexes, insensate	Total contact casting
Pressure	Sacrum, heel, occiput	Initially a "bruise"	Yes	Immobilized elderly, spinal cord injury	Offloading
Arterial	Distal foot, toes	Irregular edges, little bleeding with débridement	Severe, especially with elevation and walking	Hairlessness, absent pulses, claudication, impotence	Revascularize

ulcer changing? Is it growing, developing redness, lymphangitis, exudate, or a foul order? Is the ulcer bed friable? Is it painful? Are there associated fevers or chills? Is there a personal or family history of superficial or deep vein thrombosis? Does the patient have a known clotting disorder? Is there associated edema, leg heaviness, leg aching with prolonged standing, restless legs, night cramps, skin changes (hyperpigmentation, eczema, scarring), pruritus, or burning, all suggestive of CVI [29]? Is the discomfort relieved by elevation and walking, as in CVI, or worsened, as in arterial insufficiency (although arterial and venous disease may coexist)? Is there claudication, impotence, or generalized atherosclerotic cardiovascular disease suggesting arterial insufficiency?

Physical examination

The physical examination must be thorough and not be limited to the ulcer. The patient is generally assessed with focus on overall robustness, mobility, nutritional status, and hygiene. Patients who develop chronic ulcers are generally in poor health and need a comprehensive examination. Special attention is given to the ulcer, documenting the precise location, size, and depth. The gaiter area, in particular above the medial malleolus, is typical for venous ulceration. An isolated lateral malleolus rarely results from venous disease alone and may suggest a combination of trauma (car door versus driver's ankle) and arterial insufficiency. Is the ulcer mobile or is it fixed to deeper layers of tissue? The ulcer base is evaluated for purulent discharge and necrotic tissue and may be probed to determine if bone is contacted. One study indicated palpable bone protruding from the ulcer base was highly correlated with osteomyelitis [30]. The skin around the ulcer is assessed next. Is there evidence of surrounding inflammation, dilated venules, edema, infection, eczema (stasis dermatitis), hemosiderin deposits, lipodermatosclerosis, or atrophie blanche (white scarring at site of previous ulcer) seen in CVI? Is there callus developing at pressure points?

The examination continues with a more extensive vascular examination. Are pulses palpable? It is also important to calculate ankle brachial index (ABI), which is the ratio of lower extremity to upper extremity systolic blood pressure. Are varicose veins present? (Normally only veins in the foot and ankle are visible.) Is there evidence of superficial thrombophlebitis? This condition, particularly when it appears in the proximal greater saphenous vein, may lead to or concur with DVT in up to 40% of cases [31]. Has the patient experienced a sudden swelling in the leg suggestive of DVT? Even pregnant women (who typically develop venous varicosities) should be considered for DVT when sudden, unilateral swelling crops up.

Finally the neurologic examination is performed. The patient is carefully screened for neuropathy. Is the skin unusually dry? Is there muscle wasting? Are the motor strength, mobility, and flexibility within an expected range? Is the gait normal? Do the shoe soles reveal an abnormal wear pattern? Are reflexes normal? Is the patient able to identify movements of the toes? Is the gross sensation normal? The Semmes-Weinstein monofilament is useful for assessing subtle sensory deficits. The filament is gently pressed against the distal foot until it buckles. At this point a standardized pressure has been applied. A normal person can detect a 4.17 monofilament, which exerts 1 g of linear force. The patient who is unable to sense the 5.07 mm strand, which exerts 10 g of linear force, is at markedly increased risk for neuropathic ulceration [32].

Diagnostic testing

Blood work

No laboratory tests provide a direct indication of the status of a nonhealing ulcer. An elevated white blood cell count with increased band forms may indicate infection or inflammation. An abnormal erythrocyte sedimentation rate or C-reactive protein may suggest a deeper process, including severe cellulitis or osteomyelitis. The total protein and prealbumin (half-life 2 days) level give an indication of the nutritional status of the patient, a vital and often overlooked factor in wound healing. The d-dimer value is a nonspecific finding; when in the normal range it may suggest the absence of DVT or pulmonary embolus in a low- to moderate-risk patient [33]. A plasma zinc level may be indicated in nonhealing wounds [34]. Blood cultures are useful if sepsis is suspected.

Microbiology

All ulcers are colonized by bacteria. Colonization is described as a complex polymicrobial landscape that lives in balance with host defenses, generally without ill effect. The presence of excessive moisture, low oxygen tension, necrotic tissue, and dead space may tip this balance toward a more aggressive critical colonization leading to infection [35]. Infection causes persistent inflammation and leads to formation of microthrombi, causing further ischemia, increased friability, and necrosis [36].

Culture results of superficial swabbing from the ulcer base may be misleading. Other techniques, such as deep tissue sampling of an infected ulcer obtained by curettage of the ulcer base after wound débridement, deep needle aspiration, or 2-mm punch biopsy, are considered more valuable, although they may be more uncomfortable for the patient [37].

Imaging

Plain radiographs are a reasonable screening tool for a patient who has a nonhealing wound. Unsuspected foreign bodies, fractures, and gas from gangrenous infection may be visualized. The plain film may also detect osteomyelitis with its characteristic soft tissue swelling, focal demineralization, periosteal elevation, and cortical disruption. Plain radiography is not a very sensitive (60%) or specific (65%) for osteomyelitis, however. If osteomyelitis is suspected, MRI, especially when enhanced with gadolinium, is more than 95% sensitive for soft tissue and bone inflammation [38].

Ultrasound is a widely available instrument, valuable in the evaluation of the nonhealing wound. Doppler flow ultrasound has a sensitivity/specificity for identifying arterial occlusive lesions of approximately 80% to 90% [34]. Wounds of all types depend completely on the availability of fresh oxygenated blood for healing. Doppler studies are noninvasive and may be followed by either magnetic resonance angiography (MRA) or contrast arteriography if angioplasty, stenting, or bypass are considered. Contrast angiography, although still considered the gold standard [10] of pre-interventional imaging, has significant disadvantages compared with minimally invasive MRA. These drawbacks include local arterial injury, pseudoaneurysm, traumatic AV fistula formation, thrombosis, contrast allergy, and contrast nephrotoxicity.

Management of chronic nonhealing wounds

Initially emergency medical providers must address and manage the underlying causes of ulceration, in particular vascular insufficiency, continued trauma, and hyperglycemia. If the wound is progressively worsening despite aggressive care or is located in an atypical location, other possibilities should be considered. These diagnoses include underlying malignancy [39], vasculitis, atypical infection, shooter's patch (an area exploited for repeated vascular access by intravenous drug user) [40], foreign body reaction, non-accidental trauma [41], and factitious wound. The general principles of chronic wound treatment are cleanse, nourish, and protect.

Cleansing

All wounds should be cleansed as thoroughly as possible without disturbing or disrupting underlying viable tissue. Initial decontamination is performed using high-pressure irrigation as for any wound (saline lavage using a large syringe with 18-gauge needle or anti-splash attachment). Topical disinfectants, such as hydrogen peroxide, iodophors, and chlorhexidine, are not generally used in management of chronic ulcers. They may hamper wound healing by direct cytotoxic effects on keratinocytes and fibroblasts. Gentle patting of the surface with soft moist gauze may follow. Further cleaning occurs with débridement (ie, the removal of nonviable tissue and, in the latest understanding, disruption of the biofilm, a protective polysaccharide layer secreted by bacteria). In general, a lower rate of healing is achieved in wounds that are débrided less frequently [42]. In the emergency department sharp débridement is performed with steel scalpel, scissors, and forceps. Sharp débridement is aimed at removing overtly necrotic material and fibrinous exudate. If a stable eschar (ie, a hardened crust of dead tissue) has formed it may not need to be removed. Sharp débridement is selective and controllable. Care must be taken to avoid healthy tissue, and liberal use of local or regional nerve anesthesia is useful for extensive débridement.

Nourishment

Nourishment is the second feature of therapy. Wounds are nourished by blood, oxygen, moisture, food, and external factors. Most important by far is ensuring an adequate arterial blood supply to the wound. The ABI has been shown in multiple studies to be a highly predictive tool [43]. ABI has a roughly 95% sensitivity and specificity for angiographic peripheral arterial disease when less than 0.9 [44]. A value greater than 1.2 may be falsely elevated, a result of calcified lower extremity vessels. A value of between 0.7 and 0.9 indicates a mild to moderate degree of peripheral arterial disease. Anything less than 0.7 denotes significant pathology and should be referred to a specialized vascular laboratory for more sophisticated evaluation, including transcutaneous oxygen tension (TCOT) and possible angiography. ABI reflects macrovascular arterial status, whereas TCOT reveals macro- and microvascular conditions. A patient who does not have diabetes requires a minimum TCOT of 30 mm Hg to heal a wound [12]. Patients who have diabetes require a level of 40 mm Hg to heal.

Adjunctive hyperbaric oxygen therapy (HBOt) has been shown to be effective in healing wounds that are reversibly hypoxic as demonstrated by TCOT. This process can elevate local tissue oxygen tensions, resulting in improved leukocyte function, enhanced collagen synthesis, and neovascularization. It has also been shown to inhibit anaerobic bacterial activity.

Another vital nourishing factor is moisture. Studies since the 1960s have repeatedly indicated a moist environment is significantly better than dry milieu for healing [45–48]. Conversely, dehydration by air exposure, dry gauze, heat lamps, and so forth, is detrimental [28]. Topical moisturizing preparations vary widely. In general, simple petrolatum without preservatives is best. Lanolin may over time become a sensitizing agent. Other over-the-counter products may be helpful but many contain sensitizing agents and, in an individual patient, should be discontinued if skin irritation arises.

Several other nourishing factors have been studied. Topical therapies, including recombinant growth factors (which stimulate angiogenesis, collagen formation, and epithelialization), bilayer keratinocyte skin grafts, and cadaveric skin transplants, are available [49]. Vacuum assist devices clearly aid formation of granulation tissue in difficult wounds [50]. Vitamin deficiencies must be considered and addressed. A daily diet rich in protein, approximately 1.5 to 2 g/kg body weight, is critical for wound healing [51].

Protection

Protection is the third pillar of wound healing. The wound must be physically protected from additional trauma and injury and failure to do so negatively affects the healing process. Pain is an indication of underlying pathology that may be reversible. Bacteria release mediators of inflammation that sensitize pain receptors. Bacterial bioburden may be the most common reason for pain within a wound. Simple, sharp débridement often improves this discomfort. Unrelieved pain may require topical or systemic medication and may necessitate specialty pain management referral. Unmitigated pain leads to decreased patient compliance, depression, and overall worsened quality of life.

Specific recommendations

Chronic venous ulcers

The foundation of CVI ulcer therapy is compression and elevation [52,53]. A wound in the normal healing process develops swelling, a localized edema fluid. If this expected edema stagnates and accumulates, as in the case of CVI, it becomes saturated with proinflammatory factors that lead to impaired healing and secondary lymphedema, occasionally massive. Initially when a patient presents to the emergency department with uncontrolled edema, the practitioner focuses on limb volume decompression. Tubular elastic bandages are a simple and cost-effective product to get the process started. The patient should be encouraged to keep the legs elevated above chest level while sleeping and to avoid dangling legs unsupported while sitting. Elevation of the affected lower extremities offers symptomatic relief and improved healing.

Graduated compression stockings are a prescribed, measured, and expensive product used to keep edema at bay. Graduated compressive leg garments are not to be confused with the commonly available, all-purpose stockings, which offer little benefit. Patients who have arterial insufficiency, especially if the ABI is less than 0.5–0.8, may not be good candidates for compression. Stockings are divided into areas of progressively diminishing compression starting with highest pressure at the ankles (20 to 30 mm Hg in moderate disease and 30 to 40 mm Hg in more severe disease) and lowest pressure at the upper end. The stockings may be knee high or extend to the thigh. These compressive dressings can be used daily for 6 to 9 months before losing effectiveness. A word of caution: patients occasionally do not tolerate the thigh-high stockings and may roll them down for comfort. This may create a tourniquet effect and be unsafe.

Stretchy elastic bandages have been used as compressive dressings. Caution must be advised not to place them too tightly or without gradually diminishing pressure as they run upward to avoid a tourniquet effect. They are considered by some to be too unpredictable in their action. In addition, they tend to lose their elastic quality quickly.

An Unna boot is a gauze wrap impregnated with zinc oxide and calamine. As it dries, it becomes a rigid support and thus acts as a firm strut against which the calf muscles contract. This product has been available for many decades and its mechanism of action is not clearly understood. There are many varieties of multilayer compression bandage systems that provide excellent support and compression. The surrounding skin of a venous ulcer frequently exhibits signs of eczematous dermatitis that may respond to a topical steroid preparation.

Diabetic ulcers

Treatment of diabetic foot ulcers should be aimed at treatment of neuropathy, foot deformity, repetitive trauma, poor glycemic control, and arterial insufficiency. Each of these factors should be addressed in treatment. Foot ulcers are often the precursor to amputation and thus must be treated aggressively. Appropriate referrals to the endocrinologist, podiatrist, wound care specialist, and vascular surgeon should be considered.

Pressure relief is essential in the treatment of ulcers. Total contact casting (TCC) is a specialized casting method that allows continued ambulation while offloading the ulcer [54]. TCC is changed weekly but is not removable by the patient, thus ensuring compliance. Removable TCC variations have been shown to have less effectiveness because of patient nonadherence [55]. The removable TCC can be converted to nonremovable with the simple addition of wrapped cohesive bandage and plaster of Paris. Diabetic ulcers that have been resistant to other forms of therapy may heal within 6 weeks with TCC [56]. Pressure relief in less severe circumstances may be achieved with computer-designed footwear. If custom footwear is not an option for the patient, quality athletic running shoes or shoes with a larger toe box may be an alternative. All shoes should be fitted in the later afternoon when foot swelling is greatest. Therapeutic shoes bring about a dramatic decrease in ulcer recurrence rate. Foot deformities may be referred to a podiatrist to evaluate appropriateness of prophylactic surgery.

Diabetic ulcers are at high risk for polymicrobial infection with an average of 1.5 to 5.8 bacterial isolates per patient, two thirds aerobic and one third anaerobic [37]. *Staphylococcus aureus* is the most common isolate, with an increasing percentage methicillin resistant [57,58]. Group B β-hemolytic streptococcus is another common and potent pathogen. Gram-negative organisms are also pervasive. Ulcer therapy usually requires a combination of agents. Severe infection may respond to combination vancomycin plus β-lactam/β-lactamase inhibitor or vancomycin plus carbapenem [59].

If the condition is clinically appropriate for outpatient management, the patient should be instructed to monitor the condition closely and should be given appropriate referral for reevaluation and continued wound care. If that is not considered feasible, the patient should be instructed to return to the emergency department in 24 to 48 hours for reevaluation. These wounds may worsen quickly leading to osteomyelitis and bacteremia. Osteomyelitis complicates diabetic ulcers in one third to one half of severe ulcers and requires prolonged and specialized care.

Pressure ulcers

Pressure ulcer therapy begins with offloading of the lesion. For patients who are completely immobilized, particularly on a standard surface, turning and repositioning should occur on a frequent basis, at least once every 2 hours. Sophisticated and expensive dynamic air-fluidized support systems are available and may be superior to the less expensive but more readily available static support mattress overlays. There are multiple pressure-reducing devices that can be compared in effectiveness [25,60].

Aside from essential reduction of skin friction and shear forces, the wounds should be kept clean, well débrided, moisturized, possibly dressed with occlusive dressings, and free of active infection. Although moisture is an important element in wound healing, excessive moisture in the form of sweat, exudate, or incontinence is linked to wound aggravation. Topical or oral antibiotics are useful in low-grade infection, especially if *Staphylococcus*, *Pseudomonas*, *Providencia* or anaerobic species are cultured [28].

Dressings

There are many basic types of dressings, some with embedded antimicrobials, categorized into hydrogels, alginates, hydrocolloids, foams, films, and others, each with advantages and disadvantages [53,61,62]. A particular dressing is selected by a wound care specialist based on the specific features of the existing condition. If the wound is essentially dry and clean, nonadherent, soothing, water-soluble, carboxy-methylcellulose hydrogel can be applied directly to the wound [63]. This is wrapped with dry gauze. If the wound is seeping abundant exudate, an absorptive calcium alginate dressing may be more appropriate. Hydrocolloids protectively adhere to a shallow wound, promote autolysis and granulation tissue, and are impermeable to moisture, bacteria, and contamination. Absorbent, opaque, nondébriding foams and transparent nonabsorbent films also are available.

Antibiotic coverage

Antibiotic coverage should be directed primarily toward *S. aureus* (including methicillin resistant) and gram-positive *Streptococcus* (especially β-hemolytic). Many wounds have polymicrobial pathology involving anaerobes, *Enterobacter*, *Pseudomonas*, and a host of less common pathogens [58,64–66]. Appropriate antibiotic combinations found in major antimicrobial guides are then fine honed based on local community sensitivity patterns. Agents, often used in combination, include cephalosporins, β-lactam/β-lactamase inhibitor, fluoroquinolones, clindamycin, imipenem/cilastin, vancomycin, metronidazole, linezolid, and daptomycin. Duration of therapy is 7 to 10 days in mild to moderate infection and as long as necessary in more critical circumstances. Topical antibiotics used alone or in combination may be effective in low-grade infection. Silver sulfadiazine 1% cream (broad antimicrobial), mupirocin (only effective against gram-positive cocci), polymyxin (gram-negatives, including *Pseudomonas*) are generally well tolerated. Topical neomycin (effective against many gram-negative species and staphylococci but not *Pseudomonas*, *Streptococcus*, or anaerobes) and bacitracin (gram-positive activity) may be allergenic in approximately 10% of patients [67]. Patients who have arterial insufficiency or moderate to severe infection require parenteral preparations and vascular surgery consultation.

Summary

Chronic wounds are an immense source of suffering, health care expenditure, and disability for literally millions of patients. On essentially a daily basis, a patient who has either a chronic nonhealing wound or is at risk for one presents to every Emergency Department (ED) in the country. The ED practitioner is in a unique position to identify these patients, initiate appropriate care, and establish proper referrals. Specialists within the field of chronic wound management are making enormous advances implementing sophisticated care but often are unable to make contact with the population at risk. With sensitivity to these conditions, the vigilant ED practitioner can have an enormous impact on public health.

References

[1] Mustoe T. Understanding chronic wounds: a unifying hypothesis on their pathogenesis and implications for therapy. Am J Surg 2004;187(5 Suppl 1):S65–70.

[2] Singer A, Clark R. Cutaneous wound healing. NEJM 1999;341:738–46.

[3] Kruse I, Edelman S. Evaluation and treatment of diabetic foot ulcers. Clinical Diabetes 2006;24:91–3.

[4] Barone EJ, Yager DR, Pozez AL, et al. Interleukin-1 alpha and collagenase activity are elevated in chronic wounds. Plast Reconstr Surg 1998;102(4):1023–7.

[5] Charo I, Ranshohoff R. The many roles of chemokines and chemokine receptors in inflammation. NEJM 2006;354:610–21.

[6] Armstrong DG, Nguyen HC. Improvement in healing with aggressive adema reduction after debridemebt of foot infection in person with diabetes. Arch Surg 2000;135:1405–9.

[7] Levin ME. Management of the diabetic foot: preventing amputation. South Med J 2002; 95(1):10–20.

[8] Cavanagh PR, Lipsky BA, Bradbury AW, et al. Treatment for diabetic foot ulcers. Lancet 2005;336:1725–35.

[9] Campbell LV, Graham AR. The lower limb in people with diabetes. Position statement. MJ Australia 2000;173:369–77.

[10] Sumpio BE. Foot Ulcers. NEJM 2000;343:787–93.

[11] Kamal K, Powell RJ, Sumpio BE. The pathobiology of diabetes mellitus: implications for surgeons. J Am Col Surg 1996;183:271–89.

[12] Singh N, Armstrong D, Lipsky B. Preventing foot ulcers in patients with diabetes. JAMA 2005;293:217–28.

[13] Boulton JM, Kirsner RS, Vileikyte L. Neuropathic diabetic foot ulcers. NEJM 2004;351: 48–55.

[14] Reiber GE, Boulton AJM. Causal pathways for incident lower-extremity ulcers in patients with diabetes from two settings. Diabetes Care 1999;22:157–62.

[15] Levin ME. Preventing amputation in the patient with diabetes. Diabetes Care 1995;18(10): 1383–94.

[16] Murray HJ, Young MJ, Boulton AJM. The association between callus formation, high pressures and neuropathy in diabetic foot ulceration. Diabetic Med 1996;13(11):979–82.

[17] Edmonds ME, Foster AVM. Diabetic foot ulcers. BMJ 2006;332:407–10.

[18] McGuckin. Validation of venous leg ulcer guidelines in the United States and United Kingdom. American Journal of Surgery 2002;18(2):132–7.

[19] Bergan. Chronic venous disease. NEJM 2006;355(5):488–98.

[20] Eberhardt R, Raffetto JD. Chronic venous insufficiency. Circulation 2005;111:2398–409.

[21] Araki CF, Back TL, Padberg FT. The significance of calf muscle pump failure in venous ulceration. Journal of Vascular Surgery 1994;20:872–9.

[22] Tassiopoulos AK, Golts E, Labropoulos N. Current concepts in chronic venous ulceration. Eur J Endovasc Surg 2000;20:227–32.

[23] Takase S, Pascarella L, Bergan J, et al. Hypertension induced venous valve remodeling. J Vasc Surg 2004;39:1329–34.

[24] Sieggreen M, Kline R. Recognizing and managing venous leg ulcers. Advances in Skin and Wound Care July/August 2004.

[25] Staas WE Jr, Cioschi HM. Pressure sores, a multifaceted approach to prevention and treatment. West J Med 1991;154:539–44.

[26] Edlich RF, Winters KL, Woodard CR, et al. Pressure ulcer prevention. J Long Term Eff Med Implants 2004;14(4):285–304.

[27] Reddy M, Gill S, Rochon P. Preventing pressure ulcers: a systematic review. JAMA 2006; 296(8):974–84.

[28] Thomas DR. Prevention and treatment of pressure ulcers: what works? what doesn't? Cleveland Clinic 2001;68(8):704–22.

[29] Kurz X, Kahn SR, Abenhaim L, et al. Chronic venous disorders of the leg: epidemiology, outcomes diagnosis and management. Int Angiol 1999;18(2):83–102.

[30] Grayson ML, Gibbons GW, Balogh K, et al. Probing to bone in infected pedal ulcers. A clinical sign of underlying osteomyelitis in diabetic patients. JAMA 1995;273(9):721–3.

[31] Feied C, Handler J. Thrombophlebitis, superficial. Available at: http://www.emedicine.com/emerg/topic582.htm (Emedicine). Accessed January 10, 2007.

[32] Caputo GM, Cavanagh PR, Ulbrecht JS, et al. Assessment and management of foot disease in patients with diabetes. N Engl J Med 1994;331(13):854–60.

[33] Schreiber D. Deep venous thrombosis and thrombophlebitis. Available at: http://www.emedicine.com/emerg/topic582.htm (Emedicine). Accessed January 10, 2007.

[34] Freedberg I, Eisen A. Fitzpatrick's dermatology in general medicine. Vol. 2. McGraw-Hill; 2003.

[35] Bowler PG. The 100,000 bacterial growth guideline: reassessing its clinical relevance in wound healing. Ostomy/Wound Management 2003;49(1):44–53.

[36] Levin ME. Management of the diabetic foot: preventing amputation. South Med J 2002; 95(1):10–20.

[37] Pellizzer G, Strazzabosco M. Deep tissue biopsy vs. superficial swab culture monitoring in the microbiological assessment of limb-threatening diabetic foot infection. Diabetic Medicine 2001;18:822–7.

[38] Jude EB, Unsworth PF. Optimal treatment of infected diabetic foot ulcers. Drugs Aging 2004;21(13):833–50.

[39] Alam M, Ratner D. Cutaneous squamous-cell carcinoma. NEJM 2001;344(13):975–83.

[40] Tice AD. An unusual, non-healing ulcer on the forearm. NEJM 2002;347(21):1725–6.

[41] Wissow LS. Child abuse and neglect. NEJM 1995;332(21):1425–31.

[42] Steed DL, Donohoe D. Effect of extensive debridement and treatment of the healing of diabetic foot ulcers. J Am Coll Surg 1996;186:61–4.

[43] Khan NA, Rahim SA. Does the clinical examination predict lower extremity peripheral arterial disease? JAMA 2006;295:536–46.

[44] U.S. Preventive Services Task Force. Screening for peripheral arterial disease: recommendation statement. Am Fam Phys 2006;73(3):497–500.
[45] Boulton JM, Kirsner RS, Vileikyte L. Neuropathic diabetic foot ulcers. NEJM 2004;351: 48–55.
[46] Hess CT, Kirsner RS. Orchestrating wound healing: assessing and preparing the wound bed. Advances in Skin and Wound Care 2003;16(5):1–12.
[47] Seaman S. Dressing selection in chronic wound management. J Am Podiatr Med Assoc 2002;92(1):24–33.
[48] White GM, Cox NH. Diseases of the skin. 2nd edition. Mosby Elsevier; 2006.
[49] Harding KG, Morris HL, Patel GK. Healing chronic wounds. BMJ 2002;324:160–3.
[50] Evans D, Land L. Topical negative pressure for treating chronic wounds: a systematic review. Br J Plast Surg 2001;54(3):238–42.
[51] MacKay D, Miller A. Nutritional support for wound healing. Altern Med Rev 2003;8(4): 359–77.
[52] Ibegbuna V, Konstantinos TD. Effect of elastic compression stockings on venous hemodynamics during walking. J Vasc Surg 2003;37:420–5.
[53] Freedberg I, Eisen A. Fitzpatrick's dermatology in general medicine. Vol. 2. McGraw-Hill; 2003.
[54] Willliams DT, Harding KG. New treatments for diabetic neuropathic foot ulceration: views from a wound healing unit. Curr Diab Rep 2003;3(6):468–74.
[55] Armstrong DG. Activity patterns of patients with diabetic foot ulceration. Diabetes Care 2003;26:2595–7.
[56] Cavanagh PR, Lipsky BA, Bradbury AW, et al. Treatment for diabetic foot ulcers. Lancet 2005;336:1725–35.
[57] Armstrong DG, Lipsky BA. Diabetic foot infections: stepwise medical and surgical management. Int Wound J Ju 2004;1(2):123–32.
[58] Armstrong DG, Lipsky BA. Diabetic foot infections: stepwise medical and surgical management. Int Wound J 2004;1:123–32.
[59] Gilbert DN, Moellering RC. The Sanford guide to antimicrobial therapy. 36th edition. 2006.
[60] Cullum N, McInnes E. Support surfaces for pressure ulcer prevention. Cochrane Database Syst Rev 2004;(3):CD001735.
[61] Sheffield PJ, senior editor. Wound care practice 2004. Best Publishing Co.
[62] Jones V, Grey JE, Harding KG. Wound dressings. BMJ 2006;332:777–80.
[63] d'Hemecourt PA. Sodium carboxymethylcellulose aqueous based gel vs becaplermin gel in patients with nonhealing lower extremity diabetic ulcers. Wounds 1998;10(3):69–75.
[64] Lipsky BA. A report from the international consensus on diagnosing and treating the infected diabetic foot. Diabetes/Metabolism Res Rev 2004;20(Suppl 1):S68–77.
[65] Serena T, Robson M. Lack of reliability of clinical/visual assessment of chronic wound infection: the incidence of biopsy-proven infection in venous ulcers. Wounds 2006;18(7): 197–202.
[66] Swartz MN. Cellulitis. NEJM 2004;350(9):904–12.
[67] Lio PA, Kaye ET. Topical antibacterial agents. Infect Dis Clin N Am 2004;18:717–33.

ELSEVIER
SAUNDERS

Emerg Med Clin N Am
25 (2007) 223–234

EMERGENCY
MEDICINE
CLINICS OF
NORTH AMERICA

Imaging Modalities in Wounds and Superficial Skin Infections

Robert B. Blankenship, MD, FACEP[a,b,*],
Todd Baker, MD[a,b]

[a]Department of Emergency Medicine, Madigan Army Medical Center,
Tacoma, WA 98431, USA
[b]Division of Emergency Medicine, University of Washington Medical Center,
1959 NE Pacific Street, Box 356123, Seattle, WA 98195-6123, USA

Open wounds and lacerations are the most commonly encountered problems in emergency medicine, affecting 8% of adult patients [1] and 30% to 40% of pediatric patients [2] who present to emergency departments (EDs) in the United States. Emergency physicians cannot control the patient's age, preexisting comorbid conditions, or laceration width, and all of these factors can increase the risk for infection [3]. The probability of infection can be decreased by prompt detection and removal of foreign bodies complicating an open wound.

Unfortunately, detection of retained soft tissue foreign bodies remains a significant problem. Previous literature reported that 38% of foreign bodies in hand wounds were missed by the initial treating physician [4]. Considering this study, we should not be surprised that missed foreign bodies are the second leading cause of lawsuits in emergency medicine [5]. In addition to the legal ramifications, detection and removal of a foreign body is essential to avoid the many complications of a retained foreign body, which may include infection, inflammation, allergic reaction, and disability. Currently, there are several imaging modalities that the emergency medicine provider may use to aid in foreign body detection and wound management. Techniques and appropriate use of these imaging modalities for foreign bodies and soft tissue infections are discussed in this article.

* Corresponding author. Department of Emergency Medicine, Madigan Army Medical Center, Tacoma, WA 98431.
E-mail address: robert.b.blankenship@us.army.mil (R.B. Blankenship).

0733-8627/07/$ - see front matter © 2007 Elsevier Inc. All rights reserved.
doi:10.1016/j.emc.2007.01.011   *emed.theclinics.com*

Plain radiography

Although a thorough history and physical may suggest the presence of a foreign body, it is not sufficient to rule out the possibility of a foreign body. In cases in which there is a concern for potential foreign body, imaging and wound exploration should be performed. Traditionally, plain radiography has been the most commonly used modality in the evaluation for foreign bodies in extremity trauma. This approach is commonly used given the ease of obtaining and interpreting plain films, its cost, and its wide availability. Studies to date support this approach for radiopaque substances, including aluminum, that are 1 to 2 mm or greater in size, because they are reliably detected 80% to 95% of the time [4,6–8]. Caution is advised, however, because the above-reported accuracy only applies to radiopaque foreign bodies. Plain radiography has poor sensitivity in the detection of radiolucent foreign bodies, such as wood, plastic, and vegetative material, such as cactus spines [4].

CT

CT can detect radiopaque and radiolucent foreign bodies, with a much higher sensitivity for radiopaque ones. CT for radiolucent foreign bodies is much better than plain radiography yet it only has an intermediate sensitivity [9,10]. Given its increased cost, the need for ionizing radiation, and its lack of sensitivity, CT is not routinely recommended to rule out a radiolucent foreign body. CT can best be used when a foreign body is suspected but not detected by radiographs or ultrasound [11].

CT has historically been used extensively in the imaging of soft tissue infections and may be considered to be the gold standard in the detection of abscesses. Unlike ultrasound, which is best for more superficial soft tissue infections, CT can evaluate deeper structures and the extent of surrounding inflammation, and it is well accepted by surgeons. CT has also been used to diagnose and evaluate emergent wound infections, such as necrotizing fasciitis [12,13].

MRI

MRI has also proven to be accurate in the detection of foreign bodies, but it can be difficult to distinguish foreign bodies from adjacent structures, such as scar tissue, calcifications, and tendons. Furthermore, the high cost and lack of availability render MRI impractical for routine foreign body detection in the ED. Perhaps the only time one might consider obtaining an MRI from the ED in wound infections would be a case in which it was difficult to differentiate between cellulitis and necrotizing fasciitis [14–16]. MRI has good sensitivity but poorer specificity in necrotizing fasciitis, so one should include both the clinical findings and the MRI results together in formulating a treatment plan. Given the rapidly progressive nature of necrotizing fascitis it is prudent to obtain an immediate surgical consult when necrotizing fasciitis is suspected.

Ultrasound

There is a growing body of clinical data reporting that ultrasound is the imaging modality of choice in the evaluation of suspected radiolucent foreign bodies [17–19]. Much of the literature evaluating the use of ultrasound in detecting foreign bodies has been performed in cadaveric tissue, chicken thighs, turkey breasts, beef cubes, and canine models [18,20–24]. Most of these studies have determined ultrasound was accurate in the detection of foreign bodies, with rare exceptions. The sensitivity of these studies ranges from 43% to 98%, and the specificity ranges from 59% to 98%.

Most of the clinical data supporting ultrasound use in the detection of foreign bodies has been in the form of case reports and nonclinical studies [19,25–27]. There are a few clinical studies that support ultrasound's reliability in detection of foreign bodies, however. Gilbert and colleagues [28] performed ultrasounds on 50 patients suspected of having a radiolucent foreign body, and ultrasound detected 21 of the 22 foreign bodies found at operation. There were three false positives in this study. Banerjee and Das [29] performed a prospective study of 45 patients to assess the accuracy of ultrasound detection and localization of foreign bodies of the extremities, with 45 patients enrolled. Each patient had plain radiographs and ultrasounds performed. Of the 20 patients who had radiopaque foreign bodies, ultrasound detected 19. Of 25 patients who had negative radiographs, ultrasound correctly identified 7 patients who had a foreign body. Crawford and Matheson [30] evaluated 39 consecutive patients who had a suspected retained foreign body in the hand and in whom standard soft issue radiographs were negative with ultrasound. Ultrasound correctly identified 19 of the 20 patients who had a confirmed foreign body removed surgically. In this study there were also two false positive cases. At the present time there is only one clinical study that has evaluated the use of ultrasound for foreign body detection [2] in children. This study suggested that ultrasound detection of foreign bodies was comparable to plain radiographs interpreted by an attending pediatric radiologist. The study was limited, however, in that only 12 patients who had foreign body were included and the experience level of the emergency medicine faculty was unclear. Further studies are needed to prove the accuracy of ultrasound to detect foreign bodies in pediatric patients.

Performing ultrasound for foreign body detection

Before beginning to scan a patient with ultrasound it is important to elicit several key aspects in their history to assist localization of a foreign body. Knowing where the patient has a sensation of a foreign body can assist you in deciding where to begin your ultrasound search. Knowing the age and potential type of material of the foreign body is important because the sonographic appearance of a foreign body varies based on its composition and age.

The ultrasound examination should be performed with a high-frequency (7.5 MHz or higher) linear array transducer (Fig. 1). The higher the frequency of the transducer used the better the resolution is. A higher-frequency probe also decreases the near-field acoustic dead space. The near-field acoustic dead space is a term used to describe the ultrasound image immediately adjacent to the transducer. Overall the image quality in this near field is compromised, which makes visualization of a very superficial foreign body or a foreign body in a toe or finger difficult (Fig. 2). The easiest method to compensate for this limitation is to use a standoff pad. Standoff pads are made of low acoustic impedance material and they elevate the transducer from the tissue being scanned, eliminating the near-field acoustic dead space. Standoff pads are commercially available, but they can be made from a water-filled latex glove [31] or by using 250- to 500-cc bags of intravenous fluids. One can also use a water bath as a standoff. This technique obviates the need for ultrasound gel or contact between the ultrasound transducer and the patient's skin, thus eliminating discomfort [32].

When scanning the patient it is important to be slow and methodical to optimize chances of detecting the foreign body because its appearance could closely match the surrounding soft tissue or structures. The best views of the foreign bodies are obtained when the transducer is either parallel or perpendicular to the foreign body. Most foreign bodies appear echogenic on ultrasound. Wooden foreign bodies are echogenic, although they may become less echogenic over time [18]. Wooden foreign bodies may exhibit posterior

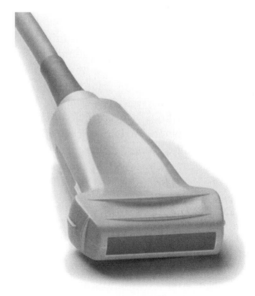

Fig. 1. A high-frequency linear array transducer. This is the 38-mm broadband (6–13 MHz) HFL38 linear array transducer.

The near-field acoustic dead space is a term used to describe the ultrasound image immediately adjacent to the transducer. Overall the image quality in this very near field is compromised which make visualization of a very superficial foreign body or a foreign body in a toe or finger difficult.

Fig. 2. The near-field acoustic dead space is a term used to describe the ultrasound image immediately adjacent to the transducer, which has sub-optimal image quality.

acoustic shadowing (Fig. 3), but this finding is not universally present [28,33]. Glass and metallic foreign bodies are also echogenic and they often have a comet tail artifact (Fig. 4). After 24 to 48 hours a foreign body can also become surrounded by a sonolucent echo secondary to possible hyperemia, edema, or inflammation (Fig. 5). This hypoechoic rim can also aid in the detection of a foreign body [18].

Sonographer experience can limit the ability to detect superficial foreign bodies of the hands and feet. Foreign bodies in patient's extremities are frequently close to normal structures, such as tendons, muscle, and bone. Without a thorough understanding of the anatomy and normal variants a sesamoid bone, scar, or calcification might be mistaken for a foreign body.

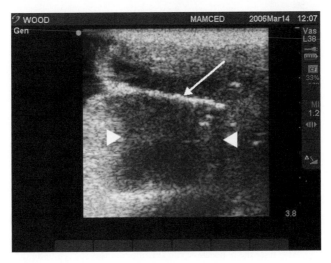

Fig. 3. Longitudinal view of a wooden foreign body (*arrow*). Note the posterior acoustic shadowing (*between arrow heads*).

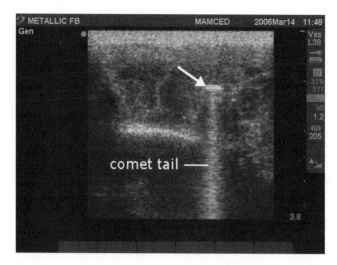

Fig. 4. Longitudinal view of a small echogenic metallic foreign body (*arrow*). Note the comet tail artifact posterior to the metallic foreign body characteristic of glass and metallic foreign bodies.

Limitations of ultrasound for foreign body detection

Ultrasound has only been studied to detect superficial bodies, so if a deep foreign body is suspected another imaging modality, such as CT or radiographs, may be more appropriate. As mentioned above there are several

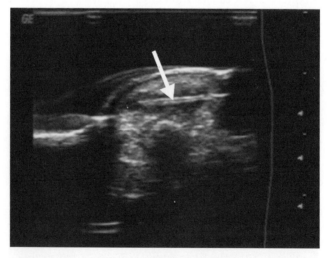

Fig. 5. Longitudinal ultrasound of a distal finger. An echogenic foreign body in long axis is easily seen (*arrow*). Also note the hypoechoic rim surrounding this foreign body that had been in the patient's fingertip for several days. A standoff was used in obtaining this image of a very superficial foreign body.

causes of false positive scans, including scars and calcifications. Additionally, air in a wound is echogenic and may be misinterpreted as a foreign body. Small amounts of air may be introduced with irrigation; therefore it may be prudent to perform ultrasound before irrigation to reduce the possibility of iatrogenic introduction of air into the wound before being examined. Although ultrasound can be used in the extremities, it can be difficult to perform on fingers or toes without a high-frequency probe and an adequate standoff pad. To carefully examine a wound for a foreign body with ultrasound an ample amount of time is required. Although there are no data to accurately conclude the average scan time for this type of ultrasound examination there is some evidence to suggest it is approximately 10 minutes [30].

Despite the above-mentioned limitations, it is clear that ultrasound is beneficial for patients who have a suspected radiolucent foreign body. Ultrasound can aid in accurate detection and localization and facilitate the removal of foreign bodies. Additionally, it can be used in the patient who has a radiopaque foreign body to localize and facilitate removal. Considering ultrasound is relatively inexpensive, can be performed at the bedside, and is readily available, it has become the initial imaging modality of choice for many experienced emergency providers for the evaluation and detection of foreign bodies in wounds.

Soft tissue infections

Soft tissue infections are common clinical entities cared for in the ED. Classically, the diagnosis of abscess or cellulitis is made clinically. In the case of a patient who has fluctuance or spontaneous drainage of pus, the diagnosis of abscess can be easily secured. Unfortunately, the differentiation between cellulitis and abscess is not always easy to decipher on a clinical basis [34–36]. Ultrasound may help the emergency medicine provider rapidly differentiate between cellulitis and an abscess, ensuring the appropriate therapy is rendered, thus reducing costs, potential complications, delays in treatment, and medical-legal risks.

Use of ultrasound in soft tissue management

Ultrasound use for the detection of abscess has been reported in the medical literature since the 1980s [37–39]. Although there are few prospective articles assessing sensitivity of this procedure for ultrasound, recent literature reports ultrasound is 98% sensitive for abscess, whereas physical examination is only 86% sensitive [35]. In addition to its use in routine skin infections, ultrasound has been shown to be useful in difficult-to-detect breast abscesses [35,40]. One ultrasound study showed the drainage of these abscesses was less invasive and allowed for improved cosmesis [41,42].

Unlike ultrasound examinations for foreign body, which can be difficult and time consuming, the accuracy of ultrasound is excellent for abscess and the examination only takes a few minutes to perform [35].

Ultrasound for superficial skin infections should be performed with a high-frequency (7.5 MHz or higher) linear array transducer. Lower-frequency probes (5 MHz), which offer more penetration, may be useful for abscesses that are suspected to be deeper. Before discussing the ultrasound findings of cellulitis and abscess, it is important to understand normal subcutaneous tissue appearance on ultrasound. The subcutaneous tissue is primarily fat, which appears hypoechoic. Connective tissue runs sporadically throughout the subcutaneous tissue and it is hyperechoic. Fascial planes have a consistent thickness and are hyperechoic on the ultrasound screen (Fig. 6). Muscle has a characteristic striated appearance that is best appreciated when seen on long axis, but it can also be appreciated when seen obliquely or on end (Fig. 7). The vasculature is easy to note because its lumen should be regular and anechoic in appearance. Veins are thin walled and easily compressible, whereas arteries have a thicker wall and are pulsatile. Depending on the depth of the window and the area being scanned, bone may be seen, which is characterized by a brightly echogenic cortex with distal shadowing.

Cellulitis

Cellulitis causes swelling of the subcutaneous tissue, which results in increased distance between the skin and the underlying fascia and bone.

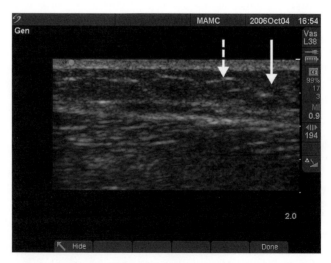

Fig. 6. Ultrasound image of normal hypoechoic subcutaneous tissue (*solid arrow*) with hyperechoic connective tissue (*broken arrow*).

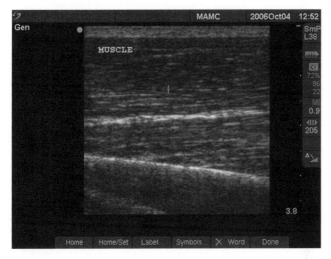

Fig. 7. Ultrasound image of muscle. Note the characteristic striated appearance seen on long axis.

This distance causes a diffuse increase in the echogenicity of the subcutaneous tissue. The edema also is seen on the ultrasound as increased hypoechoic strands between the subcutaneous tissue resulting in a cobblestone or reticular appearance (Fig. 8). At times these changes can be best appreciated by comparing the appearance of the affected soft tissue versus the unaffected side of the patient, or one can compare the skin that appears to have cellulitis versus soft tissue distal to the affected region.

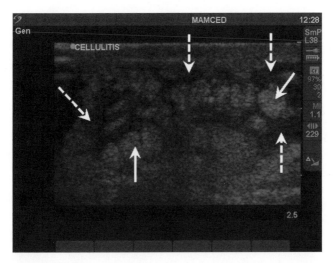

Fig. 8. Ultrasound in a patient who has cellulitis. Note the increased echogenicity of the subcutaneous tissue (*arrows*) and the hypoechoic strands of edema (*dashed arrows*).

Abscesses

Abscesses have variable sonographic appearances. The most common appearance of an abscess is a spherical or elliptical mass (Fig. 9). The mass is usually hypoechoic or may be anechoic with a surrounding echogenic rim. Alternative appearances include an isoechoic or echogenic mass. In these cases, one can look for posterior acoustic enhancement that signifies an abscess instead of a solid mass. The sonographer can also attempt to elicit motion when these masses are compressed with a transducer. Doppler ultrasound can be used to look for the characteristic hyperemia of the surrounding tissue with absence of Doppler flow inside the abscess. Some irregular pockets of pus may be difficult to differentiate from increased edema. In these cases it might be prudent to attempt ultrasound-guided needle aspiration to determine if an abscess is present. In cases in which a superficial abscess is suspected one should consider a standoff to ensure that a small abscess is not missed because of near-field acoustic dead space.

Summary

Imaging modalities are essential to understand the best care for our patients in the ED. By fully understanding which applications are best suited for each situation, one can expedite and improve the care rendered for an emergency medicine patient. Furthermore, by using the appropriate modalities one can minimize the risk for missing a foreign body or abscess or relying too heavily on a physical examination to rule out these conditions. Although further study needs to be done in the pediatric population it is

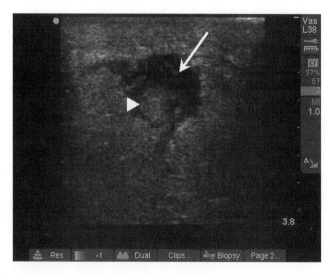

Fig. 9. Ultrasound of an anechoic abscess (*arrow*) that contains isoechoic debris (*arrowhead*).

clear that ultrasound has a significant role in the imaging of patients who have open wounds and those who have soft tissue infections. In conclusion, ultrasound can be used to evaluate for foreign body, cellulitis, and abscess. Multiple studies have demonstrated its usefulness. Further research is required to fully explore the endless possibilities of ultrasound in emergency medicine.

References

[1] McCaig LF, Nawar EW. National Hospital Ambulatory Medical Care Survey: 2004 emergency department summary. Adv Data 2006;372:1–29.

[2] Friedman DI, Forti RJ, Wall SP, et al. The utility of bedside ultrasound and patient perception in detecting soft tissue foreign bodies in children. Pediatr Emerg Care 2005;21(8):487–92.

[3] Hollander JE, Singer AJ, Valentine SM, et al. Risk factors for infection in patients with traumatic lacerations. Acad Emerg Med 2001;8(7):716–20.

[4] Anderson MA, Newmeyer WL 3rd, Kilgore ES Jr. Diagnosis and treatment of retained foreign bodies in the hand. Am J Surg 1982;144(1):63–7.

[5] Schlager D. Ultrasound detection of foreign bodies and procedure guidance. Emerg Med Clin North Am 1997;15(4):895–912.

[6] Chisholm CD, Wood CO, Chua G, et al. Radiographic detection of gravel in soft tissue. Ann Emerg Med 1997;29(6):725–30.

[7] Courter BJ. Radiographic screening for glass foreign bodies—what does a "negative" foreign body series really mean? Ann Emerg Med 1990;19(9):997–1000.

[8] Valente JH, Lemke T, Ridlen M, et al. Aluminum foreign bodies: do they show up on x-ray? Emerg Radiol 2005;12(1–2):30–3.

[9] Ginsburg MJ, Ellis GL, Flom LL. Detection of soft-tissue foreign bodies by plain radiography, xerography, computed tomography, and ultrasonography. Ann Emerg Med 1990; 19(6):701–3.

[10] Russell RC, Williamson DA, Sullivan JW, et al. Detection of foreign bodies in the hand. J Hand Surg [Am] 1991;16(1):2–11.

[11] Flom LL, Ellis GL. Radiologic evaluation of foreign bodies. Emerg Med Clin North Am 1992;10(1):163–77.

[12] Wysoki MG, Santora TA, Shah RM, et al. Necrotizing fasciitis: CT characteristics. Radiology 1997;203(3):859–63.

[13] Becker M, Zbaren P, Hermans R, et al. Necrotizing fasciitis of the head and neck: role of CT in diagnosis and management. Radiology 1997;202(2):471–6.

[14] Schmid MR, Kossmann T, Duewell S. Differentiation of necrotizing fasciitis and cellulitis using MR imaging. AJR Am J Roentgenol 1998;170(3):615–20.

[15] Beltran J. MR imaging of soft-tissue infection. Magn Reson Imaging Clin N Am 1995;3(4): 743–51.

[16] Rahmouni A, Chosidow O, Mathieu D, et al. MR imaging in acute infectious cellulitis. Radiology 1994;192(2):493–6.

[17] Turner J, Wilde CH, Hughes KC, et al. Ultrasound-guided retrieval of small foreign objects in subcutaneous tissue. Ann Emerg Med 1997;29(6):731–4.

[18] Jacobson JA, Powell A, Craig JG, et al. Wooden foreign bodies in soft tissue: detection at US. Radiology 1998;206(1):45–8.

[19] Boyse TD, Fessell DP, Jacobson JA, et al. US of soft-tissue foreign bodies and associated complications with surgical correlation. Radiographics 2001;21(5):1251–6.

[20] de Lacey G, Evans R, Sandin B. Penetrating injuries: how easy is it to see glass (and plastic) on radiographs? Br J Radiol 1985;58(685):27–30.

[21] Hill R, Conron R, Greissinger P, et al. Ultrasound for the detection of foreign bodies in human tissue. Ann Emerg Med 1997;29(3):353–6.

[22] Schlager D, Sanders AB, Wiggins D, et al. Ultrasound for the detection of foreign bodies. Ann Emerg Med 1991;20(2):189–91.

[23] Blyme PJ, Lind T, Schantz K, et al. Ultrasonographic detection of foreign bodies in soft tissue. A human cadaver study. Arch Orthop Trauma Surg 1990;110(1):24–5.

[24] Manthey DE, Storrow AB, Milbourn JM, et al. Ultrasound versus radiography in the detection of soft-tissue foreign bodies. Ann Emerg Med 1996;28(1):7–9.

[25] Yanay O, Vaughan DJ, Diab M, et al. Retained wooden foreign body in a child's thigh complicated by severe necrotizing fasciitis: a case report and discussion of imaging modalities for early diagnosis. Pediatr Emerg Care 2001;17(5):354–5.

[26] Levine WN, Leslie BM. The use of ultrasonography to detect a radiolucent foreign body in the hand: a case report. J Hand Surg [Am] 1993;18(2):218–20.

[27] Pigott DC, Buckingham RB, Eller RL, et al. Foreign body in the tongue: a novel use for emergency department ultrasonography. Ann Emerg Med 2005;45(6):677–9.

[28] Gilbert FJ, Campbell RS, Bayliss AP. The role of ultrasound in the detection of non-radiopaque foreign bodies. Clin Radiol 1990;41(2):109–12.

[29] Banerjee B, Das RK. Sonographic detection of foreign bodies of the extremities. Br J Radiol 1991;64(758):107–12.

[30] Crawford R, Matheson AB. Clinical value of ultrasonography in the detection and removal of radiolucent foreign bodies. Injury 1989;20(6):341–3.

[31] Dean AJ, Gronczewski CA, Costantino TG. Technique for emergency medicine bedside ultrasound identification of a radiolucent foreign body. J Emerg Med 2003;24(3):303–8.

[32] Blaivas M, Lyon M, Brannam L, et al. Water bath evaluation technique for emergency ultrasound of painful superficial structures. Am J Emerg Med 2004;22(7):589–93.

[33] Howden MD. Foreign bodies within finger tendon sheaths demonstrated by ultrasound: two cases. Clin Radiol 1994;49(6):419–20.

[34] Tayal VS, Hasan N, Norton HJ, et al. The effect of soft-tissue ultrasound on the management of cellulitis in the emergency department. Acad Emerg Med 2006;13(4):384–8.

[35] Squire BT, Fox JC, Anderson C. ABSCESS: applied bedside sonography for convenient evaluation of superficial soft tissue infections. Acad Emerg Med 2005;12(7):601–6.

[36] Blaivas M. Ultrasound-guided breast abscess aspiration in a difficult case. Acad Emerg Med 2001;8(4):398–401.

[37] vanSonnenberg E, Wittich GR, Casola G, et al. Sonography of thigh abscess: detection, diagnosis, and drainage. AJR Am J Roentgenol 1987;149(4):769–72.

[38] Beckmann CR, Thomason JL, Sampson MB, et al. Ultrasonographic confirmation of a thigh abscess. IMJ Ill Med J 1985;167(2):126–7.

[39] Floyd JL, Goodman EL. Soft-tissue abscesses in a diabetic patient. Localization by gallium citrate Ga 67 scanning and sonography. JAMA 1981;246(6):675–6.

[40] Eryilmaz R, Sahin M, Hakan Tekelioglu M, et al. Management of lactational breast abscesses. Breast 2005;14(5):375–9.

[41] Strauss A, Middendorf K, Muller-Egloff S, et al. [Sonographically guided percutaneous needle aspiration of breast abscesses—a minimal-invasive alternative to surgical incision]. Ultraschall Med 2003;24(6):393–8 [in German].

[42] Christensen AF, Al-Suliman N, Nielsen KR, et al. Ultrasound-guided drainage of breast abscesses: results in 151 patients. Br J Radiol 2005;78(927):186–8.

ELSEVIER
SAUNDERS

Emerg Med Clin N Am
25 (2007) 235–242

EMERGENCY
MEDICINE
CLINICS OF
NORTH AMERICA

Occlusive Wound Dressings in Emergency Medicine and Acute Care

Margaret A. Fonder[a], Adam J. Mamelak, MD[b],
Gerald S. Lazarus, MD[b,c],
Arjun Chanmugam, MD, MBA[d],*

[a]Department of Dermatology, Johns Hopkins University, Baltimore, MD 21287, USA
[b]Johns Hopkins Wound Center, Johns Hopkins Bayview Medical Center,
Baltimore, MD 21287, USA
[c]Johns Hopkins University School of Medicine, Baltimore, MD 21287, USA
[d]Department of Emergency Medicine, Johns Hopkins University School of Medicine,
1830 East Monument Street, Suite 6-110, Baltimore, MD 21287, USA

Among medical professionals and patients alike, there exists a firmly entrenched belief that wounds heal best when permitted to dry out and form hard crusts, or scabs. Absorptive gauze-based dressings designed to dry the wound base have long been the most widely used dressing type. The advocacy for dry wound healing is misguided, however, because research has repeatedly demonstrated that superior healing is achieved when wounds are maintained in a moist environment under occlusive wound dressings.

Occlusive dressings are moisture-retentive wound coverings that may be either fully occlusive (impermeable to fluids and gases) or semiocclusive (impermeable to fluids but partially permeable to gases like oxygen and water vapor). Occlusive dressings have been shown to speed healing, reduce pain, and improve patient quality of life compared with gauze dressings. Despite these benefits, however, they are underutilized [1,2].

Lacerations, abrasions, and other acute wounds represent the third most common presenting complaint in emergency departments [3]. This article reviews the advantages and indications for occlusive wound dressings in the emergency department setting.

---
* Corresponding author.
E-mail address: achanmug@jhmi.edu (A. Chanmugam).

0733-8627/07/$ - see front matter © 2007 Elsevier Inc. All rights reserved.
doi:10.1016/j.emc.2007.01.012   *emed.theclinics.com*

Gauze dressings, the old standard

Gauzes (Fig. 1) are cotton or synthetic dressings designed to absorb fluid and dehydrate the wound base. The dry, hard crust that forms beneath gauze dressings acts as a physical barrier to migrating keratinocytes, impeding wound re-epithelialization [4]. Gauze also has a tendency to bond to the wound surface, which causes pain and trauma to the wound bed at dressing changes and further retards the healing process. Even gauzes designed to be nonadherent, such as petrolatum-impregnated gauze and perforated plastic film-covered gauze, sometimes adhere [4,5]. Furthermore, because of their meshlike nature, gauze dressings make wounds highly vulnerable to bacterial contamination and infection [2,6,7]. This risk is especially high for wounds covered with wet or exudate-soaked gauze dressings [4,8]. Gauzes may also shed fibers into the wound, producing a foreign body reaction that can delay healing [4,9,10]. Finally, gauze dressings must be changed every 12 to 24 hours, making them a labor- and resource-intensive approach to wound care.

Advantages of occlusive wound dressings

In 1962, Winter [11] demonstrated that porcine wounds covered with occlusive dressings re-epithelialized nearly twice as fast as similar wounds left exposed to air. Subsequent studies confirmed these effects in humans [12,13]. By preventing eschar formation and maintaining moisture at the wound surface, occlusive dressings facilitate keratinocyte migration and wound re-epithelialization [4,11]. Furthermore, moisture-retentive dressings do not adhere to the wound bed, and therefore cause less trauma to the re-epithelializing wound during changes than do gauze dressings.

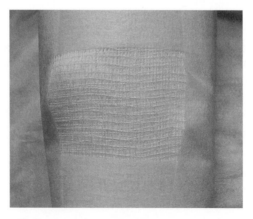

Fig. 1. Gauze dressing attached with paper tape.

Wound fluid from acute, uninfected wounds has been shown to stimulate fibroblast, keratinocyte, and endothelial cell proliferation [14,15]. Moisture-retentive wound dressings thus may also improve healing by maintaining and prolonging contact of the wound bed with wound fluids. Furthermore, the hypoxic wound microenvironment created by occlusive and semi-occlusive dressings has been shown to stimulate wound angiogenesis and collagen synthesis [16–18].

Despite initial fears that occlusive dressings would promote wound infection, they have actually been shown to decrease infection rates compared with traditional gauze dressings [2,6,7]. This effect is largely attributable to the superior barrier properties of these watertight dressings compared with gauzes [2,4,8,19]. Occlusive dressings also decrease the pH at the wound surface, creating an environment inhospitable to bacterial growth, which may contribute to the decreased rates of wound infection [16].

The goal of wound care is to restore function to wounded tissue as quickly as possible so that patients may swiftly return to their daily activities with minimal compromise of quality of life [20]. In studies, occlusive dressings outperform traditional gauzes in patient comfort, convenience, and compliance [1,21–23]. An important advantage is that because many occlusive dressings are firmly adhesive and waterproof, patients may bathe without having to re-dress the wound. Additionally, several studies have documented that occlusive dressings decrease wound pain compared with gauze dressings [14,22,24,25]. There is also evidence to suggest that moisture-retentive dressings may reduce scarring and improve cosmetic outcomes [22].

Many practitioners favor gauze dressings to moisture-retentive dressings because gauze costs less per dressing. When one considers that gauze dressings require once or twice daily changes compared with occlusive dressings that not only shorten healing times but can also be left in place for days at a time, cost effectiveness may be comparable [2,26–28].

Occlusive dressing types

There are more than a thousand moisture-retentive occlusive wound dressings on the market today [1]. The so-called "ideal wound dressing" is one that would create a moist healing environment, control exudate levels, allow gas exchange, provide thermal insulation, prevent bacterial contamination, cause minimal discomfort when in place and during dressing changes, and require infrequent dressing changes, while remaining cost effective [20,29,30]. Many modern occlusive-type wound dressings approximate these characteristics. These products include films, hydrocolloids, foams, and hydrogels [27].

Films (Fig. 2A) are thin membranes that are transparent, adhesive, and waterproof. Films are not absorptive; they manage wound exudates by moisture vapor transmission only. They are thus best reserved for wounds

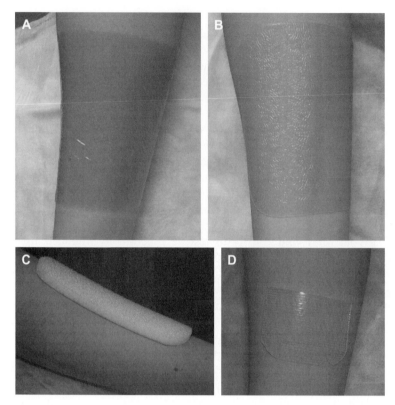

Fig. 2. Moisture-retentive wound dressings. (*A*) Film dressing. (*B*) Hydrocolloid dressing. (*C*) Foam dressing. (*D*) Sheet hydrogel dressing.

with low levels of drainage. Because they are transparent, films are ideal for wounds requiring frequent inspection, because the status of the wound can be monitored without having to remove the dressing. The adhesive on films adheres only to the dry intact skin surrounding a wound, not the moist wound surface, thus minimizing pain and wound bed trauma at dressing changes. Film dressings are highly conformable and flexible, making them ideal for treating wounds on joints and hands. They may be left in place up to 7 days or until a fluid leak occurs or the dressing separates from the wound bed [31]. For lasting wear, films should be applied with at least a 2-cm border of intact skin beyond the wound edges.

Hydrocolloids (Fig. 2B) are adhesive, conformable, semiocclusive, water-proof dressings that are thicker than films and moderately absorptive, making them ideal for treating wounds with a moderate degree of exudate or drainage. In general, wounds involving deeper dermis produce larger amounts of exudate than those located more superficially [10]. Like films, hydrocolloids may be left in place for 7 days or until a fluid leak occurs or the dressing separates from the wound bed [31]. Here also, a border of dry intact skin of at least 2 cm is necessary for dressing adherence. When in contact with a moist wound surface, hydrocolloids form a hydrophilic gel that helps to maintain a moist environment for healing and prevents dressing adherence to the wound base [32]. Patients should be advised that this discharge may become malodorous or purulent-appearing after several days of wear, but is not a sign of infection.

Foams (Fig. 2C) are moderately absorbent dressings composed of a soft, cushion-like material. Some foams are adhesive, whereas others must be secured by an adhesive secondary dressing such as a transparent film. Foams may be used to dress wounds with moderate amounts of exudate and should be changed approximately every 3 days [4,31].

Hydrogels (Fig. 2D) are moisture-donating water-based gels available in sheet form attached to a semipermeable film backing or in amorphous form from a tube. Hydrogels are nonadhesive and must be secured by a secondary dressing. They are ideal for dressing dry wounds or wounds with low levels of exudate. In our experience, patients often report marked reductions in wound pain when hydrogel dressings are applied, and sheet hydrogels produce the most pronounced pain-reducing effects. Hydrogel dressings should be changed every 1 to 3 days [4].

When to use occlusive dressings

Abrasions, lacerations, minor burns, and chronic ulcers are among the wound types most commonly seen in emergency departments. When used appropriately, moisture-retentive dressings can have benefits for each of these wound types. Before applying dressings to any wound, standard protocols of patient stabilization, assessment for deep tissue injury, wound cleansing, debridement of devitalized tissue and debris, and wound closure should be followed.

Abrasions are superficial wounds caused by frictional forces that rub or scrape away portions of the epidermis and sometimes dermis. These wounds can be extremely painful. Occlusive dressings are ideal for this wound type [33,34]. To achieve maximal benefits for re-epithelialization, the dressing should be applied within 2 hours of wounding and left in place for at least 24 hours [35]. Because superficial wounds generally produce little exudate, a hydrogel (for pain relief) covered by an adhesive film might be a suitable regimen for many abrasions.

Lacerations are wounds caused by sharp cutting forces or blunt trauma [33,34]. These wounds may be closed primarily with staples or sutures or left to heal by secondary intention. Occlusive wound dressings are ideal for treating lacerations, whether sutured or left open [5,36,37], and may even be used to temporarily cover wounds returning for delayed primary closure [20]. The choice of dressing type should be based on the degree of wound exudate observed and expected. Some experts maintain that occlusive dressings can be left in place over sutured wounds until it is time for suture removal as long as the dressing remains adhered and there are no fluid leaks [20].

Minor burns may benefit from the use of occlusive dressings also. Hydrocolloid dressings have been shown to speed the re-epithelialization of superficial and deep partial-thickness burns, with less pain and lower overall cost than conventional treatment with silver sulfadiazine cream [38,39].

Chronic wounds, such as venous stasis ulcers and decubitus ulcers, are commonly treated with occlusive dressings with well-documented improvements over gauze dressings in rate and quality of healing and cost efficacy [27,28,40].

Precautions

Although occlusive dressings have many benefits for wound healing, certain precautions must be taken with their use. First, occlusive dressings are not appropriate for use over infected wounds. Additionally, many occlusive dressings (eg, films, hydrocolloids) are firmly adhesive, a feature that helps to form a waterproof seal at the skin surface and facilitates long wear times but can also cause stripping or tearing of fragile skin if dressings are applied and removed too frequently [18]. Caution must also be exercised when using moisture-retentive dressings to treat highly exudative wounds, because fluid pooling can lead to irritation or maceration of the surrounding skin [31]. Macerated tissue is pale, friable, and prone to breakdown, potentially causing wound enlargement. The accumulation of significant fluid collections beneath an occlusive dressing is a sign that a dressing change is warranted. Finally, occlusive dressings are not appropriate for use over puncture injuries or sinus tracts. These types of deep wounds must be encouraged to heal from the base upward to eliminate dead space and prevent abscess formation, and thus require loose packing with gauze ribbons rather than a surface dressing [41].

Summary

Occlusive-type wound dressings have numerous benefits for the treatment of many wounds encountered in the emergency department, including faster healing, reduced risk for infection, and decreased pain and scarring. The authors encourage physicians to sample these products and incorporate them into regular practice.

References

[1] Eaglstein WH. Moist wound healing with occlusive dressings: a clinical focus. Dermatol Surg 2001;27:175–81.
[2] Ovington LG. Hanging wet-to-dry dressings out to dry. Home Healthc Nurse 2001;19: 477–83.

[3] Nourjah P. National Hospital Ambulatory Medical Care Survey: 1997 emergency department summary. Adv Data 1999;304:1–24.
[4] Cho CY, Lo JS. Dressing the part. Dermatol Clin 1998;16:25–47.
[5] Ma KK, Chan MF, Pang SM. The effectiveness of using a lipido-colloid dressing for patients with traumatic digital wounds. Clin Nurs Res 2006;15:119–34.
[6] Hutchinson JJ, McGuckin M. Occlusive dressings: a microbiologic and clinical review. Am J Infect Control 1990;18:257–68.
[7] Hutchinson JJ, Lawrence JC. Wound infection under occlusive dressings. J Hosp Infect 1991;17:83–94.
[8] Colebrook L, Hood AM. Infection through soaked dressings. Lancet 1948;252:682–3.
[9] Hess CT. When to use gauze dressings. Adv Skin Wound Care 2000;13:266–8.
[10] Richardson M. Procedures for cleansing, closing, and covering acute wounds. Nurs Times 2004;100:54–9.
[11] Winter GD. Formation of the scab and the rate of epithelialization of superficial wounds in the skin of the young domestic pig. Nature 1962;193:293–4.
[12] Hinman CD, Maibach HI. Effect of air exposure and occlusion on experimental human skin wounds. Nature 1963;200:377–8.
[13] Rovee DT, Kurowsky CA, Labun J, et al. Effect of local wound environment on epidermal healing. In: Rovee D, Maibach H, editors. Epidermal wound healing. Chicago: Year Book Medical Publishers; 1972. p. 159–81.
[14] Madden MR, Nolan E, Finkelstein JL, et al. Comparison of an occlusive and a semi-occlusive dressing and the effect of the wound exudate upon keratinocyte proliferation. J Trauma 1989;29:924–31.
[15] Katz MH, Alvarez AF, Kirsner RS, et al. Human wound fluid from acute wounds stimulates fibroblast and endothelial cell growth. J Am Acad Dermatol 1991;25:1054–8.
[16] Varghese MC, Balin AK, Carter DM, et al. Local environment of chronic wounds under synthetic dressings. Arch Dermatol 1986;122:52–7.
[17] Knighton DR, Silver IA, Hunt TK. Regulation of wound-healing angiogenesis—effect of oxygen gradients and inspired oxygen concentration. Surgery 1981;90:262–70.
[18] Alvarez OM, Mertz PM, Eaglstein WH. The effect of occlusive dressings on collagen synthesis and re-epithelialization in superficial wounds. J Surg Res 1983;35:142–8.
[19] Mertz PM, Marshall DA, Eaglstein WH. Occlusive wound dressings to prevent bacterial invasion and wound infection. J Am Acad Dermatol 1985;12:662–8.
[20] Wijetunge DB. Management of acute and traumatic wounds: main aspects of care in adults and children. Am J Surg 1994;167:56S–60S.
[21] Andersson AP, Puntervold T, Warburg FE. Treatment of excoriations with a transparent hydrocolloid dressing: a prospective study. Injury 1991;22:429–30.
[22] Rubio PA. Use of semiocclusive, transparent film dressings for surgical wound protection: experience in 3637 cases. Int Surg 1991;76:253–4.
[23] Michie DD, Hugill JV. Influence of occlusive and impregnated gauze dressings on incisional healing: a prospective, randomized, controlled study. Ann Plast Surg 1994;32:57–64.
[24] Nemeth AH, Eaglstein WH, Taylor JR, et al. Faster healing and less pain in skin biopsy sites treated with an occlusive dressing. Arch Dermatol 1991;127:1679–83.
[25] Barnett A, Berkowitz RL, Mills R, et al. Comparison of synthetic adhesive moisture vapor permeable and fine mesh gauze dressings for split-thickness skin graft donor sites. Am J Surg 1983;145:379–81.
[26] Jones AM, San Miguel L. Are modern wound dressings a clinical and cost-effective alternative to the use of gauze? J Wound Care 2006;15:65–9.
[27] Fonder MA, Lazarus GS, Cowan DA, et al. Treating the chronic wound: a practical approach to the care of non-healing wounds and wound care dressings. J Am Acad Dermatol, in press.
[28] Bolton L, McNees P, van Rijswijk L, et al. Wound-healing outcomes using standardized assessment and care in clinical practice. J Wound Ostomy Continence Nurs 2004;31:65–71.

[29] Seaman S. Dressing selection in chronic wound management. J Am Podiatr Med Assoc 2002; 92:24–33.

[30] May SR. An algorithm for wound management with natural and synthetic dressings. In: Krasner D, editor. Chronic wound care: a clinical source book for healthcare professionals. King of Prussia (PA): Health Management Publications, Inc; 1990. p. 301–8.

[31] Kannon GA, Garret AB. Moist wound healing with occlusive dressings. Dermatol Surg 1995;21:583–90.

[32] Fletcher J. Understanding wound dressings: hydrocolloids. Nurs Times 2005;101:51.

[33] Young T. Wound care in the accident and emergency department. Br J Nurs 1997;6:395–401.

[34] Small V. Management of cuts, abrasions and lacerations. Nurs Stand 2000;15:41–4.

[35] Eaglstein WH, Davis SC, Mehle AL, et al. Optimal use of an occlusive dressing to enhance healing. Arch Dermatol 1988;124:392–5.

[36] Falanga V. Occlusive wound dressings. Why, when, which? Arch Dermatol 1988;124:872–7.

[37] Hollander JE, Singer AJ. Laceration management. Ann Emerg Med 1999;34:356–67.

[38] Hermans MHE. Hydrocolloid dressing (Duoderm) for the treatment of superficial and deep partial thickness burns. Scand J Plast Reconstr Surg 1987;21:283–5.

[39] Wyatt D, McGowan DN, Najaran M. Comparison of a hydrocolloid dressing and silver sulfadiazine cream in the outpatient management of second-degree burns. Trauma 1990;30: 857–64.

[40] Singh A, Halder S, Menon GR, et al. Meta-analysis of randomized controlled trials on hydrocolloid occlusive dressing versus conventional gauze dressing in the healing of chronic wounds. Asian J Surg 2004;27:326–32.

[41] Cho M, Hunt TK. The overall clinical approach to wounds. In: Falanga V, editor. Cutaneous wound healing. London: Martin Dunitz, Ltd; 2001. p. 141–54.

**ELSEVIER
SAUNDERS**

Emerg Med Clin N Am
25 (2007) 243–248

EMERGENCY
MEDICINE
CLINICS OF
NORTH AMERICA

Index

Note: Page numbers of article titles are in **boldface** type.

248

Moving?

Make sure your subscription moves with you!

To notify us of your new address, find your **Clinics Account Number** (located on your mailing label above your name), and contact customer service at:

E-mail: elspcs@elsevier.com

800-654-2452 (subscribers in the U.S. & Canada)
407-345-4000 (subscribers outside of the U.S. & Canada)

Fax number: 407-363-9661

Elsevier Periodicals Customer Service
6277 Sea Harbor Drive
Orlando, FL 32887-4800

*To ensure uninterrupted delivery of your subscription, please notify us at least 4 weeks in advance of move.

ELSEVIER